Voice Update

Voice Update

Proceedings of the 1st World Voice Congress, Oporto, Portugal, April 9–13, 1995

Editor:

M. Pais Clemente
Department of Otorhinolaryngology
Oporto Medical School/Hospital de S. João
Oporto, Portugal

1996

ELSEVIER

Amsterdam – Lausanne – New York – Oxford – Shannon – Tokyo

International Congress Series No. 1097
Advances in the Biosciences Volume 97
ISBN 0-444-82230-5

This book is printed on acid-free paper.

Published by:
Elsevier Science B.V.
P.O. Box 211
1000 AE Amsterdam
The Netherlands

In order to ensure rapid publication this volume was prepared using a method of electronic text processing known as Optical Character Recognition (OCR). Scientific accuracy and consistency of style were handled by the author. Time did not allow for the usual extensive editing process of the Publisher.

Printed in the Netherlands

Preface

The *First World Voice Congress* took place between April 9 and 13, 1995 in the city of Oporto, Portugal.

It was an historical landmark, with the participation of otolaryngologists, phoniatricians, voice-speech pathologists, logopedists, voice teachers and coaches, voice scientists, singers, actors and other professionals concerned with medical, scientific and artistic aspects of voice science, voice care, pedagogy and vocal arts.

There was great interest and enthusiasm for this meeting with more than 1,000 participants from 44 countries. The highest academic level was achieved by inviting voice specialists from all over the world who are well known for their outstanding contributions in the field of voice.

The *First World Voice Congress* was sponsored by the newly established association, the World Voice Consortium, which has the following main objectives: to promote voice care and research, to stimulate education, to disseminate information and to initiate and coordinate meetings on voice.

The *First World Voice Congress* had an outstanding scientific program covering all fields of voice. The program included clinical voice evaluation, diagnosis, medical, surgical and other treatments of voice in benign, premalignant and malignant laryngeal lesions, in neurogenic, endocrine, systemic and functional voice disorders, in laryngeal trauma due to scarring and webbing and other professional voice issues.

This book contains most of the presentations at the *First World Voice Congress* and covers some of the aspects related to voice science and care. Some free papers, workshops and poster presentations are also included to complete this proceedings.

This book reflects the voice update state-of-the-art and I wish to extend my deepest gratitude to all the contributors and their co-workers who have worked with great dedication to present their articles in order to make this "Voice Update" possible.

I also believe this book contains valuable information to stimulate knowledge for all of those who are involved with professional voice care and/or interested in the field of voice science and the vocal arts.

M. Pais Clemente, editor

Introduction voice update

Voice update is without precedence. It represents the state-of-the-arts of phonatory know-how as of April 9, 1995, presented by top voice experts from almost 50 countries. The value of this text goes far beyond learning about the latest research or about clinical know-how typically featured in a journal form. The value of *Voice Update* is unique because the editor has selected papers which often summarize a life-long experience and has elected to address voice issues and voice problems from a global perspective. Consequently, the information presented is quite uniform in style, form and quality. In addition, it is neatly packaged into specific sections, which flow smoothly, giving an easy and a rather palatable reading experience.

The voice evaluation section highlights the unequivocal value of objective approaches, but spares no warnings about overinterpretation and the other pitfalls involved in clinical data collection. These papers are quite useful to both surgical and therapeutic approaches, and the way the information is presented gives a truly unique and refreshing view of objective measures in voice diagnostics.

Medical treatment of dysphonia is outweighed by surgical treatment approaches. Although this represents a natural bias, it also gives the reader food for thought of how to improve on noninvasive treatments in the future.

Postlaryngectomy voice rehabilitation is treated concisely and comprehensively. The section on the therapy aspects of dysphonia is refreshing because treatment avenues presented are based for a change on physiologic models, giving new ways of conducting therapeutic voice restoration. Similarly, the section on integrated treatment of dysphonias shows clearly how to manage successfully challenging functional cases in a multidisciplinary setting design.

The section on professional voice represents both voice teacher and voice science viewpoints. This combination shows elegantly how art and science integrate to better our knowledge of processes governing artistic voice production.

The section on future development of voice, science and care highlights pragmatic and scientific directions and challenges of this continuously expanding field. The future is quite open and much needs to be done. The free paper section completes this reading and brings into focus pertinent scientific and clinical aspects concerning voice.

In all, although at times a laborious task, I felt a sense of accomplishment after reading *Voice Update*. I also felt that this publication illuminates well the intrinsic goal of the World Voice Consortium, namely promotion of voice care and science.

Krzysztof Izdebski, F.K., M.A., Ph.D., C.C.C-SPL, FASHA
San Francisco, California, July 1996

World Voice Consortium

List of Contributors

R. Eugenia Chavez de Bartelt, M.D.
Phoniatrics and Audiology Consultory, Mexico City, Mexico

Mara Behlau, Ph.D.
Associate Professor, Department of Otolaryngology and Human Communication Disorders, Universidade Federal de S. Paulo, Escola Paulista de Medicina, Director Centro de Estudos da Voz, S. Paulo, Brasil

Michael S. Benninger, M.D.
Chairman Department of Otolaryngology – Head and Neck Surgery, Henry Ford Medical Hospital, Detroit, Michigan, USA

Janina K. Casper, Ph.D.
Associate Professor, Department of Otolaryngology and Communication Sciences, State University of New York Health Science Center
Syracuse, New York, USA

M. Pais Clemente, M.D., Ph.D.
Chairman and Professor Otorhinolaryngology, Department of Otorhinolaryngology, Oporto Medical School/Hospital de S. João, President Portuguese Institute of Voice, Chairman World Voice Consortium, Oporto, Portugal

Philippe H. Dejonckere, M.D., Ph.D.
The Institute of Phoniatrics, University Utrecht, Utrecht, The Netherlands

Özkul M. Doğan, M.D.
Assistant Professor, SSK Tepecik Educational Hospital, ENT Clinic, Izmir, Turkey

Philip C. Doyle, Ph.D., CCC-(S), SLP-(C)
Director Vocal Production Laboratory, Department of Communicative Disorders, The University of Western Ontario, London, Ontario, Canada

Vicki L. Hammen, Ph.D.
Assistant Professor, Department of Audiology & Speech Sciences, Heavilon Hall, Purdue University West Lafayette, Indiana, USA

Thomas M. Harris, F.R.C.S., M.A.
Consultant Laryngologist
Lewisham Hospital and Queen Mary's Hospital Sidcup, UK

Ingo F. Herrmann, M.D.
ENT Department, European Hospital, Rome, Italy

Frans J.M. Hilgers, M.D., Ph.D.
Department of Otolaryngology – Head & Neck Surgery, The Netherlands Cancer Institute, Amsterdam, The Netherlands

Minoru Hirano, M.D.
Dean School of Medicine, Kurume University, Kurume, Japan

Krzysztof Izdebski, F.K., M.A., Ph.D. CCC-SPL
Chairman Pacific Voice and Speech Foundation, Associate Clinical Professor, Department of Otolaryngology – Head and Neck Surgery, University of California, Davis Medical School, San Francisco, California, USA

Oskar Kleinsasser, M.D., Ph.D.
Chairman and Professor, ENT Department, Philips University, Marburg, Germany

M. Nasser Kotby, M.D.
Director Unit of Phoniatrics and Disorders of Communication, Department of Otolaryngology – Head and Neck Surgery, Ain Shams University, Cairo, Egypt

Rebecca Leonard, Ph.D.
Associate Professor, Department of Otolaryngology – Head and Neck Surgery, University of California, Davis Medical School, Sacramento, California, USA

Hermann LeRoux, B.M., M.M., T.L.D., P.D.M.
Chairman Voice Department, San Francisco Conservatory of Music, San Francisco, California, USA

Christy L. Ludlow, Ph.D.
Voice and Speech Section, National Institute on Deafness and other Communication Disorders, Bethesda, MD, USA

Hans F. Mahieu, M.D., Ph.D.
Professor, Department of Otorhinolaryngology – Head & Neck Surgery, Academisch Ziekenhuis, Vrije Universiteit Amsterdam, The Netherlands

Anita McAllister
Department of Speech Pathology, Danderyd Hospital, Danderyd, Sweden

G. Motta, M.D., Ph.D.
Chairman and Professor, Institute of Otolaryngology and Phoniatrics, University of Naples, Naples, Italy

Thomas Murry, Ph.D., CCC-SLP
Professor, Department of Otolaryngology – Head & Neck Surgery, University of Tennessee, Memphis, Tennessee, USA

G. Niedzielska, M.D.
Department of Pediatric Otolaryngology, Phoniatrics and Audiology Medical School, Lublin, Poland

Desiderio Passali, M.D., Ph.D.
Chairman and Professor Department of Otorhinolaryngology, University of Sienna, Sienna, Italy

Rui S. Penha, M.D, Ph.D.
Chairman and Professor, Department of Otorhinolaryngology, Hospital Egas Moniz, Faculty of Medical Sciences, New University of Lisbon, Lisbon, Portugal

Paulo Pontes, M.D.
Professor Escola Paulista de Medicina, Director Instituto da Laringe, S. Paulo, Brazil

Antoni Pruszewicz, M.D., Ph.D., Dr. h.c.
Chairman and Professor, Department of Phoniatrics and Audiology, K. Marcinkowski University School, Poznan, Poland

Lorraine Olson Ramig, Ph.D, CCC-SP
Associate Professor, Department of Communication Disorders and Speech Science, The University of Colorado, Boulder, Colorado, USA

Ank C. Reinders
The Hague, The Netherlands

Lucille S. Rubin, Ph.D.
Executive Director, President Professionally Speaking, Voice Faculty, Theatre School, Circle-in-the Square, New York, New York, USA

Robert T. Sataloff, M.D., D.M.A.
Chairman Board of Directors, The Voice Foundation, Acting Chairman Department of Otolaryngology Graduate Hospital, Professor of Otolaryngology Thomas Jefferson University, Philadelphia, Pennsylvania, USA

Ronald C. Scherer, Ph.D
Senior Scientist Wilbur James Gould Voice Research Center, The Denver Center for the Performing Arts, Denver, Colorado, USA

Harm K. Schutte, M.D., Ph.D.
Voice Research Laboratory at University of Groningen, Department of Medical Physiology, Faculty of Medicine, Groningen, The Netherlands

Alberto Staffieri, M.D.
ENT Clinic, University of Udine, Udine, Italy

W. Steiner, M.D., Ph.D.
Chairman and Professor, Department of Otorhinolaryngology, Georg August University, Gottingen, Germany

Joseph C. Stemple, Ph.D.
Institute for Voice Analysis and Rehabilitation, Dayton, Ohio, USA

R.E. (Ed) Stone, Jr., Ph.D.
Associate Professor, Vanderbilt Voice Center, Department of Otolaryngology, Vanderbilt University Medical Center, Nashville, Tennessee, USA

Gijsbertus J. Verkerke, Ph.D.
University of Groningen, Faculty of Medicine, Centre for Biomedical Technology, Groningen, The Netherlands

J.J. Alvarez Vicent, M.D., Ph.D.
Chairman and Professor,Department of Otolaryngology, Hospital 12 de Octubre, Madrid, Spain

Co-workers

Y.A. Abu-Ras
Unit of Phoniatrics, Alexandria University, Alexandria, Egypt

A.H. Ackerstaff
Department of Otolaryngology — Head and Neck Surgery, The Netherlands Cancer Institute, Amsterdam, The Netherlands

Tatar Alper
SSK Tepecik Educational Hospital ENT Clinic, Yenişehir-Izmir, Turkey

Ranjinidevi Ambalavanar
Voice and Speech Section, National Institute on Deafness and other Communication Disorders, Bethesda, Maryland, USA

Petra Ambrosch
Department of Otorhinolaryngology, Georg August University, Gottingen, Germany

E.M. Aref
Unit of Phoniatrics, Assuit University, Assuit, Egypt

A.J.M. Balm
Department of Otolaryngology – Head and Neck Surgery, The Netherlands Cancer Institute, Amsterdam, The Netherlands

Julie Barkmeier
Voice and Speech Section, National Institute on Deafness and other Communication Disorders, Bethesda, Maryland, USA

S.S. Bassiony
Unit of Phoniatrics, Ain Shams University, Cairo, Egypt

Altar Bedri
SSK Tepecik Educational Hospital ENT Clinic, Yenişehir-Izmir, Turkey

Luisa Belussi, M.D., Ch.D.
Department of Otorhinolaryngology, University of Siena, Siena, Italy

Henk J. Busscher
Scientific and Applied Surface Advice B.V. (Sasa B.V.), Thesinge, The Netherlands

R. Canessa
Institute of Otolaryngology and Phoniatrics, University of Naples, Naples, Italy

Eduardo Cardoso, M.D.
Department of Otorhinolaryngology, Oporto Medical School, Hospital S. João, Oporto, Portugal

Vitor Cardoso
Department of Otorhinolaryngology, Oporto Medical School, Hospital S. João, Oporto, Portugal

Pascal Carrive
School of Psychology, University of New South Wales, N.S.W., Australia

U. Cesari, M.D.
Institute of Otolaryngology and Phoniatrics, University of Naples, Naples, Italy

Laudelina Pais Clemente, M.D.
Department of Otorhinolaryngology, Oporto Medical School, Hospital S. João, Oporto, Portugal

Martin P. De Vries
Faculty of Medicine, Centre for Biomedical Technology, University of Groningen, Groningen, The Netherlands

Julia Edgar
Voice and Speech Section, National Institute on Deafness and Other Communication Disorders, Bethesda, Maryland, USA

S.R. El-Sady
Unit of Phoniatrics, Ain Shams University, Cairo, Egypt

E. Esposito, M.D.
Faculty of Medicine "Federico II", Naples, Italy

Maria Emília Elias, M.D.
Research Fellow, American Institute for Voice and Ear Research, Philadelphia, Pennsylvania, USA

E. Fresnel-Elbaz, M.D.
Service ORL et Chirurgie Cervico-Faciale, Fondation A. de Rothschild, Paris, France

Kerry J. Flom, Ph.D.
Director Clinical Studies and Internal Evaluations, Oncor, Gaithersburg, Maryland, USA

Jesus A. Guimera
Hospital Virgen de Aranzazu, San Sebastian, Spain

R.T. Gregor, M.D.
Department of Otolaryngology – Head and Neck Surgery, The Netherlands Cancer Institute, Amsterdam, The Netherlands

Carol Grigg, M.S.
Department of Audiology and Speech Sciences, University of Washington, Seattle, Washington, USA

Dinah Harris
Voice Clinic at Queen Mary's Hospital, Sidcup, UK

Sara Harris
Voice Clinic at Queen Mary's Hospital, Sidcup, UK

Reinhardt J. Heuer, Ph.D.
Senior Research Scientist, American Institute for Voice and Ear Research, Philadelphia, Pennsylvania, USA

Allen D. Hillel, M.D.
University of Washington, Seattle, Washington, USA

Jacob Lieberman
Voice Clinic at Queen Mary's Hospital, Sidcup, UK

Carla P. Moura, M.D.
Department of Otorhinolaryngology, Oporto Medical School, Hospital S. João, Oporto, Portugal

S. Motta, M.D.
Institute of Otolaryngology and Phoniatrics, University of Naples, Naples, Italy

Uğur Ömer
SSK Tepecik, Educational Hospital ENT Clinic, Yenişehir-Izmir, Turkey

A.A. Orabi
Unit of Phoniatrics, Ain Shams University, Cairo, Egypt

Rui Pratas, M.D.
Department of Otorhinolaryngology, Oporto Medical School, Hospital S. João, Oporto, Portugal

Gerhard Rakhorst
Faculty of Medicine, Centre for Biomedical Technology, University of Groningen, Groningen, The Netherlands

Sara A. Recio
ENT-Department, European Hospital, Rome, Italy

Marc Remacle, M.D.
Professor Cliniques Universitaires de Mont-Godinne, Université Catholique de Louvain, Yvoir, Belgium

Manuel Ribeiro, M.D.
Department of Otorhinolaryngology, Oporto Medical School, Hospital S. João, Oporto, Portugal

M. Lima Rodrigues, M.D.
Department of Otorhinolaryngology, Oporto Medical School, Hospital S. João, Oporto, Portugal

Deborah C. Rosen, R.N., M.S.
Otolaryngologic Nurse Clinician, American Institute for Voice and Ear Research, Philadelphia, Pennsylvania, USA

Jeffrey S. Sanfor
Oncor, Gaithersburg, Maryland, USA

B.E.G.M. Scholtens
Department of Otolaryngology – Head and Neck Surgery, The Netherlands Cancer Institute, Amsterdam, The Netherlands

Elisabeth Sederholm
Department of Speech Pathology, Danderyd Hospital, Danderyd, Sweden

Joseph R. Spiegel, M.D., F.A.C.S.
Associate Professor of Otolaryngology, Thomas Jefferson University, Philadelphia, Pennsylvania, USA

N. Straziuso
Institute of Otolaryngology and Phoniatrics, University of Naples, Naples, Italy

Kaptaner Stuat
SSK Tepecik, Educational Hospital ENT Clinic, Yenişehir-Izmir, Turkey

Katarina Svanberg, M.D.
Department of Oncology, Lund University Hospital, Lund, Sweden

Sune Svanberg, Ph.D.
Division of Atomic Physics, Lund Institute of Technology, Lund, Sweden

Fernando Vales, M.D.
Department of Otorhinolaryngology, Oporto Medical School, Hospital S. João, Oporto, Portugal

Henny C. Van der Mei
University of Groningen, Faculty of Medicine, Materia Technica, Groningen, The Netherlands

Aalze Veenstra
Faculty of Medicine, Centre for Biomedical Technology, University of Groningen, Groningen, The Netherlands

Ingrid Wang, M.D.
Department of Oncology, Lund University Hospital, Lund, Sweden

Ronald R. Ward, M.D.
Chief Department of Otolaryngology – Head and Neck Surgery, Kaiser Permanent Medical Center, San Francisco, California, USA

Patricia Waugh, M.S.
Department of Audiology and Speech Sciences, University of Washington, Seattle, Washington, USA

Sandra R. Wolman, M.D.
Oncor, Gaithersburg, Maryland, USA

Gayle E. Woolson, M.D.
Professor Department of Otolaryngology – Head and Neck Surgery, University of Tennessee, Memphis, Tennessee, USA

Contents

Surgical treatment of dysphonias

Dysphonia in organic benign, premalignant and malignant lesions

Dysphonia following laryngeal trauma, scarring and webbing

Treatment of neurogenic dysphonias

Laryngeal frameworks surgery

Voice restoration and rehabilitation postlaryngectomy

Future developments in voice science and care

Free papers, workshops and poster presentations

Voice evaluation

Voice Update.
M. Pais Clemente, editor.

The wonderful world of communication in nature

Rui S. Penha
Department of Otorhinolaryngology, Hospital Egas Moniz, Faculty of Medical Sciences, New University of Lisbon, Portugal

Abstract. Of all species that inhabit the earth, the Homo Sapiens had the slowest development. The genesis of language and speech remains obscure. The most consistent explanation proposes that the first symbolic sounds were accompanied by hand gestures and facial expressions. There are around 4,000 different languages and dialects, and all children learn their native language, no matter how complex it is. There are mental and linguistic structures that allow children to acquire language, and all of them master the basics between the ages of 4 and 6 years. The sequence by which language appeared is possibly the following: First there were gestures associated with babbling. From babbling there were holophrases. Then gestures became more precise and associated with more precise sound symbols. Finally, gestures and holophrases were replaced by gestures and words.

Another form of communication extensive to many animal species, including man, is play behaviour. Play teaches to make sound judgements and is a rehearsal for the challenges and ambiguities of life. Similar to speech, play is a key to an individual's development and her/his social relationships.

Key words: Bible, language, modern, prehistoric, speech.

In the beginning, the Lord created the heaven and the earth. And the earth was without form and void. And the Lord said: Let there be light. And there was light. And the Lord saw the light, that it was good and the Lord divided the light from the darkness. And the Lord called the light Day, and the darkness He called Night. And the Lord made the firmament in the midst of the waters. And the Lord said: Let the waters under heaven be gathered together into one place, and let the dry land appear. And the Lord saw it was good (Genesis, chapter 1 [1–10]).

And the Lord took the man, and put him into the garden of Eden to dress it and to keep it. And the Lord commanded that man could eat from every tree, except from the tree of knowledge of good and evil: for the day you will eat from it, you should surely die. (Genesis, chapter 2, [15–25]). After the flood, Noah lived 350 years. And all the days of Noah were 950 years and then he died. (Genesis, chapter 9, [28–29]).

And the whole earth was one language and one speech. And it came to pass as they journeyed from the east, that they found a place in the land of Shinar, and they dwelt there. And they said: Go to, let us build us a city and a tower, whose top may reach into heaven. And the Lord came down to see the city and the tower which the children of man builded. And the Lord said: Behold, the people is one and they have

Address for correspondence: Rui S. Penha MD, PhD, Serviço de Otorrinolaringologia, Hospital Egas Moniz, R. da Junqueira 126, 1300 Lisboa, Portugal.

all one language, and this they began to do. And now, nothing will be restrained from them, which they have imagined to do. Go to, let us go down and then confound their language, that they may not understand one another's speech. So the Lord scattered them abroad from thence upon the face of all earth. Therefore the name of Babel was given to the tower. (Genesis, chapter 11 [1–9]).

It is interesting to notice that since the beginning of the Old Testament there was always a straight communication between man and the Lord. However, how that communication was done is still unclear. Many questions arise in our minds like how could a man live as long as Noah? and what really happened at the tower of Babel? Did it really exist? What is the truth behind this allegory? There has always been an attempt to correlate archeological findings with the stories from the Bible, however, remnants of the ark of Noah were never found, neither those of the tower of Babel.

What we know is that in the early times of the evolution of Man, the development of the visual acuity and the decrease in the sense of smell became a milestone for the increase of the mental capabilities. When stereoscopic vision was added, coupled with an increase in the flexibility of the hand, the way to the future was opened. The opponent thumb in the hand became added to the development of the brain.

Some authors believe that the human species left life in the trees to start living on the ground. Nevertheless, it is possible that the arborigenous stage of development is a form of adaptation in the life of monkeys, a stage never known by the human species. Anyway, life in the large uncovered plains made Man carnivorous and exposed to better nutrients as compared to that of leaves and fruits. Nevertheless, this relatively weak animal without claws or strong canines to kill animals and survive, developed the need to make tools. Tool development further increased visual acuity and manual dexterity, and consequently lead to further development and growth of the brain.

The genesis of language and speech remains obscure. It is not sure how this great invention was born. The great monkeys may produce emotional expressions and are prone to dance and beat rhythms to express their humor. It is possible to teach certain monkeys to say one or two words, however, that is as far as they can go.

The most consistent explanation for the use of spoken language refers to the fact that the first symbolic sounds were accompanied by hand gestures and facial expressions. It is curious to observe that the Aborigines from Australia and the Indians from North America keep a language based on signs. The Aruntas communicate by a language that includes 450 signs. People who are born deaf and who are not rehabilitated, communicate by gestures which may be understood universally.

The sequence by which language appeared is possibly the following: First there were gestures associated with babbling. From babbling there were holophrases with no sense but helping to express an event or feeling. Then the gestures became more precise and associated with more precise sound symbols. It is thought that specific thoughts were born at this stage. Finally, gestures and holophrases were abandoned, giving rise to signs and words. From this moment on, language expanded rapidly with developing syntax, vocabulary, numeration and analytic thoughts.

The anatomy of our brain supports the thesis that language derives from gestures. There is no particular center of language in the brain. Language is controlled by a large area in the cortex that starts just anterior to the visual cortex, crosses the auditory cortex and extends up to the end of the motor cortex. This area is always in the left cortex of the right handed and in the right cortex of the left handed.

According to William Stokoe, who is a full professor for teaching the deaf in Gallaudet, Washington, gestural communication is not a relation of incoherent gestures, but a language with multiple components, such as the figures created with the hands and fingers as well as their spacial orientation. Ursulla Bellugi, a neurologist who has studied sign language of the deaf for 26 years, found that it is processed in the brain in the same way as language.

Of all species that inhabit the Earth, the Homo Sapiens had the slowest development. Children usually remain for many years in a state of physical immaturity and are dependant on the care and protection of others to survive. There is certainly a difference in the rhythm of development among the species.

A couple of psychologists raised their son Donald together with a chimpanzee named Gua. Donald and Gua were cared for in the same way, wearing the same clothes, eating the same food, and receiving the same level of love, care and education. The great hereditary difference and rate of maturation lead Gua to reach its maximal genetic potential long before Donald. Only at the age of 9 months, when the study was over, Donald reached Gua in certain developmental areas, such as following verbal commands, but started bypassing Gua in the development of language. Nevertheless, Donald remained way behind Gua in respect to physical mobility. Attempts to teach Gua to speak, however, resulted in failure. At the age of 3 years, Gua could only say three words, and this was considered the end point of language development for the chimpanzee. On the other hand, a 3-year-old child may already disclose a vocabulary of 900 words

Chomsky proposes that the 4,000 known languages are based on the same genetically determined principles that he describes as “invariable properties”, “universal language characteristics” or “universal grammar”. According to the same author, language results from the relation among predisposed mental structures, maturation and interaction with the ambient.

All children learn their native language no matter how complex it is, and all of them master the basics between 4 and 6 years of age. There are linguistic and mental structures that allow children to acquire language. Then comes the expansive communication in which the child relates to those surrounding him.

Children initially understand a language before they start speaking it. The development of language starts at 3 months and extends up to 30 months. Around 9 months of age, similar to that which happened with the Homo Sapiens, children start with echolalia in which they imitate the sounds of others. Then at the age of 1 year they start pronouncing holophrases which are sentences with a single word. At 2 years of age, children can say sentences with several words, and at the age of 3 years they have a vocabulary of around 900 words. Children learn language following a continuum of influences involving the surrounding ambient and the hereditary background. The continuum may be divided into four groups of thought:

1. Behaviourism – according to this theory children learn how to speak through operative conditioning, in which the parents and teachers selectively reinforce the child's vocalization. As such, children learn language by imitating a model, mainly the parents, associating their voice with the need for gratification.
2. Relativism and cultural determinism – according to this theory the cultural influence is considered more important than the individual differences and hereditary background. Children are considered to have an inborn predisposition to learn language. Whorf considers that each specific language influences our mental process in such a way that people with different languages have a different perception of the world and even think in a different way.
3. Interactionism – this theory considers that language develops through the interaction among hereditary background, maturation and ambiental influence. Language is considered an essential part of the human development.
4. Preformism and predeterminism – modern linguistic authors, mainly Noam Chomsky, consider that the human being has a biological inborn predisposition to learn language. This occurs naturally, similar to that which happens with walking.

In communication among animals, play behaviour is as important as sleeping and dreaming. Play is a key element in an individual's development and in their social relationship and status. Among mammals and birds, abundant play and complex play are usually associated with more developed brains. Play clearly helps in the healthy development of young animals, both physically and mentally. Conversely, if the young are prevented from playing or maltreated so that their play is abnormal, their development may also be abnormal.

Play behaviour is extensive to many animal species. Chimpanzees are among the champions of play among nonhuman primates, and the absence of play behaviour is often a sign of depression. Play also teaches to make sound judgements. Play fighting may let an animal learn when it can trust another animal and, if things get too violent, when it needs to defend itself. Interestingly, a young Japanese monkey has learned to make a snowball. No one, however, has ever seen a monkey throwing a ball. A further example is when the end seemed very near for a Canadian eskimo dog, tethered near the shore of Hudson Bay, when a 1,000 lb polar bear appeared. Surely the dog was destined to become a meal; however, the dog wagged his tail, grinned and bowed to the bear as an invitation to play. The bear accepted the dog's body language and the next minute they were playing together. Also, when two seahorses copulate for mere seconds, the female deposits as many as 200 eggs into the male's ballooning pouch. Are these not full examples of communication in the animal world? Play is, after all, a rehearsal for the challenges and ambiguities of life, and playful adults are often highly creative, even brilliant individuals.

Voice Update.
M. Pais Clemente, editor.

Laryngovideostroboscopy: its value in medical assessment

Minoru Hirano
Department of Otolaryngology – Head and Neck Surgery, Kurume University, Kurume, Japan

Key words: glottic carcinoma, laryngovideostroboscopy, mucosal wave, vocal fold scar, vocal fold paralysis, vocal fold cyst.

Introduction

Clinical applications of modern laryngostroboscopy date back to 1960 when Elimar Schoenhaerl in Germany completed the monumental basic and clinical studies titled "Die Stroboskopie in der praktischen Laryngologie" by means of an electronic stroboscope [1]. In those days, however, stroboscopic images of vibrating vocal folds were viewed under a laryngeal mirror and no recordings of the images were available.

In the late 1970s video recordings of stroboscopic images of vocal folds became technically available [2], and in the 1980s several good instruments employing a telescope or a fiberscope were developed [3–6]. Laryngovideostroboscopy is now one of the routine procedures in modern laryngological practice.

The videostroboscopic instruments should be located in the regular otolaryngological office. We should conduct laryngovideostroboscopy as routinely as ordinary ear-nose-throat examinations. If one had his/her videostroboscopic unit in a separate test laboratory, he/she would not make full use of it.

Value in medical assessment

In medical assessment laryngovideostroboscopy is very useful for the following purposes:

1. The detection of early glottic carcinoma.
2. The detection of early recurrent glottic carcinoma following radiotherapy.
3. The estimation of the extent of carcinomatous invasion.
4. The detection of the scar of the vocal fold.
5. The detection of very small cysts of the vocal fold.
6. The differentiation of cysts from nodules and polyps.
7. The estimation of histopathology of nodules, polyps and Reinke's edema.
8. The estimation of the degree and prognosis of vocal fold paralysis.
9. The diagnosis of functional dysphonia.

The first stroboscopic sign of glottic cancer is a lack of mucosal wave. The amplitude of vibration is first reduced and as the cancer becomes larger the amplitude becomes zero, presenting with a nonvibrating portion. When the vocal fold is entirely involved it does not vibrate at all but stays still during phonation.

Normal vocal folds have a pliable mucosa at the edge. This portion is called the superficial layer of the lamina propria or Reinke's space. This pliable structure is essential to the occurrence of mucosal wave during vibration.

In glottic cancer the normal pliable mucosa is replaced by a stiff cancer tissue. This causes an absence of mucosal wave during phonation. When the cancer is small it presents with some vibratory movements, but without mucosal wave. As the cancer becomes larger the structure becomes unable to vibrate.

Table 1 shows stroboscopic findings of 67 patients with glottic T1a cancer. There was no mucosal wave at the lesion in all cases. The amplitude of vibration at the lesion was zero in 25 patients, presenting with a nonvibratory segment, and it was small in 42 patients. In addition, in those 42 patients, the carcinomatous lesion was small enough to vibrate but was stiff and disturbed an occurrence of mucosal wave.

The findings for the macroscopically unaffected portion are also clinically important. In 13 patients, the entire vocal fold looked affected. In the remaining 54, a part of the vocal fold looked normal or unaffected, but the mucosal wave was absent at the unaffected portion in 27 cases, indicating a subepithelial cancer invasion.

When radiotherapy is chosen for the treatment, this finding may not be clinically important because the entire vocal fold is usually irradiated. When surgery, especially endolaryngeal microscopic laser surgery, is employed as the treatment modality, the stroboscopic finding relative to the mucosal wave is very important to determine the extent of removal. From an oncological point of view, we have to have a sufficient safety margin, but from a functional point of view, we want to have a sufficient but minimal safety margin.

Stroboscopic signs of vocal fold scars are basically the same as those of glottic carcinoma. In the case of scars, however, the vocal fold often looks quite normal under normal light. Stroboscopic examination is the only existing modality to detect small scars of the vocal fold. The stroboscopic sign of very small vocal fold cysts is localized by the limitation of vibratory movements followed by a lack of mucosal wave. Very small cysts can often be diagnosed only by means of videostroboscopy. For vocal nodules, polyps and Reinke's edema, videostroboscopy is useful to estimate the histopathological feature.

Table 1. Stroboscopic findings for glottic T1a cancer.

	Mucosal wave		Amplitude	
	Lesion	"Unaffected" portion[a]	Lesion	"Unaffected" portion[a]
Normal	0	2	0	2
Small	0	25	42	45
Absent or zero	67	27	25	7

(n = 67). [a]In 13 patients, the entire vocal fold looked macroscopically affected and no unaffected portion was noted.

Nodules presenting with normal or slightly limited mucosal wave are often edematous whereas those presenting with limited or no mucosal wave are frequently fibrous. Edematous nodules can be successfully treated with voice therapy, but fibrous nodules frequently call for surgical intervention. Polyps showing normal or slightly limited mucosal wave are frequently edematous again. Small edematous polyps can be occasionally treated successfully with voice therapy. When no mucosal wave is observed on a whitish polyp, it is often histologically fibrous. Reddish polyps are histopathologically vascular and hemorrhagic and they do not present with mucosal wave on their surface. Fibrous and hemorrhagic polyps usually call for surgical treatments.

In the case of Reinke's edema, lesions with great or normal mucosal wave are usually edematous and have serous fluid, whereas lesions with small or limited mucosal wave are frequently more fibrous and have a mucous or gelatinous content. In the former, postsurgical voice recovery usually takes place quickly, whereas in the latter, the voice tends to recover slowly. Stroboscopic findings, therefore, can allow one to predict, to some extent, how soon or late the voice will recover following surgery.

As for the degree and prognosis of vocal fold paralysis, favorable stroboscopic signs are complete glottic closure and the presence of mucosal wave, whereas incomplete glottic closure and absence of mucosal wave are unfavorable signs. Needless to say, electromyography (EMG) is more reliable than stroboscopy. EMG is, however, not available in many laryngological clinics.

Finally, it should be emphasized that diagnosis of functional dysphonia can be made only when minor organic lesions have been excluded by means of laryngovideostroboscopy.

References

1. Schönhärl E. Die Stroboskopie in der praktischen Laryngologie. Stuttgart: Georg Thieme, 1960.
2. Yoshida Y, Hirano M, Nakajima T. A videotape recording system for laryngostroboscopy. J Jpn Bronchoesophagol Soc 1979;30:1–5.
3. Hirano M, Yoshida Y, Yoshida T, Tateishi O. Strobofiberscopic video recording of vocal fold vibration. Ann Otol Rhinol Laryngol 1985;94:588–590.
4. Yanagisawa E, Godley F, Muta H. Selection of video cameras for stroboscopic videolaryngoscopy. Ann Otol Rhinol Laryngol 1987;96:578–585.
5. Sataloff RT, Spiegel JR, Carroll LM, Schiebel BR, Darby KS, Rulnick R. Strobovideolaryngoscopy in professional voice users: results and clinical value. J Voice 1988;1:359–364.
6. Watanabe H, Shin T, Matsuo K, Oda M, Fukaura J. A new computer-analyzing system for clinical use with a strobo-videoscope. Arch Otolaryngol Head Neck Surg 1986;112:978–981.

Voice Update.
M. Pais Clemente, editor.

Laryngeal imaging with stroboscopy: its value in therapeutic assessment

Rebecca Leonard and K. Izdebski

Department of Otolaryngology – Head and Neck Surgery, University of California, Davis Medical School, Sacramento, California, USA

Abstract. The voice pathologist's management of dysphonic patients has been enhanced and advanced by the use of laryngeal imaging techniques. Visualization of selected vocal tract dynamics during speech and nonspeech tasks improves our understanding of hyperfunctional, maladaptive vocal practices, and enables the clinician to identify specific conservational practices which may form the basis of voice therapy. This paper will consider a rationale for the inclusion of imaging in the voice pathologist's armamentarium, review particular objectives and tasks of the voice pathologist's image study, and discuss applications of the information obtained to remedial treatments.

Key words: laryngeal imaging, rationale, voice therapy.

Traditionally, speech pathologists have evaluated phonatory function and voice without the advantage of laryngeal observation. We have relied on what our own ears tell us about voice, what patients tell us about their dysphonia, and what physicians report regarding the state of the larynx. Listening is vital to our craft and, certainly, the sound of voice will always be the determining factor in judgments of its health. But the voice pathologist is obliged to understand, comprehensively, the disorder he or she is charged with treating, including those vocal tract structures and dynamics which have rendered the voice aberrant. Perceptual impressions of voice, supplemented by acoustic, aerodynamic, and perhaps other measures of phonatory function, provide valuable insights into the nature of dysphonia. But, in our opinion, a voice evaluation which does not include laryngeal imaging is incomplete and introduces, unnecessarily, elements of guesswork, mystery and error to the voice pathologist's task.

The intent of this paper is to discuss the value of laryngeal imaging in voice and phonatory function evaluation. In particular, we will consider tasks and objectives for an imaging study, and how information obtained benefits the clinician in treament planning. The imaging study performed by the voice pathologist – referred to here as "phonoscopic" exam [1] – requires that laryngeal structures be examined at rest, and during the performance of vegetative, vocal and speech behaviors. As on a voice evaluation, measures of fundamental frequency range and speaking levels, estimates

Address for correspondence: Rebecca Leonard, Department of Otolaryngology – Head and Neck Surgery, University of California, Davis Medical Center, 2521 Stockton Blvd., Sacramento, CA 95817, USA.

of intensity variability and maximum phonation duration are obtained. In addition, sampling of voice quality across a variety of speaking contexts, i.e., reading, conversation, phonatory modes (i.e., whisper, falsetto), and phonetic environments (i.e., all-voiced utterances, mixed voiced and voiceless utterances), is imperative.

Examination with both rigid and flexible endoscopes is ideal. Subtle details of hyperfunction may be apparent only with rigid endoscopy, which provides perhaps the best information regarding the effects of pathology on phonation, and conversely, of phonation on pathology. But examination of the larynx during speaking tasks – possible only with the flexible scope – is critical for the elaboration of hyperfunctional practices which may be producing or exacerbating pathology.

The voice clinician has at least four objectives for the initial imaging study. Briefly, they must: 1) match specific laryngeal behaviors – adaptive and maladaptive – to particular vocal qualities; 2) differentiate voice qualities which sound similar but are produced differently and, conversely, appreciate small changes in laryngeal dynamics which produce large acoustic and perceptual differences. Furthermore, 3) we must map the most efficacious vocal "space" for an individual patient, i.e., identify ranges of respiratory and phonatory function which are most conducive to the restoration or maintenance of vocal good health; and finally, if tissue pathology is present, we need to, 4) evaluate the effects of pathology on phonation, and conversely, assess the effects of particular phonatory behaviors on pathology. It is important to note that these objectives represent the domain of the voice pathologist, and may differ significantly from the laryngologist's primary objectives for an imaging exam. We would add that, in our own experience, the successful achievement of these goals has significantly advanced our clinical practice. Let us consider how the accomplishment of each can contribute to the treatment plan for an individual patient.

As noted, our first task on phonoscopic examination is to identify specific laryngeal behaviors which produce unique voicing characteristics. This determination should be made for maladaptive, or inappropriate vocal practices, as well as for behaviors which are believed appropriate. For example, assume that a patient, during connected speech tasks, demonstrates a laryngeal posture similar to the one shown in Fig. 1, in which the false vocal folds are constricted and medialized. In addition to determining how often, and in what contexts this behavior occurs, we need to know if the voice that results is consistently low-pitched, rough, and aperiodic. Similarly, does voice produced with hyperadduction of the true vocal folds, as illustrated in Fig. 2, consistently sound strained or pressed? And, on the other hand, if the patient's larynx appears similar to the one in Fig. 3, is the voice it generates always relatively normal? Sampling of phonatory behaviors across a variety of tasks and contexts enables us to make these associations, i.e., to identify laryngeal behaviors or postures which consistently produce a given vocal output.

The identification of laryngeal postures or behaviors which produce particular auditory perceptions, good or bad, is absolutely critical to a therapy which requires patients to change vocal practices. Obviously, the intent of most voice therapy is to establish or increase laryngeal behaviors which are appropriate, and to reduce or

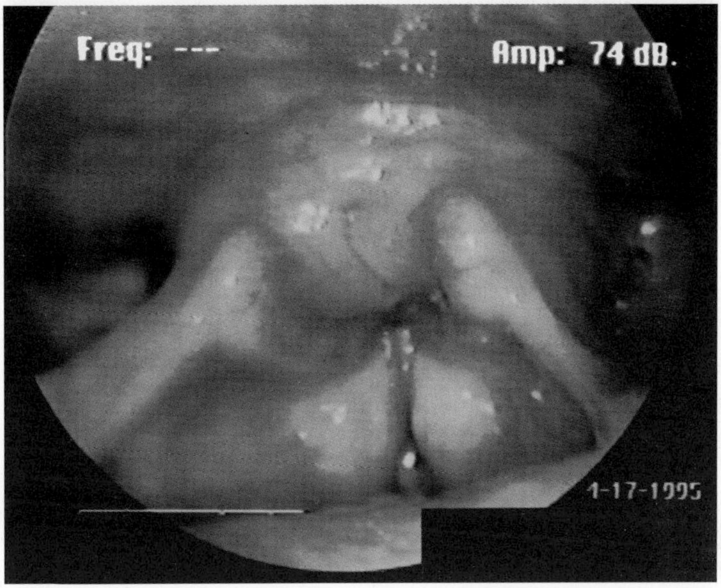

Fig. 1. False vocal folds are constricted and medialized.

eliminate those behaviors which are aberrant, or which are believed to produce pathology. Historically, we have relied on how the voice sounds, and how it feels to produce it, to form constructs of "good" voice and "bad" voice for the patient. If we

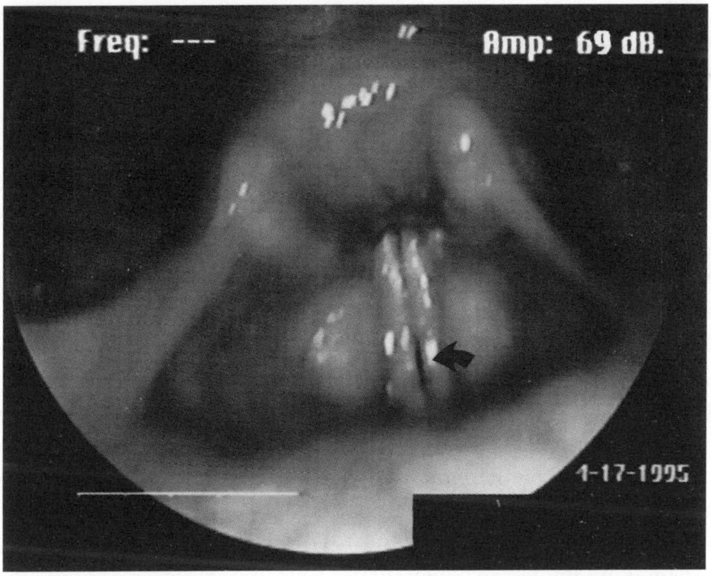

Fig. 2. True vocal folds are hyperadducted, i.e., compressed so tightly that displacement of vibratory edges during phonation is restricted to the site indicated by the arrow.

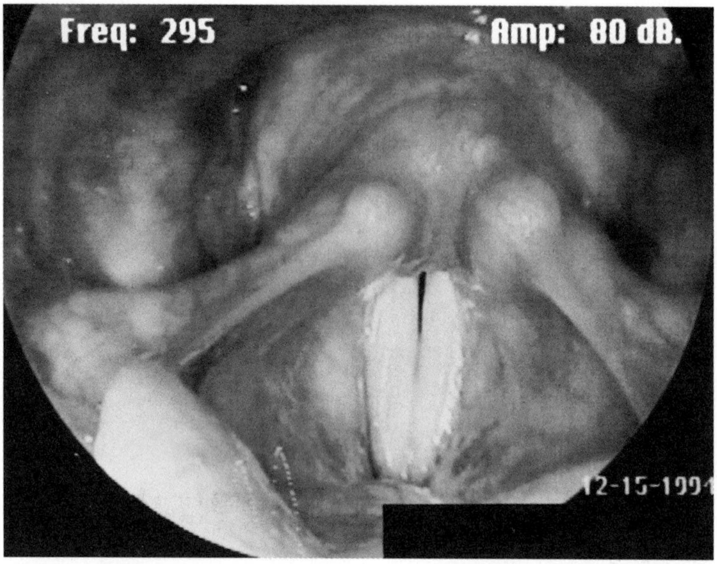

Fig. 3. Normal true vocal folds producing normal phonation and voice quality.

can obtain visual confirmation that a given vocal practice in an individual patient consistently produces a particular vocal output, then we can have greater confidence that our therapeutic instruction to the patient regarding voice that matches a given sensory template (i.e., "sounds" like, or "feels" a particular way) is valid.

This visual confirmation is particularly important in view of evidence that very different laryngeal postures may sometimes produce vocal qualities which sound similar. This is a phenomenon addressed by the second objective of our imaging study. Consider, for example, the posture of laryngeal structures shown in the next few figures. In Fig. 4, false folds are constricted and medialized during voicing; in Fig. 5, voice is being produced very differently – the true folds are abducted slightly and tensed; both the larynx and supraglottic structures have assumed a posture during phonation which might be characterized as sphincteric in Fig. 6; and in Fig. 7, vocal fold behavior appears appropriate for normal vibration, but stiffness caused by scarring along the vibratory edges produces voice which is markedly dysphonic.

These four postures differ markedly from each other visually, and involve quite different laryngeal dynamics. However, they may actually produce voices which sound quite similar. In fact, disorders of the four patients who demonstrated these particular postures during speech were all characterized as "whisper" dysphonias by listeners presented only with audio recordings. Similarities in their voices, notwithstanding each patient's therapy plan, should be tailored to the unique vocal tract dynamics associated with each dysphonia. If the voice clinician does not have the advantage of imaging the larynx, such differences may be obscured, and the potential success of therapy jeopardized.

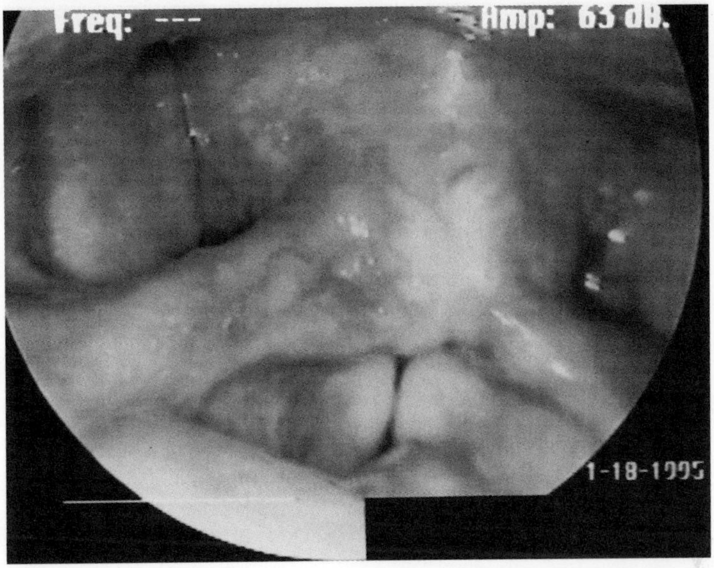

Fig. 4. False vocal folds are constricted, medialized and involved in producing voice.

In another situation, it may be especially important for the clinician to recognize when a very small alteration in laryngeal dynamics produces a large change in voice quality. On the left in Fig. 8, for example, limited pulmonary support used to drive vocal fold vibration produces irregular and only partial closure between the folds during a vibratory cycle. As illustrated on the right in Fig. 8, a very slight increase

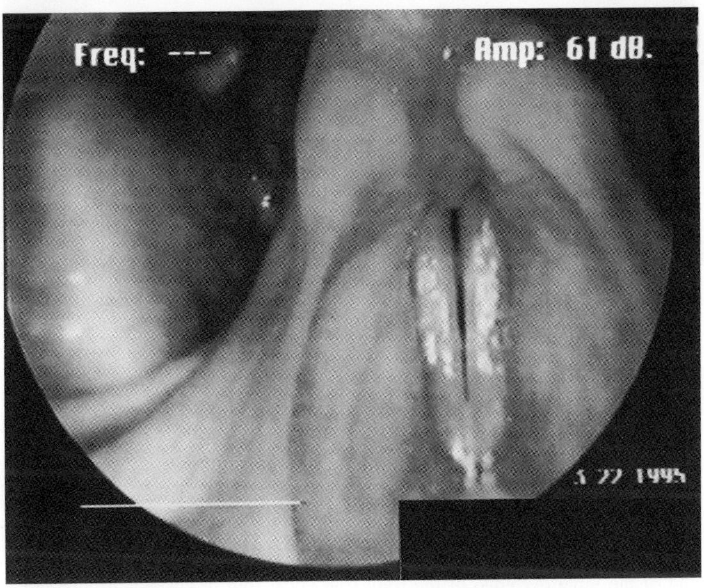

Fig. 5. True vocal folds are slightly abducted and tensed during phonation.

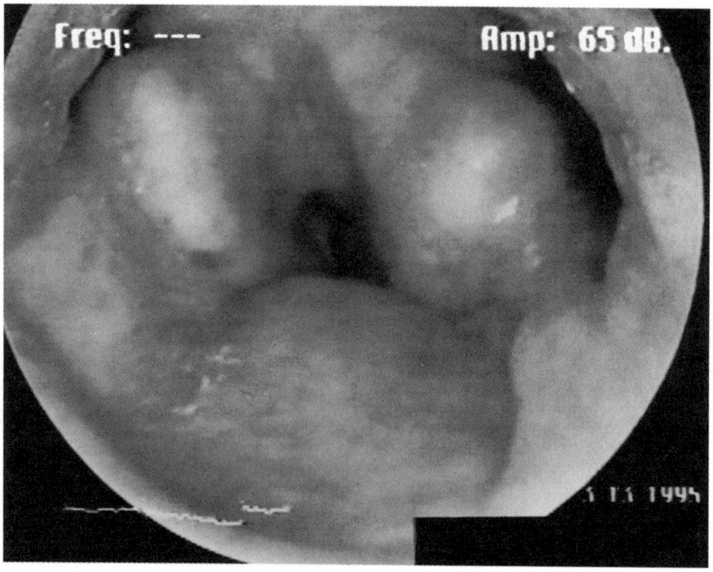

Fig. 6. True and false vocal folds, and supraglottic structures, are constricted during phonation; pattern is referred to as "sphincteric".

in respiratory effort results in greater closure between the folds during voicing, improved vibratory behavior, and notably, improved voice quality. Again, extensive sampling of voice while visualizing the larynx enables the clinician to make such

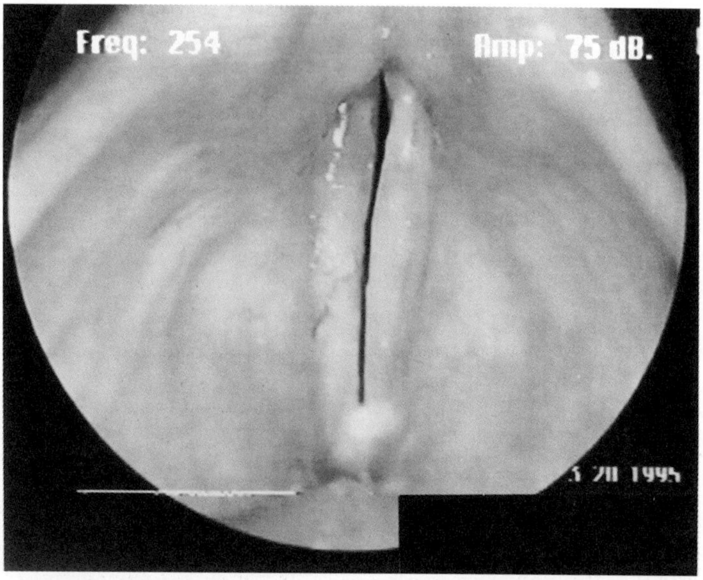

Fig. 7. Scarring of the vibratory edge of the right true vocal fold produces stiffness and aberrant voice quality.

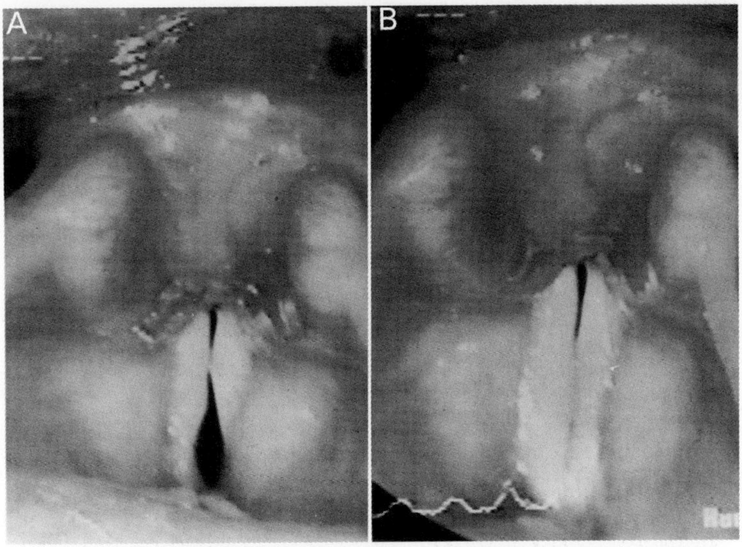

Fig. 8. **A**: True vocal folds close only partially in a patient with compromised pulmonary support during voicing. **B**: Improved respiratory support results in greater closure between true vocal folds during a cycle of vibration.

observations and, ultimately, to incorporate them into a comprehensive treatment plan for an individual patient.

A third, major objective of the voice pathologist's imaging exam is the mapping of an idealized "vocal space" for each patient. What we mean by this is that, for any patient whose vocal behavior we want to change, we need to plot a set of respiratory and phonatory coordinates that represents the best place, vocally, for this patient to be. In some cases, we may need only to "break through" a maladaptive vocal practice, such as plicae ventricularis, and we will rather quickly achieve a normal vocal space, i.e., a space where perceptually appropriate voice, extending over typical ranges of phonatory function, is possible (schematized at the top in Fig. 9). In other cases, for example, where there is actual laryngeal pathology present, our task may be to identify and map that vocal space which seems to represent the best set of phonatory function targets for our patient – targets most consistent with our ultimate objective of establishing, or restoring, normal phonatory function.

For purposes of illustration, consider the three lines at the bottom of Fig. 9 representing frequency, intensity and lung volume or pulmonary support. Sampling voice across different contexts and tasks is likely to reveal a range of, for example, vocal frequencies which can be produced relatively effortlessly by the patient, that is, as shown on the left in Fig. 10, with gentle adduction of the true folds and easy onset of phonation. Outside of this range, however, voice production may become more effortful. On the right in Fig. 10, the same patient's fundamental frequency is just three semitones higher than it was on the left, and it is apparent that some

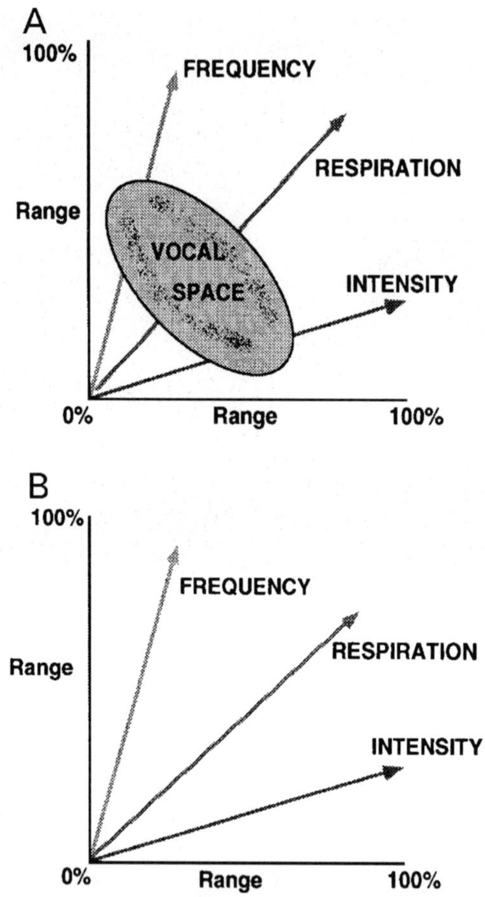

Fig. 9. **A**: Schematic composite representing frequency, intensity and expiratory ranges associated with least effortful, most economical phonation in normal speaker, normal phonatory capability. **B**: Schematic representation of possible ranges of frequency, intensity and expiration for voice production in normal speaker, normal phonatory capabilities.

constriction of the false folds, which we interpret as a sign of excessive effort, is present. This subtle increase in effort may or may not be apparent in listening to the voice; in our experience, visual evidence of effort may sometimes precede auditory or perceptual evidence. By the end of our phonoscopic evaluation, we should be able to plot a range of frequencies where voice is produced most easily and economically based on both visual and auditory evidence. Similar plots of other phonatory function parameters, in particular, vocal loudness and respiratory levels, are also completed.

A schematic representation of the combined plots enables us to define a dysphonic patient's typical (and possibly limited and hyperfunctional) vocal space, as illustrated in Fig. 11 (top) and to compare it to an "idealized" or normal vocal space (Fig. 11, middle). The comparison permits insights into which parameters, or combination of

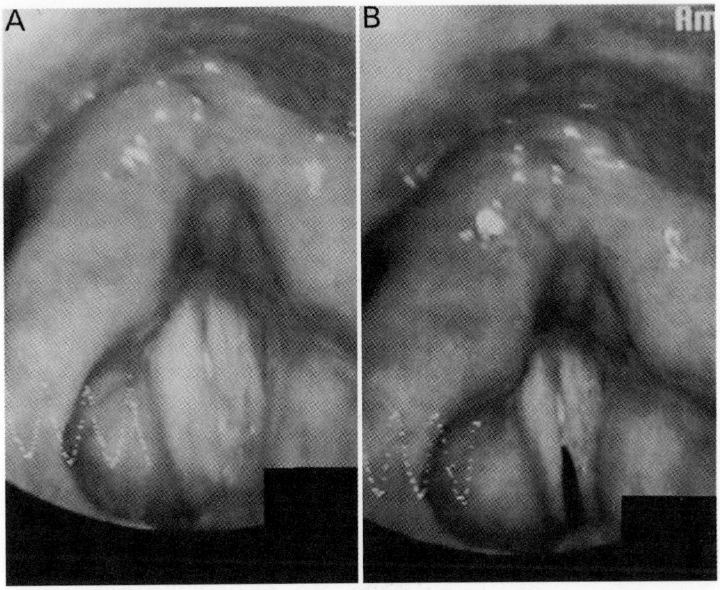

Fig. 10. **A**: Voice produced at a given fundamental frequency is produced with normal appearance of true vocal folds. **B**: At a fundamental frequency three semitones higher, evidence of slight false vocal fold constriction is apparent.

parameters, addressed in what order, might comprise reasonable treatment objectives for our patient, and the most efficacious vocal space, as illustrated at the bottom in Fig. 11, for his/her particular phonatory capabilities.

The fourth objective of the voice pathologist's imaging exam is important if laryngeal pathology accompanies the dysphonia. It requires a careful elaboration of the effects of pathology on phonation, and conversely, of phonatory effects on pathology. As just one example, notice on the left in Fig. 12, with a patient phonating at typical pitch and intensity levels, the greatest contact between the true vocal folds occurs at the exact location of a lesion on the left fold. When the patient is instructed to speak as if there is a very thin "cushion" of air between the folds, however, as illustrated on the right in this figure, contact between the folds is significantly altered and, perhaps, less likely to exacerbate existing pathology.

Once again, extensive sampling of the patient's typical phonatory function behaviors in the presence of pathology reveals a great deal about how pathology is being exacerbated and maintained by the patient. Equally important, direct observation of the larynx during voicing permits the clinician to explore strategies for modifying maladaptive vocal behaviors, and the patient's potential for adopting new vocal practices. Such information can then be incorporated in a comprehensive treatment plan which is tailored both to voice, and to the precise vocal tract dynamics responsible for producing it.

In summary, the objectives noted here are, in our opinion, of paramount

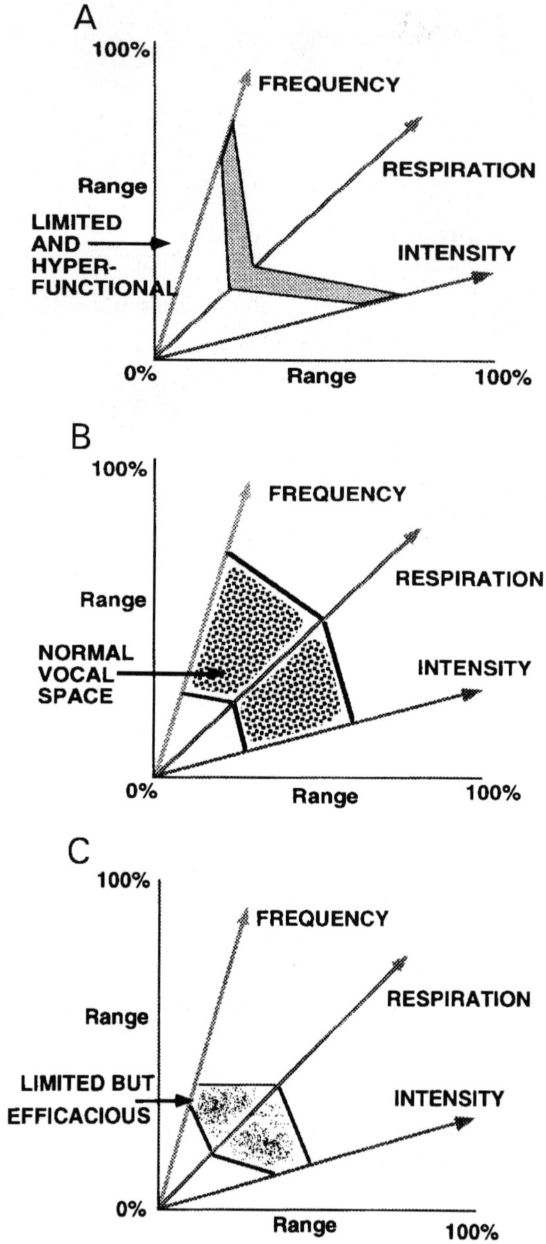

Fig. 11. **A**: Hypothetical description of a "vocal space" which is both limited and hyperfunctional, i.e., ranges of frequency, intensity and respiratory support typically utilized by patient may produce excessive/abusive vocal behaviors. **B**: Vocal space hypothesized to be "ideal" for normal speaker, i.e., ranges (not maximal) of frequency, intensity and respiratory support hypothesized as most efficient and least effortful for normal speaker with normal voice. **C**: Restricted vocal space representative of optimal, i.e., least effortful, most economical, portions of frequency, intensity and respiratory ranges for dysphonic speaker.

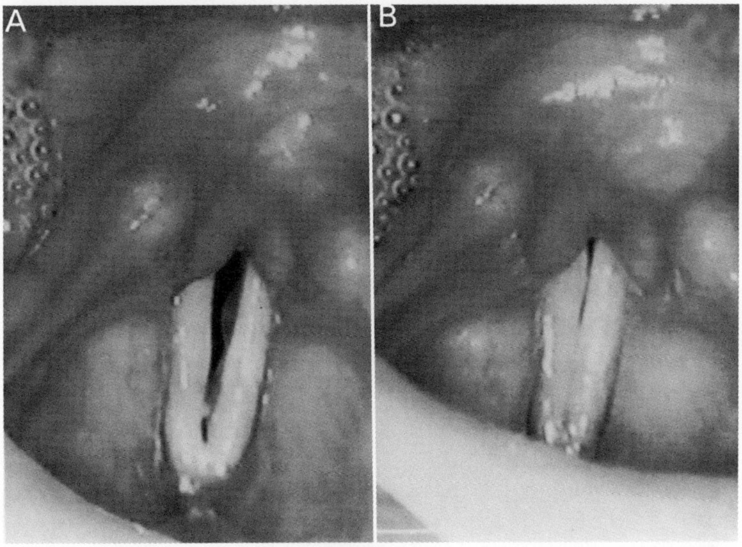

Fig. 12. **A**: At typical frequency and intensity levels, greatest contact between true vocal folds is at the site of pathology. **B**: Small change in phonatory function the alters pattern of contact between true folds.

importance to the voice pathologist charged with treating the dysphonic patient. The fullest realization of each requires visualization of the larynx and vocal tract structures during phonation, and we believe that no other measures of phonatory function, many of which are quite valuable in their own right, can adequately substitute for the information obtained from an imaging study. If the objectives described here can be achieved, they eliminate much of the guesswork from the voice clinician's task, and enable our therapies to be more precisely focused on the complex dynamics of dysphonia – not just its sound, or our perceptions of the factors responsible for it, but on a more accurate model attained from a more comprehensive perspective of voice, and the complex of structures and dynamics that produce it.

Reference

1. Izdebski K, Ross JC, Klein JC. Rigid transoral laryngovideostroboscopy (phonoscopy). In: McFarlane S (ed) Seminars in Speech and Hearing. 1990;11(1).

Voice Update.
M. Pais Clemente, editor.

Phonetogram — voice range profile: assessment of voice capacities and its clinical value

H.K. Schutte
Voice Research Laboratory, Department of Medical Physiology, Faculty of Medicine, University of Groningen, Groningen, The Netherlands

Abstract. Voice range profile measurement is being used more and more as a practical clinical tool in the process of voice evaluation. In principle it means a graphical representation of a patient's or person's vocal capabilities concerning the fundamental frequency range and dynamic range on several arbitrarily chosen pitches. The examination of these two most important aspects of the voice has, in fact, been routinely done since interest in the voice started in the early days of phoniatrics and voice care. These two features are represented in the phonetogram after being measured in an objective and instrumental way. This information represents the capacity of one's voice, and needs to be evaluated against the vocal needs and demands put on the voice. A teacher with low vocal capacities might encounter the fact that daily occupational life presents him/her with great voice-straining demands, which could develop into a voice disorder. The voice range profile might then be used as a tool for explanation. This is usually called functional disorder where the balance between capacities and demands is lost. For a proper voice evaluation the next two steps are necessary: laryngeal examination with stroboscopy to reveal possible organic causes, and a careful exploration of the vocal demands by history taking.

Key words: fundamental frequency, laryngoscopy, sound pressure level, stroboscopy, vocal demands.

In this contribution, information is given about the advantages and clinical value of the phonetogram. The IALP Voice Committee decided a few years ago that the term voice range profile would describe the procedure in a better way. In this presentation, we will use both terms.

Phonetography, or the registration of a voice range profile, has become more popular in the past 25 years. Since the early publications in America, and the first in Europe by Calvet, much information about the procedure has been published. The value in clinical practice has been criticized as well as promoted by several authors [1–12].

Fundamentally, a voice range profile is based on measuring two characteristic factors of a voice. This is the fundamental frequency of the phonation, and the sound pressure level of the softest and loudest phonation over the whole range of fundamental frequencies. It was found on a practical basis that measuring four fundamental frequencies per octave gives enough information about the individual

Address for correspondence: Prof Dr H.K. Schutte, Voice Research Laboratory, Department of Medical Physiology, Bloemsingel 10, 9712 KZ Groningen, The Netherlands. Tel.: +31-50-632750 (secr.), +31-50-632688 (office). Fax: +31-50-632751. E-mail: h.k.schutte@med.rug.nl voice capacities in a clinical session. It should be stressed that, when we started to use the phonetogram as a clinical tool in daily practice, we restricted ourselves to measuring only these two characteristics of a voice. We were absolutely aware of the fact that the voice quality is a very important factor in the evaluation procedure of one's voice. However, measuring the voice quality in a reliable way is not easy, especially since there is no widely accepted way of instrumental measuring and description.

The sound pressure level is measured at a distance of 30 cm in front of the mouth, and to be able to do a reliable comparison between different phonetograms the same vowel configuration of the vocal tract, mostly the vowel /a/, is used.

Figure 1 shows a normal phonetogram of a nonpathological nontrained male voice. The fundamental frequency range is about 2.5 octaves and the sound pressure level range at the region of the speaking voice fundamental frequency is about 40 dB; the maximal sound pressure level (SPL) is about 110 dB at the maximal region of the chest voice, and in the higher region of the falsetto voice the maximal SPL is about the same.

Before presenting a couple of phonetogram examples a few comments are given on the procedure used to register a phonetogram. It appeared practical to start a phonetogram registration in the middle of the range which can be expected. But, of course, this is not very critical or essential. A pitch prompter, purposely made, was used, but any musical instrument with defined fundamental frequencies is suitable. More important is the fact that the examiner is able to hear whether the pitch is correct and can sing the proper pitch to help the testee. If the pitch is not correct, slight differences can be accepted, or the pitch produced is determined and the SPL value(s) registered. Usually high pitches are tested first, then the starting pitch is retested and the lower pitches follow. It showed also to be of value, if using a SPL meter, to register the highest value seen on the meter, while producing the loudest tone and the lowest value for the softest tone. In computerized phonetography this decision is made by the software programming. Between the lower and higher region in the phonetogram, usually in the untrained voice, a transition area is found where the maximal sound pressure level shows a dip. This appears to be related to the

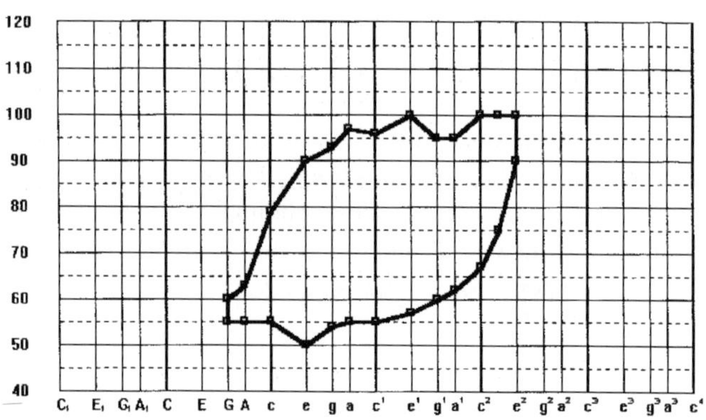

Fig. 1. A normal phonetogram of a nonpathological nontrained male voice.

transition from the chest register to other registers.

In formal singing voice training, much effort is invested to learn the proper use of the top of the chest register – the head register region. This aspect can be seen in comparing phonetograms taken before and after formal professional training, as is shown in Fig. 2. In the head register especially, the maximal SPL contour shows a better equalization.

The difference between a trained and an untrained voice with the same fundamental frequency range can be seen in a comparison of Fig. 3 with Fig. 2B. In the untrained voice, especially, the possibilities of falsetto voice production are hardly developed, whereas the region for the speaking voice, in both voices, appear to be well developed and not much different from each other. The trained voice appears to have more capacities in the higher region, whereas daily singing training supposedly also has lead to a usable falsetto voice.

The next phonetogram, in Fig. 4, is a small phonetogram. For a proper interpretation of the results we need to know under which (daily) conditions the patient has to use the voice. If she needs to use her voice in a profession like teaching in large classrooms, the voice, in general, is too weak. At a normal pitch level for speaking she cannot reach louder as about 75 dB. To raise the loudness of the voice she has

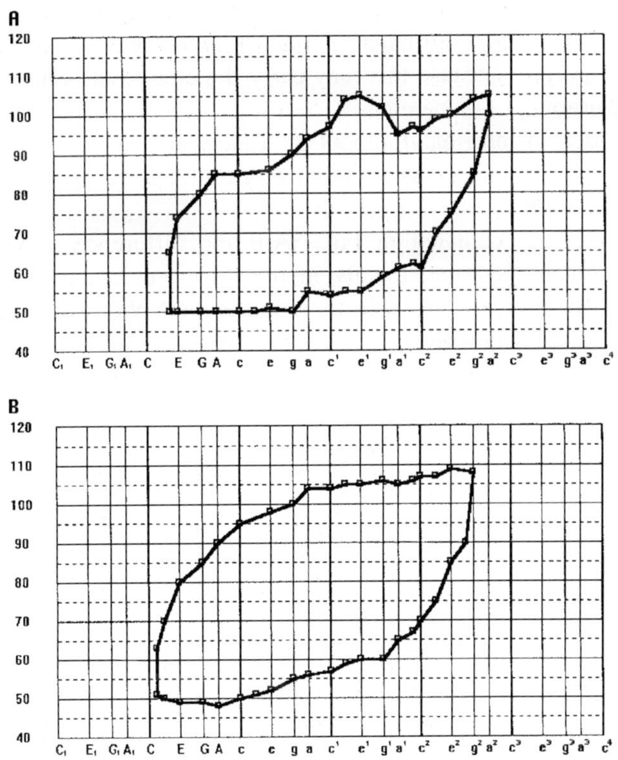

Fig. 2. **A,B**: Phonetograms showing the difference between phonetograms taken before and after formal singing voice training.

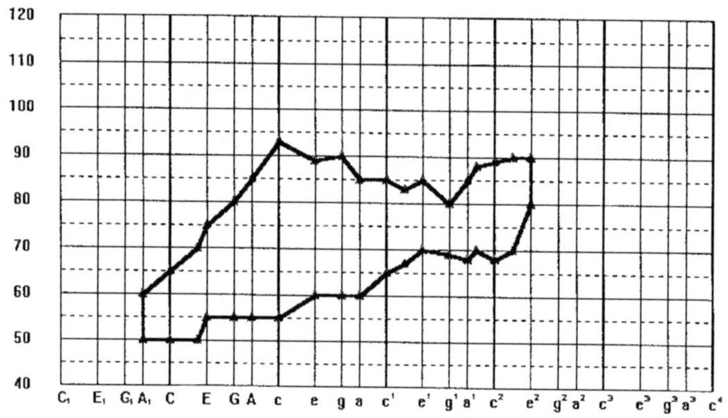

Fig. 3. A phonetogram comparing the voice capacities of a trained singer (Fig. 2B) and an untrained test person, both having about the same fundamental frequency range.

to use higher pitches, which makes her sound unnatural. The falsetto part of her voice on the right side in the phonetogram cannot contribute to reducing her voice problem.

In a diagnostic procedure the next step should be a visual examination, including stroboscopy of the larynx. In many cases, such as that presented in Fig. 4, the glottis does not close completely during a glottal cycle in phonation. This should be evaluated very carefully because this may carry the clue to the cause, and may give directions for therapy.

The combination of information about the functioning of the vocal folds and the phonetogram reveals small details and also gives information about the importance of some observations.

In the phonetogram depicted in Fig. 5A,B the difference in vocal capacities between male persons is found mainly in the lower region, in the region of the speaking voice. Both voices are able to produce loud phonations and both cover almost the same range. One voice, however, received a formal singing voice training;

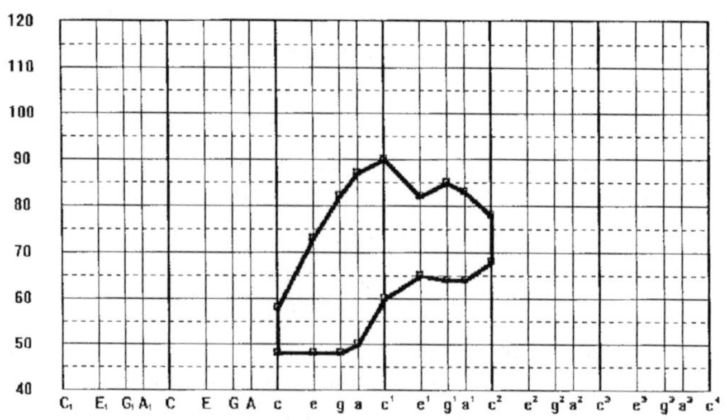

Fig. 4. A phonetogram of a female teacher having problems to sufficiently reach the back part of the classroom with her voice. Laryngoscopy showed an incomplete dorsal glottis closure.

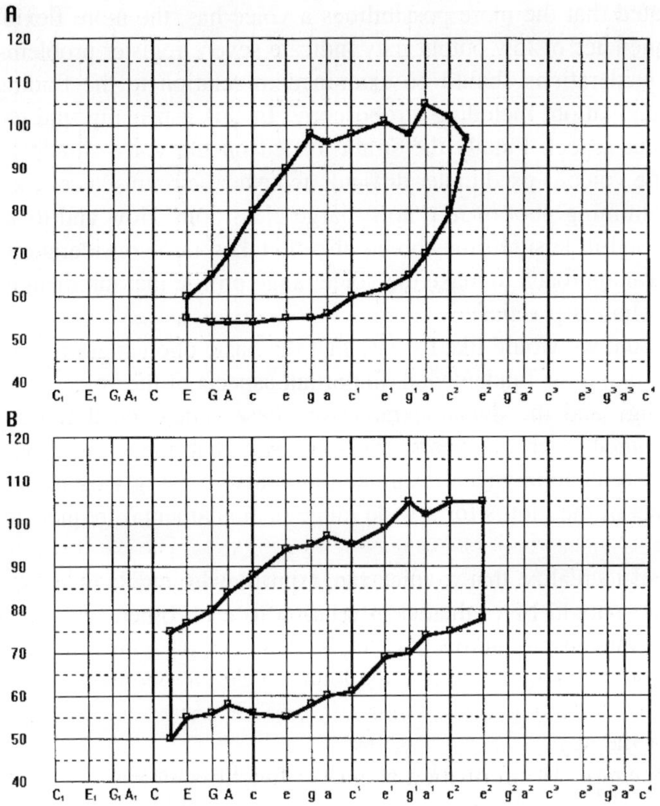

Fig. 5. **A,B**: Phonetograms comparing two different male voices, a trained and an untrained voice with almost the same ranges. Only in the low frequency region is a clear difference found, closely related to a better closure of the glottis at the dorsal part, leading to louder phonatory possibilities.

the phonetogram shows this aspect in a better equalization of the loud phonation contour and a more explicit dynamic range in the lower region of the voice.

Inspection of the larynxes reveals why there is such a difference: the trained singer shows a constitutionally well-developed larynx and full muscular vocal folds, whereas the other vocal folds are much thinner, and moreover, do not close completely in phonation, especially in the lower part of the frequency range. In this high muscular tension, to obtain a good glottis closure conflicts with the need for a relaxed musculature to produce the lower fundamental frequencies. This less complete closure may also be measured by electroglottography, which shows considerable differences in the values for the closed quotient, being higher in the trained singer [13].

Let us summarize the steps for the interpretation of the results of phonetography. It is important to determine, partly based on the type of profession, the regions of interest in the phonetogram. A high fundamental frequency range might be of interest in the case of singing, as well as the region of register transition. For the speaking voice, the region of higher frequencies is less important, although, as a general rule, it may be stated that the more possibilities a voice has, the more flexible the voice will be. Frequencies of low output may indicate severe register problems in singing. All these considerations should be examined in relation to the findings of laryngological examination, including stroboscopy. In this especially, the glottis closure is an important aspect. Finally the strain loaded on the voice should be evaluated. How much the voice is used under difficult acoustical circumstances like teaching in a covered swimming pool or in a noisy large classroom. How and to what purpose the voice is used in leisure time should also be taken into consideration. Principally this is a general approach to make the voice range profile measurement an invaluable tool in daily clinical practice.

In conclusion, we would like to state that the basic phonetogram shows the voice capacities for two most fundamental, important aspects of the voice: the fundamental frequency range and the dynamic range on these fundamental frequencies. From experience gained over the years, we may say that the clinical value is high, especially if a reliable laryngeal examination is also done, giving information about closure aspects of the glottis for a wide range of fundamental frequencies and sound pressure levels.

It is crucial to realize that a voice range profile, laryngological aspects and the voice demands should be evaluated in relation to each other, which gives the best from all three diagnostic approaches.

References

1. Coleman RF, Henn Mabis J, Kidd Hinson J. Fundamental frequency-sound pressure level profiles of adult male and female voices. J Speech Hear Disord 1977;20:197–204.
2. Gramming P, Sundberg J. Spectrum factors relevant to phonetogram measurement. J Acoust Soc Am 1988;83:2352–2360.
3. Gramming P. The Phonetogram. Thesis Malmö, 1988.
4. Klingholz F, Martin F. Die quantitative Auswertung der Stimmfeldmessung. Sprache Stimme Gehör 1983;7:106–110.
5. Klingholz F, Martin F, Jolk A. Das dreidimensionale Stimmfeld. Laryngol Rhinol Otol (Stuttgart) 1986;65:588–591.
6. Klingholz F. Das Stimmfeld: Eine Praktische Anleitung zur Messung und Auswertung. Verlag J Peperny München, 1990.
7. Schultz-Coulon H-J, Asche S. Das "Normstimmfeld" – ein Vorschlag. Sprache Stimme Gehör 1988;12:5–8.
8. Schultz-Coulon H-J. Stimmfeldmessung. Heidelberg: Springer-Verlag, 1990.
9. Schutte HK. Over het fonetogram. Tijdsch Logoped Foniatr 1975;47:82–92.
10. Schutte HK. Untersuchungen von Stimmqualitäten durch Phonetographie. HNO Prax (Leipzig) 1980;5:132–139.
11. Schutte HK, Seidner WW. Recommendation by the Union of European Phoniatricians (UEP): standardizing voice area measurement/phonetography. Folia Phoniatr 1983;35:286–288.
12. Sulter AM, Wit HP, Schutte HK, Miller DG. A structured approach to voice range profile (Phonetogram) analysis. J Speech Hear Res 1994;37:1076–1085.
13. Schutte HK, Seidner WW. Registerabhängige Differenzierung von Elektroglottogrammen. Sprache Stimme Gehör 1988;12:59–62.

Voice Update.
M. Pais Clemente, editor.

Electroglottography: a useful method in voice investigation

P.H. Dejonckere
The Institute of Phoniatrics, Universiteit Utrecht, Utrecht, The Netherlands

Abstract. Electroglottography (EGG) yields straightforward information about variations in vocal fold contact related to the vibratory behavior during phonation. It is entirely noninvasive, easy to handle, and impervious to ambient noise. It has many clinical (investigation and therapy) and research applications, especially in combination with other methods of investigating phonation.

Key words: electrolaryngography, fundamental frequency, jitter, registers, vocal fold, voice quality.

Introduction

Electroglottography (EGG), or electrolaryngography, is an entirely noninvasive, easy to handle method for monitoring some aspects of the oscillatory activity of the vocal folds during phonation. EGG has attracted in the past great interest from many voice scientists and clinicians, resulting in an abundant literature. Nevertheless, EGG is far from being generally accepted in clinical work on voice disorders. There is still intense work going on, aiming at the development and refinement of the method to make it optimally suitable and relevant for use in daily practice with voice patients, especially in combination with laryngostroboscopy [1], and in the frame of some applications as fundamental frequency (Fo) analysis and phonetography [2].

Physical and physiological bases

The basic principle of the device was first described by Philippe Fabre [3] and later applied by himself to the investigation of vocal fold vibration [4]. If a given current is flowing through a bodily structure (i.e., the neck, at the level of the thyroid cartilage), the voltage that is developed will be proportional (according to Ohm's law) to the resistance. Any airspace between two electrodes, placed on both sides of the thyroid, has to be bypassed by the electric field lines, thereby narrowing the conducting path. So, when during the vibration cycle, the conductance decreases, this is to be interpreted as an opening of the glottis, while when the vocal fold tissues make contact, the conductance increases (Fig. 1). For a number of reasons (e.g., for minimizing variations in surface contact between the electrodes and the skin), all electroglottographs work with a high frequency sinusoidal signal. Of course, all of them are

Address for correspondence: Prof P.H. Dejonckere, The Institute of Phoniatrics, Universiteit Utrecht, P.O. Box 85500, 3508 GA Utrecht, The Netherlands.

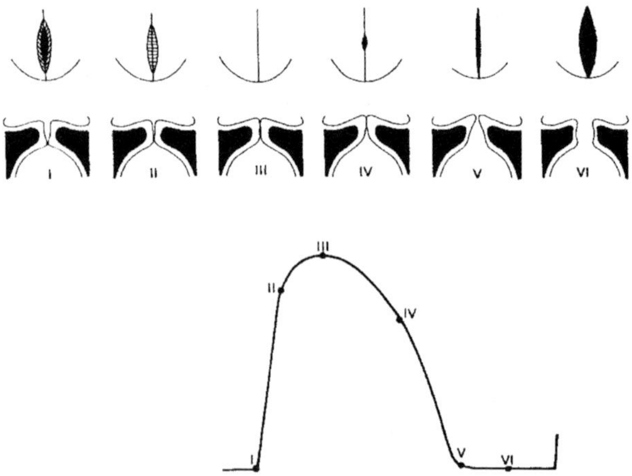

Fig. 1. Schematic relation between the EGG signal and the glottal shape (after Lecluse).

also designed to operate at, and limit current to, safe levels (max 10 mA at 0.5 V).

Only about 1% of the total impedance through the neck is modulated by the vocal fold vibrations.

Most EGG instruments possess a control circuit to compensate for the slow changes of signal level due to the varying neck resistance. However, the time constant, determining the rapidity with which the control system responds to changes of the signal, also affects the shape of the EGG waveform (a larger time constant produces a flatter open phase!). This is of importance when one is interested in the morphology of the EGG signal [5]. The type of high pass filtering used to process an EGG signal must be known in order to properly interpret the details of the waveform.

There is now sufficient evidence to assume that the electroglottographic signal, reflecting the changes in overall conductance between the electrodes, represents variations in the area of contact between the vocal folds, with some limitations in linearity ([6]; further review of the literature in [2]). Figure 1 presents the schematic relation between the EGG signal and the glottal shape. Modeling of the contact area waveform also brought about a better understanding of waveform features [7]. The electroglottograph is, of course, unable to record the absolute magnitude of vocal fold contact.

Applications in phoniatric practice

Differentiation of vocal registers

Vocal fry, or pulse register, is characterized by very long closed phases, as well as, in some cases, by dicrotic waveforms. In chest (or modal register), the classic, regular EGG wave is observed, with its easy to identify steep closing slope. In falsetto, the

EGG wave can be sinusoidal and of very low amplitude, if the changes in contact surface are limited to the extremities of the glottic spindle, or very pointed (short closed phase) if there happens to be a brief closure of thinned vocal fold edges [8,9]. The EGG nicely shows the ability of trained singers to equalize the transitions between registers without voice breaks.

Documentation of voice quality

In the quantitative description of the EGG waveform, the relative importance of the closed phase has attracted great interest as it seems to grow when the voice changes from a breathy or hypokinetic to a strained, hyperkinetic voice quality. However, the exact duration of the closed phase may be difficult to measure because of ambiguities in the definition of the precise moments of closure and opening of the vocal folds. In order to avoid this difficulty, one can use a surface quotient (as illustrated in Fig. 2) [10]. Furthermore, the SPL level needs to be carefully controlled, as it considerably influences the duration of the closed phase, in normal as well as in pathological voices. The duration of the closing time has been found useful in patients with voice disorders [2]. In most cases a lesion of one or both vocal folds affects the speed of closure, resulting in longer closing times in the EGG waveform.

Analysis of the EGG waveform can provide relevant information concerning pathophysiological mechanisms in some kinds of dysphonia [10,11].

Measurement of (EGG) jitter and EGG shimmer

For the purpose of extracting fundamental frequency, the electroglottographic waveform is, in most cases, considerably simpler due to its lesser number of overtones in use than in the acoustic waveform. The (filtered) EGG signal can be used for frequency and amplitude perturbation analysis, especially during sustained phonation [12]. Once more, vibration patterns without contact of vocal folds are not suitable.

Fo studies

The analysis of intonation contours is a common method in linguistic phonetics, and

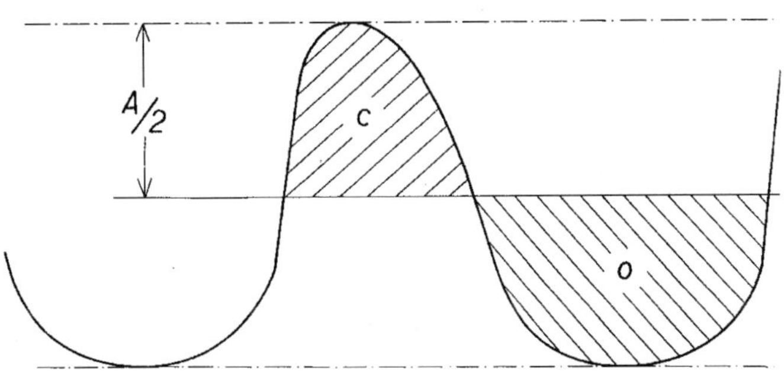

Fig. 2. Surface quotient (area C/area O) for quantifying the EGG signal. The tighter the closure, the higher the C/O quotient.

has clinical applications in e.g., neurologic voice disorders such as Parkinsonism, or prelingual deafness. Distributions of Fo (scatter plots) and statistical perturbation measures appear very useful to describe normal and abnormal (i.e., rough, creaky) voice characteristics (i.e., aperiodicity, jitter) [13]. The computed mean speaking fundamental frequency is a critical parameter for evaluation of severity and treatment effects in case of Reinke's oedema [14].

Tracheo-oesophageal voices

EGG has also been proposed for investigating the vibration mechanism in case of reconstructive laryngectomies (neoglottis) or button voices [15].

Biofeedback

The EGG waveform itself, as well as the extracted Fo intonation curve, when displayed in (quasi) real time on an oscilloscope or computer screen, have been found to be useful as a biofeedback tool in therapeutic management of many types of dysphonia, or in case of prosodic alteration [16,17].

Conclusions

Advantages

Electroglottography (EGG) yields straightforward information about variations in vocal fold contact, related to the vibratory behavior during phonation. It is entirely noninvasive, easy to handle, and impervious to ambient noise. It has a lot of clinical (investigation and therapy) and research applications, especially in combination with other methods of investigating phonation.

Limitations

As EGG is designed to monitor vocal fold contact (not movement, per se), it is unable to monitor noncontact types of vibratory events.

When examining abnormal larynges, the exact pattern of vocal fold vibration may be basically different to that expected for a normal voice. Thus, interpretation of the EGG signal using a model of normal vibration may be entirely inappropriate. As a rule, there is no unique relationship between a pathological EGG and a given anatomical or physiological condition.

References

1. Karnell MP. Synchronized videostroboscopy and electroglottography. J Voice 1989;3:68–75.
2. Colton RH, Conture EG. Problems and pitfalls of electroglottography. J Voice 1990;4:10–24.
3. Fabre P. Sphygmographie par simple contact d'électrodes cutanées, introduisant dans l'artère de faibles courants de haute fréquence détecteurs de ses variations volumétriques. J Comptes-rendus Soc

Biol (Paris) 133:639–641.

4. Fabre P. Un procédé électrique percutané de l'accolement glottique au cours de la phonation: glottographie de haute fréquence. Premiers résultats. J Bull Acad Méd 1957;141:66–69.
5. Rothenberg M. Some relations between glottal air flow and vocal fold contact area. In: Ludlow C, Hart M (eds) Proceedings of the Conference on the Assessment of Vocal Pathology. Rockville: American Speech Language Association, 1981;88–96.
6. Childers DG, Smith AM, Moore GP. Relationships between electroglottograph, speech, and vocal cord contact. J Folia Phoniatr 1984;36:105–118.
7. Titze IR. Interpretation of the electroglottographic signal. J Voice 1990;4:1–9.
8. Kitzing P. Photo- and electroglottographical recording of the laryngeal vibratory pattern during different registers. J Folia Phoniatr 1982;34:234–241.
9. Roubeau B. Mécanismes vibratoires laryngés et contrôle neuro-musculaire de la fréquence fondamentale. J Thèse, Paris (Université de Paris Sud Orsay) 1993;153.
10. Dejonckere P, Lebacq J. EGG and vocal fold nodules. J Folia Phoniatr 1985;37:196–200.
11. Dejonckere P. Control of fundamental frequency and glottal impedance with increasing sound pressure level in normal and pathological voices. J Voice 1994;3:10–16.
12. Haji T, Horiguchi S, Baer T, Gould WJ. Frequency and amplitude perturbation analysis of electroglottograph during sustained phonation. J Acoust Soc Am 1986;80:58–62.
13. Fourcin A. Electrolaryngographic assessment of vocal fold vibration. J Phonetics 1986;14:435–442.
14. Kitzing P. Phoniatric aspects of microlaryngoscopy. J Acta Phoniatrica Latina 1987;9:31–41.
15. Lecluse FLE, Tiwari RM, Snow GB. Electroglottographic studies of Staffieri neoglottis. J Laryngoscope 1981;91:971–975.
16. Fourcin A, Abberton E. The laryngograph and the voiscope in speech therapy. In: Loebell E (ed) Proceedings XVIth International Congress of Logopedics and Phoniatrics, Interlaken. Basel: Karger, 1976;116–122.
17. Baken RJ. Clinical Measurement of Voice and Speech. London: Taylor & Francis Ltd, 1987.

Voice Update.
M. Pais Clemente, editor.

The role of a voice laboratory in the study of voice disorders

R.E. Stone Jr.
Vanderbilt Voice Center, Department of Otolaryngology, Vanderbilt University Medical Center, Nashville, Tennessee, USA

Abstract. In spite of the proliferation of vocology laboratories in the USA, clinicians still seem to question the purposes of gathering objectively derived data and fail to recognize the potential clinical roles of the vocology laboratory. The laboratory may function to serve certain clinical needs such as:

1. Providing a means for interpreting degree of abnormality for specific aspects of a patient's vocal function.
2. Documenting vocal change within patients.
3. Facilitating vocologists' understanding of voice production, techniques and vocalization styles.
4. Enhancing delivery of clinical services.

In spite of such benefits, initial outlay of capital funds and personnel costs impede implementation of a voice laboratory.

Prior to 1980 clinical practitioners usually contented themselves with listening to researchers talk at conventions about customized approaches to acoustic and aerodynamic analysis of phonation. Now, in the mid 1990s, laryngologists and speech-language pathologists as well as some teachers of singing arts and sciences themselves are presenting papers made possible by commercially available data collection instruments and programs[1] in their practice locations. This earlier stage in the study of phonation is possibly best appreciated by considering that prior to 1984, less than a dozen stroboscopes for studying vocal fold behaviors could be identified (Fig. 1). These were located in university training programs for speech-language pathology and in otolaryngology environments. This number grew to an estimated 300 by 1993, and by mid-1995, approximately 700 stroboscopes dotted the country. About half are placed in speech pathology settings and half in medical doctor-only facilities.

Stroboscopy is not the only area of growth in studying phonation. In the past decade, study of aerodynamic aspects of voice has emerged as a potential for routine

Address for correspondence: R.E. Stone Jr., PhD, Vanderbilt Voice Center, Department of Otolaryngology, Vanderbilt University Medical Center, 1500 21st Ave. So Suite 2700, Nashville, TN 37212, USA. Tel.: +1-615-343-9630 (desk), +1-615-343-SING (clinic). Fax: +1-615-343-0872.
E-mail: ed.stone@mc.mail.vanderbilt.edu

[1]KAY Elemetrics, Inc., 2 Bridgewater Lane, Lincoln Park, NJ 07035-1488, USA. Tel.: +1-(800)-289-5297. Kelleher Medical, Inc., 9710 Farrer Ct., Suite N, Richmond, VA 23236, USA. Tel.: +1-(804)-323-4040. GW Instruments, TIGER Electronics, Inc. P.O. Box 85126, Seattle, WA 98145, USA. Tel.: +1-(206)-499-5758.

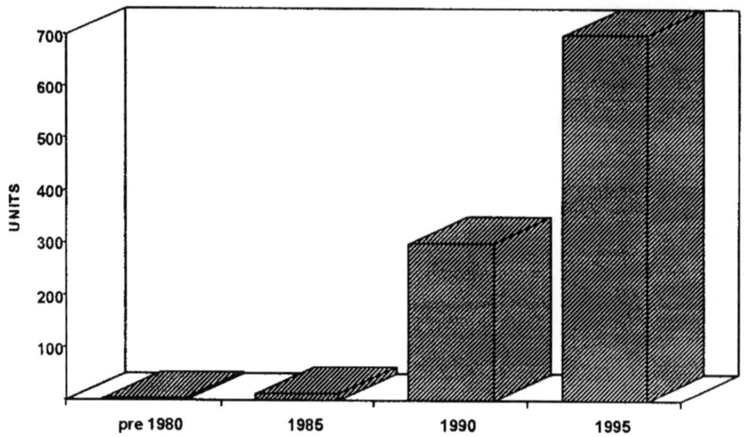

Fig. 1. Growth of stroboscopy, 1993—1995. (Parameter: estimated number of stroboscope units in use.)

study. Vocologists have increased their attention to acoustic voice analysis systems with the addition of three clinically useful commercial products within the past 5 years. Introduction to the USA of new laboratory hardware and user-friendly software from France for clinical assessment of both acoustic and aerodynamic assessment of voice production is anticipated in the near future[2].

The instructions necessary to operate such equipment and software are set forth in manuals from the distributors and are not included here. Baken [1] reviews the various "tests" that have evolved since the availability of laboratory instrumentation and supplements Hirano's [2] presentation of normal and abnormal test measurement values that may be expected. Such information does not need repeating here. Instead, some of the purposes of performing such measurements are explored to emphasize the value of such testing to the clinical vocologist.

The laboratory's role in interpreting the degree of vocal abnormality

Laboratory studies benefit the clinician's assessment of a client's vocal performance. Few individuals would quibble over Dr Hirano's comment [3] that if a person cannot hear a dysphonia and cannot see a pathology to explain the aberrancy, it probably is not of great medical consequence. Accordingly, clinicians may not need objective tests to establish the presence of some aberrant characteristics of the voice or larynx. Yet, in lieu of universally objective voice analysis by clinicians, objective tests have helped define degrees of vocal aberration, the goals for which were set forth by the noted theoretician and researcher Dr Fujimura [4]:

[2]Soremed, 4 Boulevard Carnot, Aix-en-Provence, France 13100. Tel.: +33-4221-6758.

> We are trying to quantify objectively the deviations from normal conditions... By comparing the individual data to the normal distribution... Quantifying the degree of variation from the normal distribution to quantify the degree of pathology.

Data from our laboratory can be used to illustrate Dr Fujimura's stated goals. Note in Table 1 that the mean vital capacity for normal males has been established as 4,430 ml with 68% of our normal subjects falling within ±1,027 ml. The patient's mean vital capacity averaged across three trials was 4,131 ml with a standard deviation of 259 ml. We find, therefore, that the patient's difference from normal expressed by a Z-score of –0.3 is relatively unimportant. During the reading of a 9-s portion of the Rainbow Passage, the patient's phonation quotient was 163 ml, which represents 2.9 SD less than the mean of normals. On testing flow rate during an extended phonation time task, the patient's mean was 1.6 SD below the mean for a group of normal subjects. This tends to objectively substantiate and specifically describe what subjectively might be perceived as "pressed phonation" in this individual.

Unfortunately, such use of statistical summaries of patients' behavior depends upon the measures of a parameter assuming the characteristics of a normally distributed function. When data for normals do not represent normally distributed functions, the laboratory has more difficulty fulfilling the role of showing the significance of aberrant laryngeal behaviors. This may occur, for example, when interpreting a patient's jitter values. Stone and Rainey [5] found that for Visi-Pitch assessment of jitter in a group of normal males the mode was 0.64%, the mean was 0.987%, and the median was 0.865%. In a normally distributed function these measures should be the same. Distribution of jitter scores for this sample was undeniably skewed (Fig. 2). Clearly, applying normal descriptive statistics to summarize this distribution is not appropriate. Consequently, determining the extent to which a patient's jitter values might represent aberrancy compared to this normal group appropriately, cannot be accomplished with parametric statistics.

The laboratory's role in documenting vocal change over time (trials)

Third party payers may have contributed to the current interest in "outcome studies". Clinicians are asked to illustrate the effectiveness of intervention provided by a client with objectively derived data. Here, instrumentation provided by the voice laboratory

Table 1. Aerodynamic measures in different tasks.

Task	T1	T2	T3	PT mean	PT SD	Normal mean	Normal SD	Z-score
Vital capacity (ML)	3832	4284	2477	4131	259	4430	1027	–0.3
Reading (P.Q)	148	171	169	163	13	362	76	–2.9
MPT (ml/s)	42	22	40	35	11	178	79	–1.6

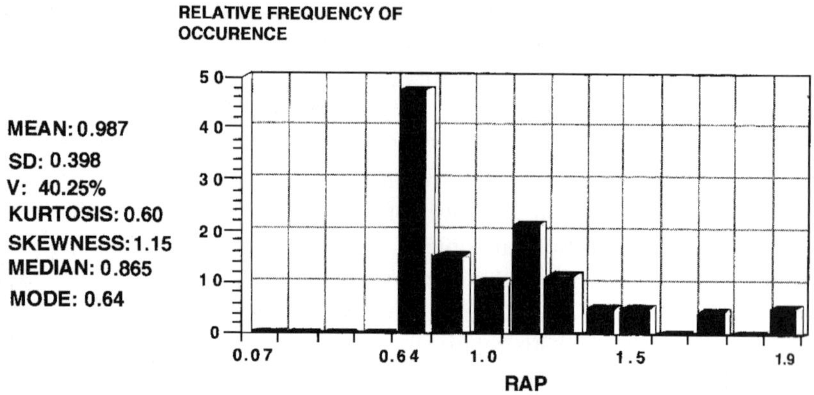

Fig. 2. Descriptive statistics of jitter measurements from a group of normal adult voices. (This parameter does not resemble a normally distributed function and, therefore, application of parametric statistics may be inappropriate.)

is of great assistance. Consider, for example, the trend in improvement in extended phonation time over 15 samples from one patient (Fig. 3). Such data would substantiate the claim of a clinician seeking, for example, to justify phonatory challenge therapy [6] for Parkinson patients.

Yet another aid the laboratory provides may be illustrated by considering early instruction for laryngectomees to develop increased duration of sound. Early in intervention the patient achieves short productions and changes so slightly from one production to another that stopwatch measurement cannot be accomplished. The non-laboratory-based clinician, therefore, is fraught with the problem of validly reinforcing trials and verifying the small increments of progress. Failing to see progress contributes to frustration of the client. Possibly this is one reason many laryngectomees abandon learning standard esophageal voice production. On the other hand, a clinician with instrumentation to measure productions, for example in tenths

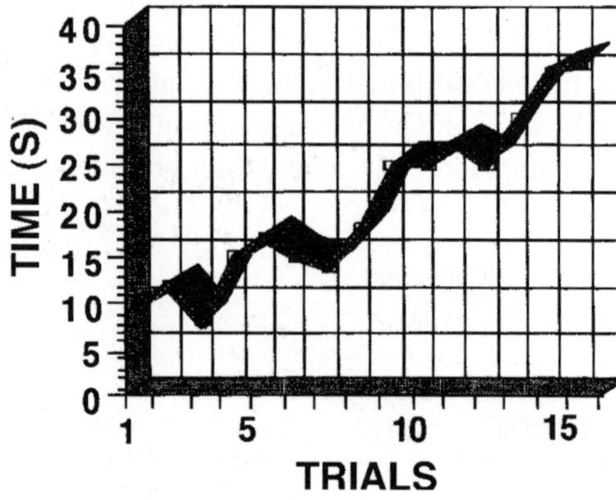

Fig. 3. Changes in duration of prolonged phonation times as a function of trials for one individual.

of seconds, is confidently able to point out progress in sustained phonation times.

The clinician desiring to report to peers on therapeutic effectiveness of a procedure or technique faces a significant problem without laboratory instrumentation. Over the past few years it has become increasingly difficult to elicit acceptance for publication of those papers describing intervention success without objectively based evidence. Reviewers expect postintervention improvements to be demonstrated in various parameters such as restoration of mucosal wave, decreased air flow rates, and normalization of acoustic measures.

Objective measurements of phonation also benefit medicolegal assessments of treatment. Such legal issues as the resolution of disability are moving toward the requirement of objectively based indications of declined laryngeal function and objective evidence of failure to benefit from intervention. Thus, routine assessment of patient behaviors for representing patient response to intervention is one of the major roles of clinical voice laboratories.

The laboratory's role in understanding physiology of voice production

In the USA, voice laboratories have contributed to our understanding of the voice and its production since the 1920s. Dr Seashore coordinated a group at the University of Iowa whose research efforts included the study of graphic displays of singing. Much that is known about vibrato today can be attributed to this group [7,8]. The ultra high-speed photography laboratory at Northwestern afforded opportunity in the 1940s for Drs von Leden and Moore to contribute substantially to our understanding of vocal fold behavior during phonation in normal and abnormal voice production. The work of Dr Fant and Dr Sundberg from the Royal Institute of Technology in Sweden continues to aid our understanding of the acoustics of voice [9,10] and various styles of singing [11].

While at the Royal Institute of Technology, Cleveland [12] used laboratory instrumentation to study the potential role of vowel formants in contributing to the classification of singing voices. Table 2, developed from Cleveland's data, shows that tenors, baritones and basses, respectively, had lower spectral positions for the means of Formants 1–4. These results have not been replicated, nor have there been any studies reported regarding female voice classifications. Investigation of such issues identifies a continuing role of the voice laboratory.

From the joint efforts of Dr Sundberg and the clinicians at the Vanderbilt Voice Center, results of studying subglottal pressures in a small group of elite country/western singers were recently announced [13]. They found that the subglottal pressures used in speech-like activities were similar to the pressures in singing. This is illustrated in Fig. 4 in which the majority of singing subglottal pressure estimates, Ps, for a subject that lies between the loud and soft functions for productions of /pæ/ in isolation and in limerick patterns.

The underlying motivation of the study was to learn what these performers of "gold-record" status do physiologically to aid the pedagogy used with aspiring artists in correcting and/or instructing their singing.

Table 2. Differences in formant frequencies of /a/ as a function of voice classification.

/a/	F1	F2	F3	F4
Tenor	609	994	2576	2909
Baritone	530	944	2400	2849
Bass	503	900	2386	2527

Note: values given in Hz. (From T.F. Cleveland, JASA 1977;61(6):1622–1629.)

The laboratory's role in enhancing delivery of behavioral intervention

With the ability to measure aerodynamic, electromyographic, photographic and acoustic parameters, the dialogue between clinician and patient can be less abstract and more reality based. As reported by Mathews [14], the dialogue may, then, convey themes known to foster maintenance of clinical skills outside the clinic environment. She found that patients' success in maintaining clinical benefits in speech is linked to their descriptions of speech that, in part, are physiologically based. Patients' knowledge of what to do and not to do is fostered by instrumentation-based intervention and, according to Mathews' work, this engenders therapeutic success.

The use of laboratory instrumentation at times also may serve as an instructional facilitative technique. For example, keeping airflow rate at a certain point on a display panel during a phonatory task can serve as a "distraction". This refocusing of attention away from oneself and one's speech habits seems to incline the patient toward new and closer-to-normal phonation. Thus, laboratory monitoring may need

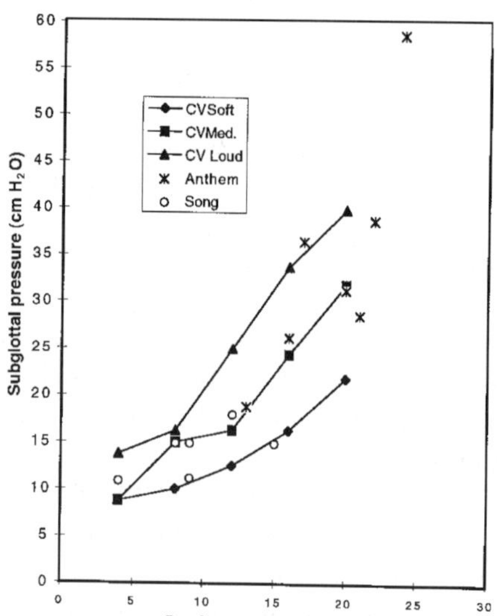

Fig. 4. Changes in subglottal pressure estimates for one subject as a function of fundamental frequency for singing- and speaking-like activities.

to be added to the list of such voice modification techniques as humming, yawn-sigh, chewing, etc.

Laboratories employed in intervention therapy can provide didactic characteristics necessary in learning theory. With reliable and valid measures that can be obtained in real time, decisions about dispensing reinforcers will enjoy validity, accuracy, and immediacy. The more accurate and consistent the decision to dispense reinforcement, the quicker the patient learns new behaviors. It has long been known that behaviors exhibited immediately before the dispensing of reinforcers is the behavior that is reinforced. Thus, if a clinician cannot immediately judge and reinforce target behaviors, he may risk reinforcing behaviors that are extraneous and unwanted. Instrumental monitoring of the patients' behavior and perception of success, such as that provided by deflection of a tracing or other feedback displays, enables immediate reward for the desired behavior, sometimes without interference or interpretation by the clinician.

Patients monitoring their vocal productions during instruction have been noted in our facility to exhibit longer work periods and increased rates of performance. Children as well as adults seem to enjoy hours of interacting with instruments and computers. This is possibly best evidenced by the plethora of computer games that have become available over the past few years. Apparently, the intrigue associated with behaviorally controlling instrumentation counters the fatigue often connected with repetitive tasks. We have found that individuals performing repetitions of extended phonation time tasks will tire of the activity in fewer trials without instrumental feedback displayed on a computer screen and the visual incentive of trying to better their previous performances. The educated patient can also keep his/her own records of performance through "scripts" that may be written to transfer data from laboratory applications to carefully designed spreadsheets. Consequently, the patient can see even small increments of improvement from one session to another, which fosters optimism. When patients are optimistic about their intervention they seem to be better workers and stick with given tasks longer.

Emission rate of behavior is also enhanced by the use of the voice laboratory as an intervention environment. Time-outs to apologize for errors in performance are decreased, probably because the patients recognize that instruments do not process and respond to such comments. Unrewarded, the apologetic behavior subsides and leaves more time for instruction and supervised practice. Furthermore, instrumental based intervention tends to invoke fewer "rapport" building activities that in face-to-face situations often focuses on social niceties but have little to do with altering behavior. These niceties often detract from the business of altering vocal skills by involving dialogue between the clinician and client in dialogue about activities that do not relate to voice and its production.

We have conducted informal time-studies of the activities directed by some clinicians outside the laboratory setting. Some clinicians may spend up to 68% of the therapy time spent in activities not directly related to behavioral change. When incorporating instrumental monitoring of performance with Parkinson patients in a Silverman Approach [6] we find that social interaction and rapport activities can typically occupy less than 16% of the therapy session.

Liabilities of the voice laboratory

Cost

In spite of the improved understanding of voice quality and the effectiveness of intervention therapy that the voice laboratory can provide, it presents some liabilities. The major ones are equipment costs and personal time of the clinician involved to do the analyses.

Basic instrumentation and software costs for aerodynamic studies can range from about US$ 5,700–46,000. Acoustic software and computer boards might well run between US$ 1,400 and 5,000. These coupled with good microphones that run from several hundred dollars up to over a thousand dollars make for a substantial investment. Unless a noise-canceling microphone[3] is used, a sound booth may be necessary to record patients' voices without contamination of ambient room noise.

Other equipment must be considered. Implementing electromyography in the laboratory incurs an expense ranging between US$ 5,000 and 40,000. Support equipment such as acoustic filters, tone generators, frequency counters, and oscilloscopes might easily increase the equipment budget by US$ 10,000–20,000. Adding acoustic recording and monitoring devices such as DATs, amplifiers, and speakers assumes an additional US$ 2,000–5,000 or more. Stroboscopy, the backbone of a voice laboratory, involves expenditure of in excess of US$ 40,000 for the most commonly used device. Other basic pieces of equipment would include one or two computers with a printer which may be available for approximately US$ 3,000 each.

Overall, laboratory equipment costs may range from around US$ 72,000 to 163,000 for a complete laboratory excluding costs of sound treating a recording facility or purchasing a sound-treated enclosure. Unfortunately, the equipment costs are not the only deterrent to the implementation of a voice laboratory.

Personnel and their time commitment running the voice lab are a significant cost. A laboratory providing comprehensive services will require maintenance, trouble shooting, and other technical assistance. In an academic medical facility such services may be available through the Biomedical Department. Academic programs may utilize the services of the voice scientist and his support personnel or individuals from the physics department. Laboratories in private practices may choose to contract the audiovisual services available in the community for support.

The commitment of a person to perform the assessments must be budgeted for as well. Conservative estimates of time can be anticipated:

- stroboscopic examination, 40–80 min;
- airflow assessment, 20–40 min;
- acoustic recording, 5–10 min; and
- acoustic analysis, 15–30 min.

---

[3]LightSPEED Technologies, Inc. 15812 SW Upper Boones Ferry Rd., Lake Oswego, OR 97035, USA. Tel.: +1-800-732-8999.

One finds that for just one patient, a time commitment for a comprehensive laboratory testing might range from over 1 and 1.5 to just under 3 h. Such a time commitment not only limits the number of patients that can be evaluated but also incurs a substantial expense for the patient.

Lack of standardized procedures

Absence of universally accepted assessment procedures in laboratory assessment and intervention, handicaps interpretation of results and confounds interlaboratory communication. For example, no published studies have yet determined the optimal microphone placement for voice recordings. Reported variations in distance from microphone to lips range from less than two inches (approximately 5 cm) to over three feet (approximately 39 cm). Yet, Titze [15] reported substantial variability in jitter measures when the microphone is directionally varied by seemingly small amounts around the sound source.

The number of trials that should be obtained for a given assessment has not reached universal acceptance. Stone [16] reported that even after eight trials only 50% of the subjects in his study of normals gave their maximum durations of phonation out of 15 tokens. Scherer [17] concluded that a greater number of trials to sample vocal behavior adequately is required for dysphonic voices than for nondysphonic voices before no new information is gained across trials.

Maximum phonation time and s/z ratio are often listed as meaningful indicators for clinical assessments. Still, standard settings have yet to be established for fundamental frequency, vocal intensity levels, or degree of mouth opening during assessment.

No group has emerged to recommend sets of vocal behaviors that should be tested except in the case of aerodynamic assessment using the Nagashima Phonatory Function Analyzer. In 1989, a conference attended by nearly every user of this instrument met and derived a set of parameters for testing. Those include vital capacity assessment and, during phonation, measurement of air flow rate, flow volume, fundamental frequency, vocal intensity and duration during several tasks. Tasks the users agreed upon involved the following:

1. Vital capacity assessment,
2. A 9-s reading of the Rainbow Passage beginning with "... These take the shape...".
3. Maximum phonation time.
4. 2-s productions of sustained */a/* at:
    a) pitch range limits; and
    b) intensity range limits.
5. Laryngeal diadochokinetic productions of:
    a) */a/*; and
    b) */ha/*.

Software has been developed at the Vanderbilt Voice Center[4] that replaces the inefficient traditional hand measurements of the graphic writeouts enabling computer analysis of the data.

On the acoustic side, there is great variability demonstrated in terms of the number of descriptors that might be used. For example, Kay Elemetrics' Multidimensional Voice Profile system provides for analysis of up to 21 descriptors. Other software available through Tiger Electronics and G.W. Instruments provides for less than 12 descriptors.

Conclusion

In answer to the question "What is the role of the voice laboratory in the study of voice disorders?" we have indicated that the voice lab will provide an atmosphere and the capability of specifying degrees of patients' vocal abnormalities. The voice laboratory may contribute to specifying efficacy of interventions. It promotes the use of clinically effective activities and fosters communication between clinician and patient that nurtures maintenance of learned behaviors. Although implementation of laboratory practices is costly, we feel that the laboratory holds promise for improved delivery of services and is necessary to better understand voice production.

References

1. Baken R. Clinical Measurement of Speech and Voice. Boston: College Hill, 1987.
2. Hirano M. Clinical Examination of Voice. New York: Springer-Verlag, 1981.
3. Hirano M. Proceedings of the Conference on the Assessment of Vocal Fold Pathology. ASHA Reports 1982;11:29.
4. Fujimura I. Proceedings of the Conference on the Assessment of Vocal Fold Pathology. ASHA Reports 1982;11:29.
5. Stone RE, Rainey CL. Intra- and intersubject variability in acoustic measures of normal voice. J Voice 1992;5:189–196.
6. Ramig LO, Bonitati C, Lemke J, Horii Y. Voice treatment for patients with Parkinson disease: development of an approach and preliminary efficacy data. J Med Speech Lang Pathol 1994;2: 191–209.
7. Schoen M, The pitch factor in artistic singing. Psychol Monogr 1922;31:230–259.
8. Tiffin J, Seashore H. Summary of the Established Facts in Experimental Studies in the Vibrato up to 1932. University of Iowa Studies in the Psychology of Music. I. 1932;344–376. Cited in Zemlin W. Speech Hear Sci. Englewood Cliffs: Prentice-Hall, Inc. 1968;205.
9. Fant G. Acoustic Theory Of Speech Production. The Hague: Mouton, 1970.
10. Sundberg J. The Science of the Singing Voice. DeKalb: Northern Illinois University Press, 1987.
11. Sundberg J, Gramming P, Lovetri J. Comparisons of pharynx, source, formant and pressure characteristics in operatic and musical theater singing. J Voice 1993;7:301–310.
12. Cleveland TC. Acoustic properties of voice timber types and their influence on voice classification. J Acoust Soc Am 1977;61:1622–1629.
13. Cleveland TC, Stone RE, Sundberg J, Iwarsson J. Subglottal pressure in six professional country singers. 1995;(In preparation).

---

[4]Written for PC computers and available from the author.

14. Mathews. An Analysis of the Relationship between the Degree of Maintained Fluency Improvement of Former Portland State University Stuttering Clients and the Overall Language Themes They Used. Master's Thesis. Portland State University, 1981.
15. Titze I. Effect of microphone type and placement on voice perturbation measurements. J Speech Hear Res 1993;36:1177–1190.
16. Stone RE. Issues in clinical assessment of laryngeal function: contradictions for subscribing to maximum phonation time and optimum fundamental frequency. In: Bless D, Abbs J (eds) Vocal Fold Physiology: Contemporary Research and Clinical Issues. San Diego: College-Hill Press, Inc., 1982;410–424.
17. Scherer R. Required number of tokens to determine representative voice perturbation values. 1995;(Submitted).

Voice Update.
M. Pais Clemente, editor.

Differential diagnosis of AD-AB-Ductor spasmodic dysphonia, vocal tremor and ventricular dysphonia by auditory and phonoscopic observations

Krzysztof Izdebski[1,2] and Ronald R. Ward[1,2,3]

[1]*Pacific Voice and Speech Foundation, San Francisco;* [2]*Department of Otolaryngology, Head and Neck Surgery, University of California, Davis, Sacramento; and* [3]*Kaiser Permanente Medical Center, San Francisco, California, USA*

Abstract. Differential diagnoses of ADDuctor, ABDuctor Spasmodic Dysphonia, vocal tremor, mixed ADDuctor spasmodic dysphonia with vocal tremor and ventricular dysphonia are discussed here from physiologic and acoustic points of view. Symptoms are described in accordance to their generation as predicted by physiologic models. Symptomatic findings are also supported by objective acoustic and phonoscopic verification. Clinically useful differential diagnosis criteria and specific tests facilitating differentiating among and between these voice disorders are provided.

Introduction

Contemporary treatment of adductor (ADD SD), abductor spasmodic dysphonia (ABD SD), mixed adductor spasmodic dysphonia with tremor (MxADDSDVT), and vocal tremor (VT) is based on destructive procedures such as right laryngeal nerve (RLN) section [1–9] or chemical denervation of selected intrinsic laryngeal muscles by intramuscular injections of botulinum toxin type A (Botox) [10–19]. Treatment of ventricular dysphonia (VeD) that failed to respond to voice therapy may also involve surgery, resulting in the ablation of the false vocal folds [20].

Consequently to avoid improper treatment, precise and accurate diagnosis of these voice conditions is of paramount importance. Also, all current surgical approaches do not cure the underlying etiology, but merely treat symptoms. Therefore, surgical intervention may result in creating a new type of dysphonia – albeit less taxing than the original underlying dysphonia. This new postoperative dysphonia often requires intensive voice therapy [2,7]. Therefore, precise understanding of how the original voice qualities are changed as a result of surgery is of paramount importance to practicing voice clinicians, because the new postoperative dysphonia must be explained to the patient, and patients must be aware that lengthy voice therapy may be needed postoperatively.

Moreover, a systematic and objective description of pretreatment symptomatology of these disorders is of importance. Ability to establish symptom patterns can explain

---

Address for correspondence: Dr K. Izdebski, 350 Parnassus Ave, Suite 501, San Francisco, CA 94117, USA.

among others: 1) the variability of symptoms; and also 2) can be useful in discussing long-term efficacy of treatment method; 3) can be helpful in predicting long-term effects of treatment on symptom elimination; 4) can be useful in establishing a pattern of posttreatment phonatory quality profile; 5) can be useful in choosing surgical site(s) selection; 6) can be useful in guiding drug dosing; 7) can be useful in validating symptom recurrence; 8) can be useful in guiding timing or salvage surgery or reinjection; and 9) can be useful in explaining and substantiating the role of posttreatment voice therapy in prolonging the surgical results. Also, a prior knowledge of how the specific voice symptoms fit a given voice disorder will empower the clinician with a base for establishing differential diagnoses, hence in designing the most efficacious treatment plan.

Models

The diagnostic criteria presented here are derived from physiologic models of ADD SD, ABD SD, VT and VeD. These models try to explain the symptomatology of each condition by implicating specific phonatory processes as being responsible for a generation of specific symptom pattern. Models presented here are based on our extensive objective investigations of thousands of dysphonic patients over the past 2 decades. These objective investigations included systematic, acoustic, phonoscopic, glottographic, aerodynamic and electromyographic studies.

ADD SD model

The ADD SD model is based on objective evaluation of over 1,000 cases of patients referred to us with the provisional diagnosis of ADD SD [21]. Of these, about 50% were diagnosed as representing ADD SD. In general, the proposed model [22] states that symptom generation in ADD SD is based on the misprocessing of sensory information from the glottis by the brainstem basal ganglia. Such misprocessing is assumed to be due to either viral or vascular damage affecting the brainstem ganglia. This misprocessing affects the fine neuromotor control of the true vocal folds during phonatory production only causing the characteristic symptomatology of ADD SD. Vegetative tasks are spared. The model of ADD SD essentially follows a focal dystonia model, but states that the presence or absence of symptoms must be governed in a predictable and systematic way. The proposed model postulates that ADD SD symptoms are organized in a systematic fashion (phonetotopic symptom generation), and that the severity or absence of symptoms is dependent on the intrinsic nature of the phonatory task executed. Therefore, symptoms will be absent when nonphonatory gestures of the glottis are performed, even if the laryngeal gestures mimic or are similar in nature to the phonatory gestures. The crucial physiologic parameters that are responsible for symptom generation and symptom variability include: 1) vocal fold contact area; 2) vocal fold collision force; and 3) glottic compression. The model postulates that any process that interrupts a sensory motor flow from forwarded to the larynx will eliminate these conditions and will result in elimination or reduction of symptoms. This includes RLN section, chemical denervation (Botox), electrical stimulation, or muscle debulking.

ABD SD model

The ABD SD model is based on the 20 cases of this condition encountered in our practices over the past 20 years. The model of ABD SD (ABD SD is also understood as a type of a focal dystonia) postulates that the patients afflicted with this condition are unable to relax in due time the laryngeal abductor musculature, that the cricothyroid continues to act or that the adductors fail to contract in time [23].

Consequently, this results in sudden air evacuation across the glottis, which in running speech is represented as sudden unvoicing or devoicing of voiced segments.

Therefore, to test properly patients suspected to present with ADD or ABD SD, specifically designed speech/phonatory tasks that reflect the activity of the laryngeal musculature must be given. Any other type of testing will fail or will give erroneous results. Because SLN may play a role, testing at lowered voice fundamental frequency gives asymptomatic results.

VT model

Pure vocal tremor model is based on over 50 cases. The VT model does not assume that vocal tremor is of dystonic nature, but proposes symptom generation sites to be located within the cerebellar system [24–26]. This model postulates a central discoordination, affecting indiscriminately all aspects of voice and nonvoice laryngeal productions. Therefore, vocal symptoms in patients with VT are present without regard to voice frequency or type of the vocal tasks produced [22,24].

MxADDSDVT model

This model is based on approximately 160 cases studied. The mixed ADDSDVT model states that patients afflicted with this condition will produce a phonatory profile consistent both with the focal dystonia model and with the cerebellar model. Therefore, vocal symptoms of ADD SD will be enhanced or reduced depending on the specificity of the motor task involved, but VT will persist independently of the task.

VeD model

The ventricular dysphonia (VeD) model presented here is based on over 60 cases studied [27]. This model postulates that symptoms are produced either in response to an inability to control true vocal fold phonatory approximation due to some peripheral lesion, or that this control is impaired due to functional conversion. If lesions are present, they usually involve anterior commissure patency, resulting in anteroposterior glottic compression, which brings the false vocal folds together during phonatory attempt. In our VeD model, the false vocal folds may actually vibrate, or may dampen the activity of the true vocal folds. The first case is usually in response to the organic lesion and gives a more periodic voice. The second is in response to functional conversion and produces a more harsh or variable voice. The voice in VeD may therefore sound overpressured with a strained/strangled quality similar to that in ADD SD, but the mechanism is diametrically opposed to that of the ADD SD.

Consequently application of the ADD SD testing or treatment paradigm will fail.

Symptomatology

The symptomatologies of the various voice disorders described here are based on acoustic, phonoscopic and acoustic investigations. Acoustic features include static and dynamic voice production and relevant connected speech. Phonation produced during nonspeech tasks (vegetative) is also tested. Visual symptoms are derived from phonoscopy [28–32].

ADD SD symptoms

Auditory symptoms

Classically, ADD SD symptoms are described as strained/strangled voice [1]. This voice quality has been termed by us "overpressured voice" [33–35]. It may be accompanied by vocal arrests. Typically, however, all ADD SD patients can laugh, sing and whisper with absent or markedly reduced symptoms.

Our model symptoms of ADD SD propose specific phonotopic symptom organization, therefore overpressure predominates in the lower voice fundamental range. Overpressure is generally present in voice range up to 1.5 octaves above the base fundamental.

Consequently, symptoms of ADD SD are most prominent within the speaking ranges of both sex groups. Symptoms are at their maximum in all-voiced speech produced at elevated loudness. Symptoms are completely eliminated or markedly reduced at higher voice frequency levels, including falsetto, whisper and during ingressive speech production. Ingressive speech is, however, symptomatic in VT. No physiologic signs are noted when patients perform vegetative tasks [22].

Consequently, sequences counting all-voiced segments are more symptomatic than sentences containing voiced/voiceless clusters. Sustained phonation at low and mid levels may be symptomatic or asymptomatic (including presence or absence of vocal arrests), but phonation at about 1–1.5 octaves above the baseline will be asymptomatic. Should arrest be present during sustained phonation, they also will predominate in the lower voice ranges and will be absent in the higher ranges. The rate of vocal arrests is similar to tremor (±5–6 Hz). The oscillatory behavior in VT is, however, more regular. The magnitude of tremor will diminish as a function of loudness, which is not the case for ADD SD arrests.

In ADD SD /s/ to /z/ distinction is symptomatic overpressure. It is present for /z/ (voiced sibilant), but not for /s/, a voiceless sibilant. This is again not valid for vocal tremor. Whistling or air blowing (out or in; a vegetative task) is also asymptomatic in ADD SD, but it will be affected in tremor.

A seemingly random symptom distribution is observed in spontaneous connected speech of ADD SD cases. This may appear to be so to an untrained listener, because spontaneous speech distributes voiced (symptomatic segments) and voiceless (asymptomatic segments) according to linguistic constraints of a given language. Therefore, the knowledge of the morpheme structure condition for the given language can be used to construct relevant test sentences capable of eliciting maximum symptoms of ADD SD [36].

When diagnosis is in doubt based on the auditory findings alone, or when phonoscopic examination is noncontributory or difficult to obtain, a diagnostic unilateral RLN block administration is advised. A predictable time frame of symptom elimination (±15 min) is achieved during successful blocking of the RLN [33,35,37].

Phonoscopic (visual) symptoms

Phonoscopic examination using both rigid and dynamic (flexible) exams are recommended. Phonoscopic examination of ADD SD patients clearly demonstrates overadduction of the glottis during selected targets production [31,32]. This can also include lateral shuddering of the vocal fold, ventricular vocal fold approximation, and/or anterior-to-posterior contraction of the entire supraglottic larynx. There are usually no organic lesions accompanied to the true cases of ADD SD. Visual signs can also be confirmed with EMG [37].

Visual signs are confined to specific speech-phonatory tasks, and are absent during vegetative tasks. This is in contrast to the VT cases.

Vocal tremor

Auditory signs

Symptoms of VT are generated by central (cerebral) disturbance. Peripheral involvement is "passive" at best and is limited to the mechanical constrains of the joint-to-muscle relation which determines the "load-and-shake" ratio. Consequently, the rate of generated shaking (tremor) will vary as a function of the muscle-joint location, being slower for large structures and faster for small structures with normal (physiologic) tremor being usually twice the rate of the pathologic tremor for a given location. This physical condition of the larynx makes the rate of pathologic vocal tremor and that of vocal arrests to be similar (±5–6 Hz), since it affects the same site. The crucial distinction between these two types of oscillations involves, however, the fact that in ADD SD only certain voice ranges are affected, while oscillation due to tremor will affect the entire vocal range, including falsetto and whisper. Vegetative or pseudolinguistic productions are also affected. Loudness increases may partially diminish the amplitude (extent) of tremor, but not tremor rate. Therefore, improper interpretation (auditory) of voice testing may give an impression that symptoms are reduced or eliminated, when in fact tremor rate remains unchanged. This will lead to improper diagnosis and easy confusion with vocal arrests present in ADD SD.

Phonoscopic signs
Similar to the case of ADD SD, phonoscopic visualization fails in general to show any organic phonatory disturbances in cases presenting with VT. Oscillation due to vocal tremor may be seen affecting glottis, pharynx, supraglottic larynx or all the other components of the vocal tract including the respiratory system singly or in combination during all vocal, speech and vegetative tasks. This is in complete contrast to symptoms of ADD SD.

MxADDSDVT

Auditory signs
When ADD SD symptoms are accompanied by vocal tremor, patients are categorized as having a form of mixed ADD SD/vocal tremor. This dysphonia is thought to include, in addition to ADD SD symptom generating site, an additional site, namely cerebellum [26]. In such a case, vocal oscillations are similar to those of tremor type and not to ADD SD [26]. To distinguish the type of oscillations as being those of AT or ADD SD type, precise measures of tremor regularity are used. Tremor-like oscillations are always more regular than vocal arrest-type oscillations of ADD SD type, although the overall rate of both types is similar (5—6 Hz for both disorders). In contrast to vocal arrests, vocal tremor oscillations will also affect indiscriminately all vocal intensity and frequency ranges, including whisper, falsetto and all vegetative tasks [22,26]. Furthermore, vocal tremor rate is not affected by the chemical block of the RLN (including the co-block of ipsi- or contralateral SLN), while tremor magnitude may be reduced by these techniques [35]. This is contrary to cases of ADD SD tremor, where blocking of the RLN results in elimination of vocal arrests.

Phonoscopic signs
Combination of the signs present in pure ADD SD and pure VT are observed phonoscopically in MxADDSDVT dysphonia. Postblock observation is crucial, and dynamic flexible observation is preferred.

ABD SD

Auditory signs
Patients suffering from abductor (ABD) SD are exceptionally rare. This condition is diagnosed when patients display sudden increases of transglottic phonatory airflow during production of speech, resulting in involuntary devoicing or unvoicing of voiced speech segments. This is best observed on voiced stressed segments that follow voiceless segments.

Clinically, the speech pattern of these patients is characterized by sudden onset of severe breathiness in phonation, making completion of a word, phrase or sentence extremely laborious if not impossible. Excessive facial struggling being compensatory in nature, may accompany moments of breathy spasms. In contrast to ADD SD, a co-symptom of vocal tremor was not noted in most of ABD SD cases studied by us, although a more rapid (±8–9 Hz) tremor may be present. Also in contrast to the ADD SD, ABD SD patients exhibit severe troubles when producing voiced/voiceless clusters.

Symptoms are absent or significantly diminished when an all-voiced sentence is produced, specifically at lowest possible voice fundamental frequency levels. Similarly, no symptoms are present during sustained phonation production. This is exactly the reverse of the ADD SD symptomatology.

Phonoscopic signs

Objective confirmation of ABD SD signs by phonoscopic observations is difficult. On occasions, a posterior glottis separation during the symptomatic event may be noted. EMG evidence usually fails to corroborate the visual signs. Likewise with previous conditions, no organic phonoscopic findings occur. If present, these are not a part of the underlying etiology.

Ventricular dysphonia

Auditory signs

Ventricular phonation (VeD) may be confused with ADD SD, because on visualization, false vocal folds may be brought into the midline in both conditions, and the voice may be presented as overpressured in both conditions. We cluster VeD symptoms produced here by active vibration of the false vocal folds or symptoms caused by hypertrophic appearance of false vocal folds without vibration. The model of symptoms generation is, however, entirely different for these two dysphonias.

VeD patients adduct false vocal folds in response to an intrinsic inability to approximate the true glottis during phonatory effort, while in ADD SD over-approximation of the false vocal folds is a part of the overpressure mechanism. In VeD cases false vocal fold approximation is usually in response to organic lesion(s) of the anterior commissure but often may result in false vocal fold approximation [27]. Overclosure of false vocal folds in ADD SD is never due to organic lesions of the anterior commissure.

Visual signs

Phonoscopic findings may include anterior commissure neoplasms, scars or other organic hindrances affecting proper closure of the glottis. The false vocal folds may be hypertrophic uni- or bilaterally at rest or may approximate to various degrees on phonatory approximation of the true vocal folds. Abnormal growth of the thyroid ala on one side may also cause false vocal fold displacement. The false vocal folds may be actually vibrating (seen stroboscopically) or may press upon the true vocal folds without actually vibrating.

In the first case, the voice is harsh but multiphonic with a high index of aperiodicity. In the second case, which is equated primarily with functional conversions, harshness predominates.

Diagnostic tasks

Differential diagnosis tasks that are useful in eliciting and varying symptoms of the described types of dysphonias are listed below. These tasks involve phonatory (static and dynamic production of voice at fundamental frequency), speech, singing, whispering, and vegetative responses. Voice is analyzed acoustically, and is recorded. Visualization (phonoscopy) is carried out with either rigid and/or flexible scopes. Other investigative techniques comprising extended battery of phonatory function studies including glottography, electromyography, delayed auditory feedback, and aerodynamics may be useful in aiding differential diagnosis.

Fundamental frequency

ADD SD
Examination of static and dynamic sustained phonation shows symptom generation in a phonetotopic manner. Symptoms are present in speech between base and 1.5 octave shifts above the base fundamental frequency. Symptoms are present with increased magnitude on speech segments loaded with voiced phonemes and are diminished on voiceless segments. Symptoms are absent in whisper and in falsetto and during vegetative phonatory production. Symptoms are also absent on vegetative, (nonspeech frequency) tasks. The two major symptoms include overpressure and vocal arrests. The rate of arrests is ±5 Hz.

MxADDSDVT
As above, but components of symptoms are not subject to complete elimination in whisper, or at the high frequency levels.

VT
As above, but symptoms affect vegetative and respiratory tasks also. Voice symptoms are frequency independent. Intensity may diminish extent of tremor but not its rate (±5 Hz).

ABD SD
Symptoms are predominately present in connected speech containing voiced/voiceless clusters. Symptoms are absent in sustained phonation, on vegetative tasks, and in all-voiced segments. Whisper and falsetto may not be clear diagnostic determinants, but symptoms tend to be eliminated during production of low voice fundamental frequency. RLN block may fail to support Dx.

VeD
Symptoms are present at all frequency and intensity levels. Symptoms are reduced or eliminated when increased airflow is produced. Application of phonoscopy, delayed auditory feedback and chemical nerve block may be diagnostically useful.

Loudness effects

Loudness will increase degree of overpressure in ADD SD. In ABD loudness will cause more pronounced air evacuation (devoicing) symptoms. Loudness increases will generally not change VT rate, but may diminish tremor amplitude. VeD symptomatology is not significantly affected by loudness.

RLN (vagal) blocking

When in doubt, diagnosis of ADD SD, VT and VeD can be supplemented by unilateral RLN block. This is accomplished using lidocaine resulting in immediate (2–3 min postinjection) paresis of the ipsilateral vocal fold [35]. ADD SD symptoms may be totally eliminated or markedly reduced during the duration of the block. The effects of the block usually last up to 20–25 min. VT symptoms are essentially unchanged by the block. The magnitude of tremor may be, however, reduced somewhat [33,35]. VeD symptoms may be eliminated altogether when VeD is of functional etiology. RLN block is not applicable when organic findings are present. RLN block will eliminate ADD SD symptoms in mixed cases without affecting the tremorous part of the syndrome.

Aerodynamics

Phonatory air consumption can be estimated clinically as a ratio of glottic closure to the maximum phonation time (MPhT) at full lung volumes. Phonation time should be measured in seconds (s), and averaged over three consecutive productions, each produced at maximum inhalatory effort and each executed as close as possible to Fo and intensity targets.

Air consumption is small (long MPhT) in ADD SD, and large (short MPhT) in ABD SD. Air consumption is increased in VT and is variable (more) in mixed ADD+VT cases than in pure ADD SD alone. Air consumption is higher in VeD speech, than it is in normative speech. It is substantially higher in VeD than in ADD SD, even when ventricular approximation is present in ADD SD. High air consumption in VeD is accompanied by a high index of aperiodicity and harsh-noisy phonation. This is not the case in pure ADD SD, ABD SD, but may be somewhat similar in mixed ADD SD with VT and when ventricular compensation is present in pure ADD SD.

Measurements of visual laryngovideostroboscopic (phonoscopic) findings

Phonoscopic imagining contributes significantly to differential diagnoses. The parameters of interest are: 1) level of closure; 2) smoothness of the glottic edge; 3) supraglottic involvement; and 4) bilateral characteristics of the mucosal wave [30–32,40]. Additional measures carried out in relative values, comprise estimates of the size of the glottic gap (degree of lateralization) of the injected vocal fold. This measure is an estimate in relative numbers of the length of each vocal fold vs. the anterior angle of the glottis. This measure is similar to the recently described technique of estimating the position of the paralyzed vocal fold by measuring anterior glottic and vocal fold angles [38,39].

Phonoscopic findings

Level of closure
This observation relates to the relative vertical alignment of the vocal fold during closure. No level closure differences observed in any of the conditions discussed above are understood as primary to the type of the dysphonia. When present, level differences are of no diagnostic value and reflect other aspects of phonatory disturbance. Level differences may, however, be present after surgical or chemical denervation.

Smoothness of the glottic edge
This observation relates to the relative smoothness of the glottic edge of the vocal fold during closure. No edge differences observed in any of conditions discussed above are understood as primary to the type of the dysphonia. When present, edge roughness is nondiagnostic and reflects other aspects of phonatory disturbance. Edge differences may, however, be present after denervation. Because Botox injection (volume) into the TA may result in convexity and displacement of the mucosal edge of the TVF, observation of the smoothness of the postinjection phonatory glottic edge needs to be carried out. Neither transitory nor chronic changes should be noted. This is valid for the phonatory edge between upper and lower phonatory lips regardless of injection sites or dosage size. Similar findings are observed following PCA and CT Botox injections.

Glottic and supraglottic involvement
Glottic or supraglottic involvement (distinct organic changes) are only associated with VeD and are not part of primary symptomatology in any of the other disorders discussed here. Supraglottic compensatory behavior in ADD SD is essentially always absent in surgically treated cases. Supraglottic component may be present when patients are not offered postoperative voice therapy support.

Glottic gap
Widening of the glottic gap is not a part of any of the conditions, except for the ABD SD, where it affects either the posterior portion of the glottis, or is present alongside the entire length of the phonatory and cartilaginous glottis.

Glottic widening is, however, present in all successfully treated patients by either mechanical (RLN section) or chemical denervation. Obtaining proper glottic widening is according to the physiologic model of ADD SD, a most crucial parameter needed to eliminate overpressure. Unilateral glottic widening (bowing the injected TA) is universally achieved in all Botox-injected patients, causing symptom reduction or elimination for the majority of patients within the first 24—36 h. In the immediate post-Botox injection state, the size of the glottic gap is greatest, and may reach up to an estimated ±2 mm. The phonatory glottis configuration seen on stroboscopic phonoscopy usually shows a fusiform-/spindle-like type approximation. The gap narrows rather rapidly in the first 2—3 weeks after injection and then remains more or less at constant levels (±1—1.5 mm) up to the time of minor symptom recurrence, which usually occurs in 3 to 3.5 months. In the last stage, the glottic gap is essentially eliminated. It is usually found not to be wider at this time than its preoperative size. This gap reduction occurs despite continuous presence of asymptotic or barely symptomatic phonation. It is difficult to establish the relation of the size of the glottic gap at this last stage to the exact moment of recurrence of symptoms. Intrasubject glottic gap assessment after consecutive injections appears to show a similar pattern. No substantial differences are noted in the glottic size as a function of dosage increases or decreases (5—15 units). Therefore we use a dose, which is primarily based on patients' preinjection symptom severity. A dose of 10 units injected unilaterally with proper localization is totally sufficient to achieve a desired glottic gap. Exceeding this dose may result in prolonged breathiness and troubles with swallowing of liquids.

Bilateral characteristics of the mucosal vibratory wave (MVW)

Observation of the MVW are paramount in interpreting postsurgical voice qualities, specifically those of aperiodicity and breathiness. All patients treated by denervation procedures show increased asymmetry of MVW between the L and R TVFs as a function of RLN sectioning or Botox injection. Dosing-to-asymmetry correlation is low, with asymmetry and the extent of the amplitude of the MVW on the injected side being more pronounced in the immediate postinjection period. With time, both the asymmetry and the amplitude variability of the MVW diminishes. The MVW eventually becomes symmetrical between the two vocal folds. This improvement can occur as early as 2 weeks postinjection, but asymmetry may also persist in some cases for as long as 2.5 months, rendering the voice hoarse and subject to sudden uncontrollable pitch breaks. Voice therapy is useful in improving this condition by eliminating involuntary pitch breaks and hoarseness through exercises aimed at controlling voice intensity.

Post-RLN and post-Botox acoustics

ADD SD

Pitch (Fo) and loudness (dB) measurements obtained at various posttreatment intervals show initial reduction in high voice Fo production and limited loudness (characterized by breathiness). Restoration of phonatory functions is generally speeded up by voice therapy. Increased air consumption connotes increased breathiness. This correlates well with the size of the glottic gap in a pattern similar to pitch restoration. Improvement in air consumption coincides with elimination of compensatory supraglottic behavior, eliminating extralaryngeal/intralaryngeal struggle, albeit of a quite different type than that of the preinjection type.

MxADDSDVT, VT

Similar physiologic patterns are observed for mixed ADDSDVT and VT cases studied. Tremor, however, persists following RLN resection, although it may be somewhat diminished in magnitude. When treated by Botox injection into the ipsi- and contralateral CT muscles, a slight increase in the glottic gap and a more asymmetrical MVW are noted. The abductory/adductory dysmotility can also be slightly more pronounced.

Consequently, Fo and loudness control can be affected slightly longer in these cases resulting in reduction but not elimination of tremor. Reduction is limited essentially to the magnitude (amplitude) of tremor, with its rate of oscillation being preserved at ±5.5 Hz.

ABD SD

We have no experience in treating ABD SD with RLN resection, and we do not recommend this form of treatment for this condition. Injection of Botox into PCA results in time-dependent ipsilateral medialization and abductory dismotility of the injected vocal fold. This medialization can be observed for a duration of up to 4 months, with gradual lateralization observed over the period of 4 months. Abductory motility judged as normal is observed at a 4-month postinjection interval. Asympto-

Table 1. Symptomatic signs and the value of specific tasks and tests applicable to the conditions described here.

	ADD SD	ABD SD	VT	MxADDSDVTR	VeD
Low voice	+	–	+	+	±
Mid-voice	+	–	+	+	±
High voice	–	–	+	+	±
Soft voice	+	+	+	+	±
Mid-voice	++	++	++	++	±
Loud voice	+++	+++	+++	+++	±
Voiced	+	+	+	+	±
Voiceless	–	+	+	+	±
Random	+	±	+	+	±
/s/	–	–	+	+	±
/z/	+	±	+	+	±
Valsalva	–	–	+	+	–
Whistle	–	–	+	+	–
Respiratory	–	–	+	+	–
Cough	–	–	+	+	–
Laughter	–	–	+	+	–
DAF	+	+	+	+	+
Xylocaine	+	?	+	+	+
Aerodynamic	+	+	+	+	+
LVS	Rigid + Flex	Rigid + Flex	Rigid + Flex	Rigid + Fles	Rigid + Flex

matic phonation may persist beyond functional recovery. In the remaining two cases, medializations of shorter duration and abductory dismotility were achieved, however, without effective symptom elimination.

Discussion

We believe that proper understanding of symptomatology of the dysphonias described here is needed to establish proper working models of each condition. Such modeling helps systematic examination of these patients and aids prediction of a posttreatment course, outcomes and long-term follow-ups. Proper evaluation of pretreatment parameters and their postoperative evaluation allows for improved design of focused and efficacious salvage treatment and therapeutic procedures. A summary of positive and negative symptoms per each condition as well as objective tests we find useful are summarized in Table 1.

References

1. Dedo HH, Izdebski K. Surgical treatment of spastic dysphonia. J Contemp Surg 1981;18:75–90.
2. Dedo HH, Shipp T. Spastic Dysphonia. A Surgical and Voice Therapy Treatment Program. Houston: College Hill Press, 1980.
3. Dedo HH, Izdebski K. Intermediate results of 306 recurrent laryngeal nerve sections for spastic dysphonia. J Laryngoscope 1983;93:916.
4. Dedo HH, Izdebski K. Problems with RLN surgery for spastic dysphonia. J Laryngoscope 1983;93:268–271.
5. Dedo HH, Behlau MS. Recurrent laryngeal nerve section for spastic dysphonia: 5–14 years preliminary results in the first 300 patients. J Ann Otol Rhinol Laryngol 1991:100:274–279.
6. Izdebski K, Dedo HH, Shipp T, Flower R. Postoperative and follow-up studies of spastic dysphonia patients treated by recurrent laryngeal nerve section. J Otolaryngol Head Neck Surg 1981;89:96–101.
7. Izdebski K. Surgical and medical treatment of spasmodic dysphonia. In: Stemple JC (ed) Voice Therapy: Clinical Studies. St. Louis: Mosby Year Book, 1993;131–147.
8. Fritzell B, Feuer E, Haglund S, Knutsson E, Schiratzki H. Experiences with recurrent laryngeal nerve section for spastic dysphonia. J Folia Phoniatr 1982;34:160–176.
9. Schiratzki H, Fritzell B. Treatment of spasmodic dysphonia by means of resection of the recurrent laryngeal nerve. J Acta Otolaryngol 1988;449(Suppl):115–117.
10. Blitzer A, Brin MF, Fahn S, Lange D, Lovelace E. Letter to the editor. J Laryngoscope 1986;96: 1300–1301.
11. Blitzer A, Brin MF. Laryngeal dystonia: a series treated with botulinum toxin therapy. J Ann Otol Rhinol Laryngol 1991;100:95–89.
12. Ludlow CL. Treatment of speech and voice disorders with botulinum toxin. JAMA 1990;264:2671–2675.
13. Ludlow CL, Naunton RF, Sedory SE, Schutz GM, Hallett M. Effects of botulinum toxin injections on speech in adductor spasmodic dysphonia. J Neurology 1988;38:1220–1225.
14. Zwirner P, Murry T, Swenson M, Woodson GE. Acoustic changes in spasmodic dysphonia after botulinum toxin injection. J Voice 1991;5:78–84.
15. Brin MF, Blitzer A, Fahn S, Lovelace RE. Adductor laryngeal dystonia: treatment with local injections of botulinum toxin (Botox). J Neurology 1988;38(Suppl 10):244.
16. Aronson AE, McCaffery TV, Litchy WJ, Lipton RJ. Botulinum toxin injection for adductor spasmodic dysphonia: patient self-ratings of voice and phonatory effort after three successive injections. J Laryngoscope 1993;103:683–692.

17. Ludlow CL, Naunton RF, Fujita N, Sedory SE. Spasmodic dysphonia: botulinum toxin injection after recurrent nerve surgery. J Otolaryngol Head Neck 1990;102:102–122.
18. Brin MF, Blitzer A, Stewart C, Fahn S. Botulinum toxin. Now for adductor laryngeal dystonia. J Neurology 1990;40(Suppl 1):381.
19. Ward R, Izdebski K, Ross JC, Dedo HH. Botox treatment of abductor spasmodic dysphonia, tremor and mixed adductor/tremor spasmodic dysphonia. In: Izdenski K (ed) Digest of the Sixth Annual Pacific Voice Conference: Organic and Neurogenic Dysphonias: Strategies and Treatment Efficacy. San Diego, USA: Singular Publishing Group, 1993;28.
20. Kosokovic F, Lenarcic-Cepelja I. Surgical therapy of dysphonia plica ventricularis. J Ann Otol Rhinol Laryngol 1977;82:408–414.
21. Izdebski HH, Boles L. Spastic dysphonia: A patient profile of 200 cases. J Ann Otol Laryngol 1984;7–14.
22. Izdebski K. Symptomatology of adductor spasmodic dysphonia. A physiologic model. J Voice 1992;6:306–319.
23. Izdebski K, Ward R. EMG verification and Botox treatment of ABD SD and vocal tremor. ASHA 1993 Annual Convention, Anaheim, USA, 1993.
24. Izdebski K, Dedo HH. Characteristics of voice tremor in spastic dysphonia: A preliminary study. In: Lawrence V (ed) Transcripts of the VIII Symposium on Care of the Professional Voice (Part III Medical/Surgical Therapy). New York: Voice Foundation, 1979;ii:17–23.
25. Ludlow CL, Bassich CJ, Connor NP, Coulter DC. Phonatory characteristics of vocal fold tremor. J Phonetics 1986;14:509–516.
26. Aronson AE, Brown JR, Litin EM, Pearson JS. Spastic dysphonia. II. Comparison with essential (voice) tremor and other neurologic and psychogenic dysphonias. J Speech Hear Dis 1968;33: 220–231.
27. von Doersten PG, Izdebski K, Ross JC, Cruz RM. Ventricular dysphonia: A profile of 40 cases. J Laryngoscope 1992;102:1296–1301.
28. Hirano M. Clinical Examination of Voice. New York, Wien: Springer-Verlag, 1981.
29. Izdebski K, Ross JC, Klein JC. Rigid transoral laryngovideostroboscopy (phonoscopy). In: McFarlane S (ed) Seminars in Speech and Hearing. 1990.
30. Hirano M, Bless DM, Videostroboscopic Examination of the Larynx. San Diego, USA: Singular Publishing Group, 1993.
31. Woodson GE, Zwirner P, Murry T, Swenson M. Use of flexible fiberoptic laryngoscopy to assess patients with spasmodic dysphonia. J Voice 1991;5:85–91.
32. Woo P, Colton R, Casper J, Brewer D. Analysis of spasmodic dysphonia by aerodynamic and laryngostroboscopic measurements. J Voice 1992;6:344–351.
33. Izdebski K, Shipp T, Dedo HH. Predicting postoperative voice characteristics of spastic dysphonia patients. J Otolaryngology 1979;87:428–434.
34. Izdebski K. Overpressure and breathiness in spastic dysphonia: An LTAS study. J Acta Otolaryngol 1984;97:373–378.
35. Izdebski K, Dedo HH. Selecting the side of RLN section for spastic dysphonia. J Otolaryngol Head Neck Surg 1980;89:423–426.
36. Seshadri R, Phua SY. Phonologic Test for Differential Diagnosis of ADDuctor and ABDuctor Spasmodic Dysphonia Using Malay and Mandarin. In: Abstract Book, First World Voice Congress, Porto, Portugal, 1995;35.
37. Shipp T, Izdebski K, Reed C, Morrisey P. Intrinsic laryngeal muscle activity in a spastic dysphonia patient. J Speech Hear Dis 1985;50:54–59.
38. Woodson GE. Configuration of the glottis in laryngeal paralysis I: clinical study. Laryngoscope 1993;103:1227–1234.
39. Woodson GE. Configuration of the glottis in laryngeal paralysis II: animal experiments. Laryngoscope 1993;103:1235–1241.

Medical treatment of dysphonias

Voice Update.
M. Pais Clemente, editor.

Treatment of dysphonias secondary to gastroesophageal reflux

Michael S. Benninger
Department of Otolaryngology — Head and Neck Surgery, Henry Ford Health System, Detroit, Michigan, USA

Key words: cough, globus, hoarseness, reflux laryngitis.

Introduction

There are many causes of acute and chronic dysphonia. The most common are related to the technique or quantity of voice use and smoking. Gastroesophageal reflux disease (GERD) can result in many upper airway disorders including chronic cough, globus syndrome, and reflux laryngitis [1]. An understanding of the mechanism of GERD has allowed for an aggressive approach to therapy which can relieve these symptoms. This paper will describe the anatomy and physiology of GERD and will describe a stepwise approach to therapy.

Anatomy and physiology of GERD

The swallowing mechanism is a complex interaction of mucosal and glandular secretions and coordinated neuromuscular activity. There are two principle sphincters of the esophagus. The upper sphincter is composed primarily of the cricopharyngeus muscle and the lower portion of the inferior constrictor. The lower sphincter is a pseudosphincter which has sphincteric action due to pressure differentials between the abdomen (+5 mmHg), the thorax (–5 mmHg) and the diaphragm. The total pressure at the lower esophageal sphincter (LES) is approximately +25 mmHg in normals and this pressure prevents the reflux of acid, pepsin, bile and pancreatic enzymes into the esophagus. There are other protective mechanisms which decrease esophageal reflux. The peristaltic activity of the esophagus is an excellent clearing mechanism for swallowing and for clearing esophageal contents. Salivation and esophageal bicarbonate secretions protect the esophageal, pharyngeal and laryngeal mucosa from injury. Furthermore, there is diaphragmatic pinching which occurs on inspiration which furthers the effectiveness of the LES. Lastly, gravity aids in the prevention of reflux when individuals are upright.

When there is a breakdown in these antireflux mechanisms, caustic materials can

---

Address for correspondence: Michael S. Benninger MD, Chairman, Department of Otolaryngology — HNS, Henry Ford Hospital, 2799 West Grand Blvd., Detroit, MI 48202, USA. Tel.: +1-313-876-3275. Fax: +1-313-876-7263.

reflux into the esophagus and pharynx. If the duration of contact is sufficient, then the normal mucosal resistance to injury is overcome and the sequelae of GERD ensue. There are three major causes of GERD: impaired motor peristaltic function of the esophagus, decreased LES pressure, and delayed gastric emptying. LES pressure abnormalities can occur because of a weak LES, a hiatal hernia, or most commonly due to transient LES relaxation (TLESR). TLESR accounts for approximately two-thirds of the GERD caused by disorders of the LES. Although TLESR does occur in normal patients, significantly greater numbers of TLESR episodes occur in patients with GERD. These are often associated with a sudden increase in abdominal pressure which overcomes the sphincteric pressure mechanism.

Delayed gastric emptying may be a factor in 60% of patients with GERD. The volume of fluid depends on the amount of food and gastric secretions and the rate of gastric emptying. Larger meals or delayed gastric emptying due to high-fat foods are associated with increased gastric contents. Increased gastric volume is associated with an increased number of TLESR episodes. In some patients decreased antral motility may be the principal cause of GERD. Esophagitis is primarily the result of acid contact time. Decreased esophageal clearance due to abnormal esophageal motility or loss of the gravitational effect which occurs in recumbent positions, and inadequate peristalsis of the lower esophagus during sleep can lead to reflux. These findings explain the major etiology of GERD which is related to the types of foods eaten and the timing of eating within a short time of sleeping. With a hiatal hernia, the LES pressure is often low, there is no diaphragmatic pinching and the intrathoracic gastric pouch acts as a reservoir of food, acid and bile. Although some have debated the role of a hiatal hernia on reflux in the absence of the other disorders mentioned above [2], experience suggests that patients with a hiatal hernia are at greater risk for GERD than others [3]. Reflux can be a significant problem in up to 50% of pregnant women. This is due to the combined effect of the increased estrogen and progesterone on LES dysfunction and the expanding uterus increasing intra-abdominal pressure.

Gastroesophageal reflux has been identified as a cause or a cofactor in many disorders of the upper aerodigestive tract other than esophagitis. Koufman has found reflux by double-probe pH monitoring in 58% of patients with globus syndrome, 45% of those with dysphagia, and 52% of individuals with chronic cough [1]. We have found that 27% of patients referred for sinusitis due to their symptoms of chronic throat clearing, cough, posterior rhinorrhea, or globus actually had no sinus pathology but rather a laryngeal disorder. Three-fourths of these were due to reflux. GERD has also been a critical factor in contact ulcers, vocal fold granulomas, Reinke's space edema and perhaps even vocal nodules [3]. An association with chronic pulmonary disease and asthma is noted but it is difficult to determine if this is a cause or an effect of the disease. Reflux may induce laryngospasm and vagally induced bronchoconstriction. Conversely reflux may occur due to the decrease in LES pressure which occurs secondary to the medications used for these pulmonary disorders, such as theophylline or systemic steroids. Therefore, reflux may be a consequence rather than a cause of asthma. Reflux has been found to be a critical factor in sudden infant death syndrome (SIDS) [4] and there is growing evidence of a relationship between reflux and laryngeal cancer as a cofactor or perhaps even the main causative agent [5]. The principal causes of pharyngeal and laryngeal cancer are smoking and alcohol use. These agents decrease LES tone and increase the likelihood of reflux [6]. The reflux exacerbates the mucosal injury caused by the smoke and alcohol and can accelerate the carcinogenic effects. Further investigation is needed to clarify the role of GERD on laryngeal cancer.

Presentation and evaluation of GERD

The symptoms of GERD are often subtle. The most common symptoms are a globus sensation, dysphonia, throat clearing and cough. The cough may be frequent and irritating or paroxysmal. Waking in the middle of the night or upon recumbency with paroxysms of cough is felt to be due to reflux laryngospasm as the larynx performs its important task of protection. Such cough may also be due to a small amount of acid aspiration. Although globus sensation and chronic throat clearing may be due to other pathologic conditions such as nodules, polyps, granulomas, allergies, etc., these symptoms should prompt a suspicion of reflux. The dysphonia is usually mild. The voice is frequently worse in the morning and improves with hydration and some voice use. It may worsen slightly after a large meal. Significant voice use results in easy fatigue. Chronic reflux may lead to more significant and chronic change in the voice. The voice is gravelly with mucous gurgling. Decreased pitch or loss of range occurs with edema. Symptoms of a heartburn are often lacking, even in patients with well documented episodes of reflux [1].

The diagnosis of GERD, and particularly reflux laryngitis, is primarily made presumptively based on the history and examination of the larynx. Any patient who complains of a globus and chronic throat clearing with or without dysphonia should be suspected as having GERD [3]. This is particularly true if they have a history of recurrent heartburn, hiatal hernia or dietary habits such as late-night eating or a diet high in fat, caffeine or alcohol. The laryngeal examination typically shows edematous or erythematous arytenoids [7] with mucosal thickening in the posterior commissure although such findings may be subtle or even absent. Contact ulcers, granulomas or Reinke's edema may be seen. Videostroboscopy may reveal edema although mucosal waveform is often normal.

Testing to confirm the diagnosis of GERD is often unnecessary. The diagnosis is often made by history and physical examination alone. The success of presumptive treatment is diagnostic. If the diagnosis is in question or the patient has not responded to imperic treatment, then further testing is indicated. A barium swallow or endoscopy may evaluate the pharynx and esophagus for mass lesions but may not show reflux even if present. A dynamic swallowing evaluation will assess the coordination and propagation of the swallow. LES monotromy or Bernstein acid perfusion tests are more specific [3]. The most definitive test is 24 h, double-probe Ph monitoring [1]. This is particularly true in cases where reflux is intermittent, although a negative test does not definitively rule out reflux, especially in cases where reflux is related to specific food or alcohol, and the patient may not use these agents in a 24-h period. Therefore, if the clinician is still suspicious of GERD, imperic treatment is indicated.

Treatment

All patients with GERD-related laryngitis benefit from humidification hydration and avoidance of throat clearing. Voice therapy is indicated should the dysphonia interfere with daily activities. Since much of GERD is due to eating habits, the principle treatment of GERD is through dietary modification (phase I treatment). The recommendations for reflux diet at the Henry Ford Hospital are noted in Table 1. Smaller meals, a low-fat diet and weight loss is recommended. The key variables are not eating within 3–4 h of bedtime, avoidance of alcohol and tobacco (particularly in the evening), and elevation of the head of the bed. For intermittent or nocturnal reflux, antacids may be of benefit just prior to retiring. Since this treatment is safe, effective, and inexpensive and is in general, good for the patient, dietary antireflux therapy is indicated in all patients with a history or physical examination consistent with GERD. We also use this regimen in all patients who have contact nodules, granulomas, or following laryngeal surgery. If patients fail phase I treatment, then prokinetic drugs or H_2-receptor blockers are initiated (phase II). Since most of GE reflux is due to either decreased LES tone or delayed gastric emptying, prokinetic medications are excellent second-line drugs. These medications increase LES sphincter tone, enhance esophageal clearance and improve delayed gastric emptying. Prokinetic medications, therefore, target the cause of GERD. They can be used for a long time without concerns regarding changes in gastric acid secretion and alteration of the gut flora. Metaclopramide was the first medication used as a prokinetic agent but is limited by its high incidence of side effects secondary to its central dopaminergic antagonism. Cisopride has become the primary prokinetic agent since it has all the virtues of metaclopramide without the antidopaminergic side effects. H_2 blockers are commonly used and can be used over long periods effectively in many patients. Concerns about chronic acid suppression have been raised.

Phase III treatment is the proton pump inhibitor, omeprazole. This medication inhibits the release of HCL acid by the stomach, and therefore, is a potent inhibitor

Table 1. Protocol for reflux pharyngitis.

1. Eat six meals/day (divide total number of calories you are currently eating by six, and consume in those quantities). You need not eat extra meals; simply more frequent meals.
2. Consume the equivalent of two tablespoons of antacid or milk between the six meals (do not consume antacid or milk instead of a meal).
3. Elevate bed legs at head of your bed by placing 8 inches of books under those legs.
4. Avoid fatty foods or liquids high in acid (i.e., orange juice).
5. Avoid coffee, tea, alcohol and cigarettes.
6. Do not eat within 3 h of going to bed.
7. Avoid tight binding clothes.
8. Avoid stooping, straining and bending.
9. Avoid (or reduce) stress.

of gastric acid secretion. Nearly all patients with GE reflux will respond to omeprazole, and therefore, should be considered if difficult, recalcitrant reflux occurs, or if significant complications such as granulomas, laryngospasm, or asthma are present. Although it is generally considered a phase III medication, its near complete response rate allows it to be both diagnostic and therapeutic and may be used in lieu of other diagnostic tests. If a patient responds appropriately, then GERD is diagnosed and other treatments such as diet and prokinetic agents can be initiated. If a patient does not respond, they are unlikely to have GERD. Omeprazole therapy is limited by concerns over long-term safety although early concerns may have been overvalued. Imiprazole should be considered postoperatively for laryngeal surgery in a patient with reflux or, at least, the early treatment of contact ulcers or granulomas.

Although infrequently needed, surgery with fundoplication may be necessary in patients with poorly controlled symptoms and along with relocation of the stomach in those with a hiatal hernia (phase IV). Laparoscopy fundoplication may allow for safer and less morbid surgery which may increase the frequency of surgical treatment. This is particularly true of those with GERD requiring continuous, and, perhaps, lifelong medication therapy.

References

1. Koufman JA. The otolaryngic manifestations of gastroesophageal reflux disease (GERD): a clinical investigation of 225 patients using ambulatory 24-hour pH monitoring and an experimental investigation of the role of acid and pepsin in the development of laryngeal injury. Laryngoscope 1991;101(Suppl 53):1–78.
2. Meyer GW, Castell DO. Evaluation and management of diseases of the esophagus. Am J Otolaryngol 1981;2:336–343.
3. Benninger MS. Medical disorders in the vocal artist. In: Benninger MS, Jacobson BH, Johnson AF (eds) Vocal Arts Medicine: The Care and Prevention of Professional Voice Disorders. New York: Thieme Medical Publishers, Inc., 1994;177–215.
4. Downing SE, Lee JC. Laryngeal chemosensitivity: a possible mechanism for sudden infant death. Pediatrics 1975;55:640–648.
5. Koufman JA. Reflux may cause laryngeal cancer. Vis Voice 1995;4:1–23.
6. Dennish GW, Castell DO. Inhibitory effect of smoking on the lower esophageal sphincter. N Engl J Med 1971;284:1136–1137.
7. Sataloff RT. Common diagnoses and treatments in professional singers. 1987;66:28–46.

Voice Update.
M. Pais Clemente, editor.

Treatment of dysphonia secondary to environmental pollution

R. Eugenia and Chavez de Bartelt
Phoniatrics and Audiology Consultory, Mexico City, Mexico

Abstract. *Background.* In recent industrial times the environmental pollution has increased significantly. Ozone, nitrogen dioxide, sulfur dioxide, carbon monoxide and dioxide are changing the physiology of the vocal folds and the airways system. Dryness, changes in the secretions viscosity, and frequent clearing during singing or speaking are the most frequent symptoms.

Method. The treatment of 100 patients with dysphonia secondary to environmental pollution were analyzed. ENT exploration, laryngeal videoendoscopy, stroboscopy, phonetogram and functional voice test were performed on each subject. Hydration methods were used. Micronebulizer, rhinotherm, inhalations at home, gargling with glycerin or iodinated solution and humidifying nose method with glycerin and petrolatum were indicated in every patient. Anti-inflammatory drugs, mucolytics and antihistamines were used. Voice exercises were needed after the dysphonia.

Results. Of those studied, 75% had no more dysphonia, 14% report occasional dysphonia, 11% showed a slight improvement, and 5% of the group needed allergy skin tests.

Conclusions. The environmental pollution increases upper airways hypersensitivity. The treatment for this kind of dysphonia has to be as broad as possible. Hydration methods are important. Professional voice users need special voice programs.

Key words: laryngeal dryness, laryngeal hydration, voice pathology.

Introduction

In industrialized societies, environmental pollution has increased due to the changes in levels of ozone, nitrogen dioxide, sulfur dioxide, carbon monoxide and dioxide. These pollutants change the physiology of vocal folds and the upper airways system. They cause dryness of the mucosa and changes in the viscosity of the secretions. The clearing mechanism of the pharynx and larynx is more frequently needed and the perceptual mechanism during singing or speaking are different.

Millions of cars, industry, 2,200 m of altitude, high temperatures and surrounding mountains make the pollution of Mexico City a special case, producing an oxidative chemical reaction.

The patient complains about problems during singing or speaking. The most frequent symptoms are dysphonia ranging from mild to severe, difficulty of controlling a clear pitch and voice color, and a feeling of obstruction due to the high viscosity secretions. The patient tries hard to have a voice as flexible as he is accustomed to and this causes a functional problem.

Address for correspondence: Chavez de Bartelt, Minerva 104-501, Col. Florida, Mexico 01030 D.F., Mexico.

The diagnosis of bilateral chorditis is made when the patient does not show an airways infection, allergy, nose pathology, vocal misuse or esophageal reflux.

The purpose of this paper is to discuss a complete phoniatrical treatment of dysphonia secondary to environmental pollution.

Material

The treatment of 100 phoniatrical patients with dysphonia secondary to environmental pollution was analyzed. They were all examined over the past 5 years. Of these, 50% were male and 50% female. Ages ranged from 15 to 75 years old.

Routine ENT explorations and laryngeal videoendoscopies with stroboscopies were made. The detailed conditions of the vocal folds mucosa, the intralaryngeal muscles and the mucous secretions were examined. Phonetogram and functional voice tests were also performed on each patient.

Method

The treatment was combined with hydration methods, medicines, voice exercises and general care methods.

The hydration methods were important in this treatment. Nasal water steam (rhinotherm, controlled warm temperature with high speed) was used in 45% of the patients and pharyngeal water steam was used in 30% twice a week, for 10–15 min each time, over 3 weeks. The use of micronebulizer with saline solution, ambroxol and tacholiquin for 10 min daily, gave more humidity to the pharynx and larynx in 75% of the group. For the nose, it was used in 45% of patients. Inhalations with boiling water and ambroxol were recommended at home, three times a day, in 90% of the patients. A vaporizer or ultrasonic nebulizer used at night increased the humidity of the upper airways system and of the environment.

The lubrication of the nasal mucosa and the air-filtration function were improved in 30% due to the application of glycerin. It created an hydrophilic exothermal reaction. The other 70% used petrolatum (Vaseline) to make an oil-in-water emulsion.

The pharyngeal mucosa was moisturized at least three times a day by gargling glycerin in 85% of the cases and the other 15% used iodinated solution. When the patient talks too much or spends more than 2 h outdoors, he has to avoid dryness of the pharyngeal mucosa by drinking water every 15 min (Table 1).

Fifty-five percent of the patients needed enzymes such as anti-inflammatory drugs. Nonsteroids like ketoprofen were taken in 10% and 25% took diclofenac. Mucolytics helped to improve the high viscosity of the secretions. Fifteen percent took carbocisteine and guaifenesin and 35% ambroxol. The other 50% did not take anything.

If the dysphonia lasted for longer than 1 week, the hypersensitivity of the patient was controlled with antihistamines like loratadine in 40% and cetirizine in 10% of the group (Table 2).

As is known, the dysphonia and the upper airways symptoms disorganize the voice

Table 1. Hydration methods.

Water steam (rhinotherm)		
Nasal 45%	Pharyngeal 30%	
Micronebulizer		
Nasal 45%	Laryngeal 75%	At home 90%
Lubrication		
Nasal	Pharyngeal (gargling)	
Glycerin 30%	Glycerin 85%	
Petrolatum 70%	Iod. solution 15%	

function. Physiological voice reorganization has been achieved in all cases. Nasal breathing and apoggio had to be practiced. Nasal phonemes helped correctly locate the sound in the nasal resonator. Scales and messa di voce exercises were also advised.

Results

In 75% of the group, dysphonia and other symptoms disappeared completely. Fourteen percent report occasional dysphonia. Eleven percent had a slight improvement.

Hydration by drinking water was necessary in all cases. Five percent of the group needed to practice allergy skin tests and a phoniatrical control was administered every 6 months to all patients.

The environmental purifiers can help to filter particles, such as dust and fungi, out of the air.

Conclusions

It is clear that the environmental pollution increases the upper airways mucosa hypersensitivity.

It is advisable to decrease the allergenic load, by avoiding allergenic food, household chemicals, smoking or staying in smoking areas for a long time, plants or animals in the bedrooms, lack of sleep, uncontrolled stress, driving for long in the sun in a polluted environment and sudden changes of temperature. In polluted areas, the

Table 2. Medicines used in the treatment.

Anti-inflammatories	Mucolytics	Antihistamines
Enzymes: 55%	Ambroxol: 35%	Loratadine: 40%
Ketoprofen: 10%	Carbocisteine – guaif.: 15%	Ceterizine: 10%
Diclofenac: 25%		
None: 10%	None: 50%	None: 50%

population needs education to preserve the humidity of the airways system and take care of health complications.

In professional voice users, the damage can be more severe and the voice care programs are more important.

The treatment of a patient with dysphonia secondary to environmental pollution, has to be as broad as possible in order to control its different noxious influences on the voice. In modern societies, it is exceptionally important to take care of the harmful consequences of the development of technology and at the same time to preserve the environment as well as where possible permitting a good vocal health.

Voice Update.
M. Pais Clemente, editor.

Treatment of dysphonias secondary to allergies

Desiderio Passàli and Luisa Bellussi
E.N.T. Department, University of Siena, Medical School, Siena, Italy

Key words: combined dysphonias, nasal topical therapy, vocal tract.

There are forms of dysphonia in which one can recognize an organic factor and others in which the functional element is prevalent, if not exclusive, i.e., the overuse or mistreatment of the voice (Table 1). However, both factors are often present and act in a combined way, being superimposed on one another and interacting in different ways. This is the case in dysphonia secondary to allergy, in which the factor "defective vocal function" can have a triggering effect, acting together with other basic or predisposing elements, such as irritating mechanisms (smoking, alcohol, air pollution), diatheses (including allergy), or psychoneurohormonal imbalances. In contrast, the dysfunctional factor can have great importance as a predisposing element in the establishment of relapsing congestive manifestations reactive to vocal trauma, on which specific phlogoses and/or vasomotor reactions (allergic or not) can easily be superimposed (Table 2).

That organic and functional factors cannot be separated and distinguished from one another in the dysphonias secondary to allergy is easily inferred from the concept of "morphofunctional unit", as a definition of all the structures that constitute the phonatory apparatus: the respiratory bellows, the laryngeal vibrator and the resonating apparatus or vocal tract. This last structure comprises, in addition to the pharyngeo-buccal cavity, the nasal cavity and the paranasal sinuses, which represent the fixed resonators. Between these structures, there is anatomical contiguity and continuity (the morphological unit), which explains the presence of descending and ascending inflammatory and infective processes. In addition, the existence of functional, i.e., cause and effect, relationships between them have been known for some time. The physiological vocal act, both that of speaking and singing, requires perfect coordination of all the muscles of the phonatory apparatus in its three sections. If there is less than perfect coordination, there occurs the pneumopharyngeo-resonance imbalance that underlies dysphonia.

Complex reflex nerve arcs are the basis of the phenomenon of resonance – the reinforcement and absorption performed by the supraglottic resonators of the pharynx. In the soft palate, in the lamina propria of the pharyngeal mucosa, in the submucosa

---

Address for correspondence: D. Passàli, Via Pó 102, 00198 Rome, Italy.

Table 1. Dysphonias.

Organic dysphonias:
- deformities of phonatory apparatus
- traumas of phonatory apparatus
- neoplasms of phonatory apparatus
- laryngeal nerve paralysis
- acute phlogosis of pharynx and larynx

Functional dysphonias:
- overuse of the voice
- mistreatment of the voice

Combined dysphonias:
- organic and functional factors cannot be separated

and in the interstitial spaces of the muscular wall, visceral receptors and proprioceptors are present in abundance. By means of a reflex arc that involves the sympathetic, parasympathetic and motor fibers of the pharyngeal plexus and the loop of Galen, these permit constant control of the muscle tone of the hypo-oropharynx, which changes in volume according to the different needs (a reduction of the impedance or absorption of the sound emitted, an increase of the resonance) [1].

As already mentioned, the nose and paranasal sinuses instead are fixed resonators and their contribution to the vocal "timbre" is represented solely by the excitation of the air contained in them. Nevertheless, experimental studies on animals have recently shown that there are also dynamic relations between the rhinopharyngeal, sinal and laryngeal cavities, the basis of which is again nervous reflexes. In fact, the presence of reflexes starting from the nasal mucosa and involving the larynx and the whole respiratory tree has been demonstrated. These nasolaryngeal reflexes are produced by contact of irritating substances with the nasal mucosa, by sharp variations in temperature or by mechanical stimuli. The efferent path of these reflexes is composed of the ophthalmic and maxillary branches of the trigeminal nerve, while the efferent branch is carried by the vagus nerve, which explains its action on the larynx by means of laryngospasm. The experimental observation that the laryngospasm can be reduced or even abolished by surgical or pharmacological vagotomy [2] confirms the role of the vagus.

Table 2. Pathogenesis of combined dysphonias.

Triggering effect	Defective vocal function.
Predisposing elements	Irritating mechanisms (smoking, alcohol, air-pollution), diatheses (allergy) and psychoneuro-hormonal imbalance.
or	
Triggering effect	Specific phlogoses (allergy).
Predisposing elements	Congestive manifestations reactive to vocal trauma (overuse, mistreatment of the voice).

The descending nasolaryngeal reflexes are flanked by some ascending laryngeo-nasal reflexes. The rich and dense sensory innervation of the larynx, in relation to the extent of the organ (2,200 myelinated fibers in the superior laryngeal nerve as opposed to the 3,000 fibers of the entire cervical vagal nerve devoted to the sensory innervation of a much more extensive area), represents the origin of some reflexes able to influence the respiratory and dynamic phonatory pattern. In particular, there are specific receptors in the laryngeal mucosa and submucosa that are sensitive to negative pressure in the upper airway, including the nasal cavity and the rhinopharynx [3]. A negative nasal pressure, such as that which occurs during an allergic crisis, produces a reflex increase of the activity of the posterior cricoarytenoid, the muscle responsible for the mobility of the vocal cords, as recorded by electromyography [4]. Topical anesthesia of the nasal mucosa abolishes this effect.

In summary, from an organic point of view, allergic rhinitis involves a continuous irritating action of the larynx, which in time is manifested as dysphonia. Furthermore, the compromise of nasal respiratory physiology, on account of the obstruction caused by edema of the mucosa and rhinorrhea, leads to oral respiration. This means the entry of cold air, irritating substances, new allergens, viruses and bacteria, which perpetuates in a vicious circle the inflammatory effects on the lower airways. The effects mediated by the nasolaryngeal reflexes, in contrast, are documentable instantly. A study conducted by the school of Naples demonstrates that positivity in the specific nasal provocation test, which we also perform routinely in our clinical practice as a third-level investigation in the diagnosis of allergic rhinitis, is demonstrable by means of rhinomametric plot and acoustic rhinometry, with an increase of nasal resistance and edema of mucosa, and that associated with it is the reactive endolaryngoscopic and sonographic picture of a functional dysphonia. In light of these pathogenetic hypotheses, the therapeutic approach to dysphonia secondary to allergy cannot and must not be limited to phoniatric treatment, but must be preceded by suitable medical therapy aimed at improving the trophism and at diminishing the impedance of the supraglottic resonators, leading the patient to talk with the minimum of phonoarticulatory effort. Modern pharmacology places at the disposition of the rhinologist topical symptomatic drugs that are quick acting, have little or no side effects (vasoconstrictors, vasoconstrictors associated with second-generation antihistamines and third-generation antihistamines) and are able to provide rapid relief of the symptomatological triad of pruritus, sneezing and obstruction [5]. Topical administration is not only able to increase the efficacy and tolerance of the drugs, but also seems not to interfere with the complex physiology of the upper airways. Even prolonged treatments with third-generation antihistamines for topical use, such as azelastine, do not adversely affect the times of mucociliary transport, while they manage to control the pruritus, sneezing and secretion and overcome the obstruction (Figs. 1 and 2).

Finally, we wish to mention that there exists today the possibility of a topical use of causal therapies and, in our case, of specific hyposensitizing therapy [6].

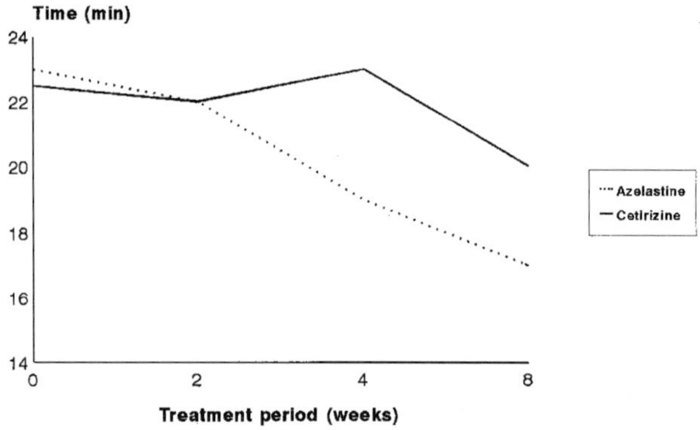

Fig. 1. Nasal mucociliary transport times in patients with perennial rhinitis treated with local (azelastine) or oral (cetirizine) administration of antihistamines.

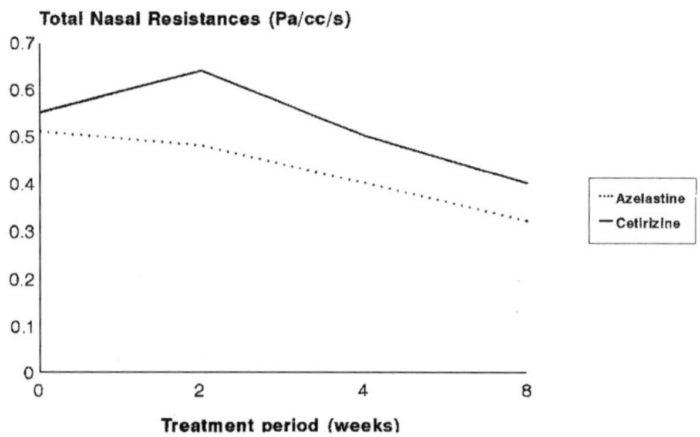

Fig. 2. Rhinomanometric findings in patients with perennial rhinitis treated with local (azelastine) or oral (cetirizine) administration of antihistamines.

References

1. Tarneaud J. Etude physiologique et clinique de la synergie pneuophonique. In: Tarneaud J (ed) Larynx et Phonatione. Paris: Presses Univ. de France, 1957.
2. De Campora E, Miconi M. Rinite ed asma. In: Passàli D (ed) La rinite allergica alle soglie del 2000. Acta ORL Ital 1994;14(43):39–45.
3. Sant'Ambrogio G, Mathew OP, Fisher ST, Sant'Ambrogio FB. Laryngeal receptors responding to transmural pressure, airflow and local muscle activity. Respir Physio 1983;54:317–330.
4. Van Lunteren E, Van de Fraaff WB, Parker DM, Mitra J, Haxhim MA, Strohl KP, Cherniack NS. Nasal and laryngeal reflex responses to negative upper airway pressure. J Appl Physiol 1984;56(3): 746–752.
5. Passàli D, Piragine F. A comparison of azelastine nasal spray and cetirizine tablets in the treatment of allergic rhinitis. J Inter Med Res 1994;22:17–23.
6. Passàli D, Anselmi M, Bellussi L. Nasal specific hyposensitizing therapy: theoretical bases and our experience. In: Passàli D (ed) Rhinology up-to-date. Roma: I.G.R., 1994;235–243.

Surgical treatment of dysphonias

Voice Update.
M. Pais Clemente, editor.

The basis of treatment of benign organically based dysphonias: anatomic and histologic correlates, physiological basis and treatment strategies

M. Pais Clemente
Department of Otorhinolaryngology, Oporto Medical School, Hospital S. João, Oporto, Portugal

Abstract. Basic principles of the anatomy, histology and physiology are reviewed very briefly emphasizing the importance of the knowledge of basic sciences for a more rational and adequate approach to the treatment of benign organically based dysphonias. A list of the most common causes of organic voice disorders is presented, describing some of the benign vocal fold mucosal disorders and benign tumors in particular. A multifactorial theory for vocal fold hemorrhage, nodules, polyps and polypoid corditis involving intrinsic and extrinsic factors is introduced which tries to interpret some of the mechanisms possibly responsible for these clinical entities. The treatment strategy for the above-described benign vocal fold mucosal diseases and benign tumors is the multidisciplinary approach, comprehending medical, surgical, voice rehabilitation or a combination of these different treatment modalities. The preferred phonosurgical technique is microlaryngoscopy with the microspot CO_2 laser because of its well-known and worldwide recognized surgical advantages. Microsurgical dissection is limited to the mucosa and the superficial layer of the lamina propria of the vocal folds, avoiding the intermediate and deep layers (vocal ligament) in order to prevent scarring with deleterious effect on sound production.

Key words: CO_2 laser, contact granulomas and contact ulcers, microlaryngoscopy, organic dysphonias, polypoid corditis, recurrent respiratory papillomatosis, vocal fold cysts, vocal nodules, vocal fold hemorrhage, vocal folds, vocal polyps.

Introduction

The treatment of laryngeal lesions implies a thorough knowledge of basic sciences applied to the laryngeal function, a perfect information of the differential diagnosis of laryngeal diseases and a complete update knowing of the different treatment modalities available. It needs teamwork, including an otolaryngologist with a differentiation in voice disorders, a speech-language pathologist, a voice teacher, a psychologist, an optical engineer and a computer technician. This team should include some co-workers interested in one or more of those areas. This is the only way to progress in the knowledge of voice science and care.

The treatment of benign organically based dysphonias will be reviewed very briefly, taking into consideration the basic sciences, its anatomy, histology, and physiology, and then relating these basic principles to different treatment strategies.

It is beyond the scope of this chapter to discuss those issues into detail and we will refer the reader to the different textbooks available.

Address for correspondence: M. Pais Clemente MD, PhD, Instituto Português da Voz, Rua Caldas Xavier, 38 - 6ºE, 4150 Oporto, Portugal.

Fundamentals of laryngeal anatomy

It is a generalized concept that the anatomical structures responsible for voice production comprehends the larynx, but practically all body systems affects the voice. Normal voice requires mechanical integrity of the respiratory tract, particularly at the level of vocal folds, and a finely tuned neuromuscular system.

We will present the fundamentals of laryngeal anatomy as an introduction to the discussion of the treatment of benign voice disorders.

The larynx is a skeletomembraneous framework constituted by the hyoid bone, the laryngeal cartilages, muscles, ligaments and laryngeal membranes adapted for different laryngeal functions, including: respiration, protection of the lower airway and phonation.

The hyoid bone should be included as a part of the laryngeal apparatus because it is attached to the larynx through the thyroid cartilage via the thyroid membrane and the extrinsic muscles of the larynx. It is also considered a lingual bone because of the tongue musculature attached to it.

The major cartilages of the larynx are the epiglottis, thyroid, cricoid and the paired arytenoids. The paired corniculate and cuneiform cartilages are small and probably serve to increase the stiffness and support of the aryepiglottic folds. The epiglottis is a leaf-like structure composed primarily of elastic cartilage.The thyroid cartilage is the largest of these and it has a shield-like shape. The cricoid cartilage is shaped like an asymmetric ring and it is the only complete skeletal ring for the airway. The arytenoid cartilages are a pair of pyramid-shaped structures that articulate with the corresponding facets of the posterosuperior surface of the cricoid cartilage. With the exception of the articulations between the cricoid cartilage and the arytenoids and also with the thyroid cartilage the skeletal structures of the larynx are attached to each other by different membranes and ligaments.

Most of the internal shape and structure of the larynx is provided by the various intrinsic muscles. The intrinsic muscles are anatomically restricted to the larynx. They modify the size of the glottic opening along with the length and tension on the vocal folds. The intrinsic muscles are paired with the exception of the interarytenoid muscle, and they act synchronously. They include the thyroarytenoid muscle (which has in its medial side the vocalis muscle), the lateral cricoarytenoid, the posterior cricoarytenoid, and the interarytenoid muscle. All these intrinsic muscles are adductors and/or tensors of the vocal folds, with the exception of the posterior cricoarytenoid muscle which is the only abductor of the vocal folds. Also belonging to this group of intrinsic muscles are the thyroepiglottic and aryepiglottic muscles and the paired cricothyroid muscles.

The extrinsic muscles of the larynx are those of the laryngohyoid complex that serve to raise, lower or stabilize the larynx. These muscles are sometimes referred to as the strap muscles [1]. They can be divided in the suprahyoid and infrahyoid groups because they are attached to the hyoid bone, which acts as a direction-changing pull. The suprahyoid group includes the muscles that elevate the larynx, like the thyrohyoid, stylohyoid, digastric, geniohyoid, mylohyoid and stylopharyngeal muscles. They also contribute to suspend the larynx, through the hyoid bone, from the skull base and mandible. The infrahyoid group contains the muscles depressors of the larynx, such as the omohyoid, sternohyoid, sternothyroid and thyrohyoid muscles. The middle constrictor, inferior constrictor and cricopharyngeus muscles are also important extrinsic laryngeal muscles. The extrinsic laryngeal muscles and pharyngeal constrictors are also associated with respiration, deglutition and phonation.

The endolaryngeal surface of the larynx is lined by a continuous mucosa which covers the false and true vocal folds, continues between the free edge of the epiglottis and the arytenoid cartilages and is referred to as the aryepiglottic folds. The reflection of the lining mucosa from the aryepiglottic folds to the lateral pharyngeal walls gives rise to the bilateral piriform sinus. The vocal fold is defined as a fold-like structure between the vocal process of the arytenoid and the anterior commissure. The vocal folds and the slit between them (rima glottidis) represent the glottis. The glottis can be divided into an intermembranous and an intercartilaginous portion by a horizontal imaginary line between the tips of the vocal processes.

The internal anatomy of the larynx consists of three compartments separated by the false and true vocal folds: the vestibule, the ventricule and the infraglottic cavity. There are also two important spaces: the pre-epiglottic space, located anteriorly to the epiglottis, and the paraglottic space which lies on each side of the glottis.

The arterial blood supply of the larynx is derived from branches of the superior and inferior laryngeal arteries and to a small extent from the cricothyroid branch of the superior thyroid artery. The venous drainage of the larynx follows the same pattern as the arterial supply.

The lymphatics of the larynx are divided into the superficial (intramucosal) and the deep (submucosal) groups [2]. The deep group can be further divided into supraglottic, glottic and subglottic.

The drainage of the supraglottic structures (aryepiglottic folds and false folds) follows the superior laryngeal and superior thyroid vessels, crosses freely from one side to the other and drains into the superior and middle groups of the jugular nodes. The epiglottis is a midline structure and thus its lymphatic drainage is bilateral. The lymphatic system of the ventricule is quite different from the other supraglottic structures, because it enters the paraglottic space and spreads through the cricothyroid membrane to the middle and inferior jugular groups, as well as the prelaryngeal (Delphian nodes), and to the paratracheal group of lymph nodes. The true vocal cords are devoid of lymphatics.

The subglottic larynx has two lymphatic systems: one system pierces the cricothyroid membrane receiving lymphatics from both sides of the larynx and disseminates bilaterally to the middle and inferior jugular groups, the prelaryngeal and paratracheal groups of lymph nodes; the other system follows the inferior thyroid vessels to end in the lower portion of the deep jugular chain as well as the subclavian, paratracheal and tracheoesophageal chains. These lymphatics following the inferior laryngeal vessels may have connections with the pretracheal nodes before entering the deep jugular nodes near the subclavian vein. These lymphatics join the jugular lymph trunks and the venous system. This anatomical network has a very important clinical significance because subglottic lesions have a more direct lymphatic route to the venous system than does lymph flowing from a malignant tumor in the supraglottic region of the larynx.

The main somatic innervation to the larynx is from the vagus nerve through the superior and recurrent laryngeal nerves on each side. The superior laryngeal nerve is primarily sensory and it divides into an internal sensory branch and an external motor branch. The internal branch provides the sensory innervation for the vallecula, epiglottis, piriform sinus, and all the internal laryngeal mucosa superior to the free margins of the true folds. Each external branch is the motor supply for just the cricothyroid muscle. The recurrent nerve gives the motor supply to all the intrinsic laryngeal muscles except the cricothyroid muscle. It also provides sensation to the subglottic region and the upper trachea.

Our recent studies on laryngeal microneuroanatomy [3] revealed the presence of neuromuscular compartments in the posterior cricoarytenoid muscle, and multiple connections between the superior laryngeal nerve and recurrent nerve, namely the communicating nerve (branch of the external superior laryngeal nerve), an additional nerve supply to the thyroarytenoid muscle (Fig. 1). Both findings have clinical significance and may explain some of the controversial aspects of the paralyzed larynx.

The receptors of the larynx can be divided into mucosal, articular and myotatic and they mediate much of the reflex activity of the larynx. The larynx also receives autonomic innervation, adrenergic and cholinergic, from the superior cervical ganglia and the vagus nerve, respectively. The primary role of this autonomic nervous system is to regulate vessel diameter and glandular secretions, thus changing the vocal fold mass and vibratory patterns.

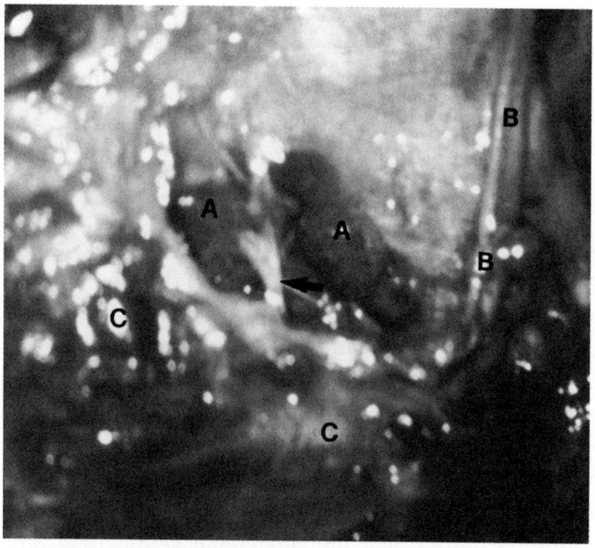

Fig. 1. Communicating nerve (arrow) supplying the thyroarytenoid muscle (A) (20×). B: External superior laryngeal nerve; C: cricothyroid muscle.

Basic histology of the vocal folds

Recent advances on the structure and biomechanical characteristics of the vocal folds have shown them to be more complicated than previously thought. In fact, the vocal folds are well adapted for transducing aerodynamic forces responsible for sound production. Any minimal changes in the histologic structure and/or viscoelastic properties of the vocal folds may affect the voice.

The membranous or vibratory portion of the vocal folds consists of mucosa and muscle: the mucosa is constituted by epithelium and lamina propria (three layers). Hirano [4] has made a great contribution for a better knowledge of the histology of the vocal folds by describing five layers:

1. The mucosa lined by squamous epithelium.
2. The lamina propria of the mucosa with its three layers
3. The superficial layer composed by loose fibers and matrix, also known as Reinke's space.
4. The intermediate layer which primarily consists of elastic fibers running approximately parallel to the edge of the vocal fold, and the deep layer constituted mainly of collagenous fibers which also run almost parallel to the edge of the vocal fold.
5. The last layer represented by the vocalis muscle with its fibers roughly parallel to the edge of the vocal fold (Fig. 2).

The structure involving the intermediate and deep layers of the lamina propria is generally known as the vocal ligament. The vocal ligament is the uppermost portion of the conus elasticus. The margin between the epithelium and the lamina propria is clear, and also from the superficial layer of the lamina propria to the intermediate layer. However, there is no defined border between the intermediate and the deep layer of the lamina propria, neither the margin between the deep layer of the lamina propria and the vocalis muscle. As the vocalis muscle is approached the number of

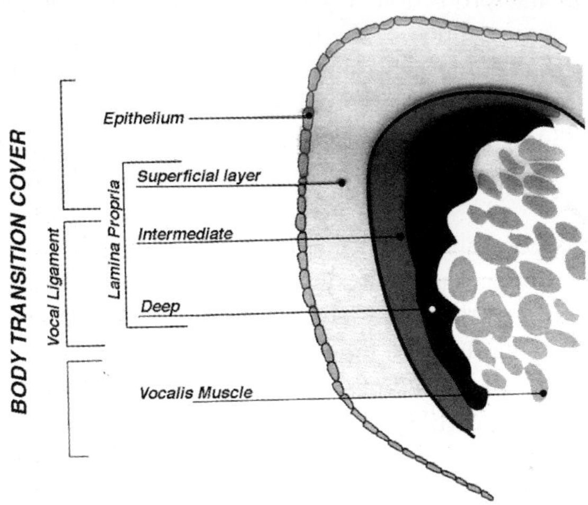

Fig. 2. Schematic cross-section of the vocal fold (Hirano).

elastic fibers decreases and that of collagenous fibers increases. Some collagenous fibers of the deep layer of the lamina propria insert into the muscle fiber bundles of the vocalis muscle.

The Reinke's space has a very important clinical and surgical significance because it is a potential space made possible by the loose adherence of the vocal fold mucosa to the underlying vocal ligament. The boundaries of this space are medially, the vocal fold mucosa, and laterally, the vocal ligament. The anterior commissure anteriorly, and vocal processes of the arytenoids posteriorly; the superior and inferior borders of Reinke's space are said to be the superior and inferior arcuate lines, the areas where the transition from squamous to columnar epithelium occurs.

Mechanically the five layers of the vocal fold act more like three layers: the cover, consisting of stratified squamous epithelium and the superficial layer of the lamina propria, a transition zone composed of the vocal ligament and the body constituted by the vocalis muscle.

According to this cover-body concept [4] the vocal folds are a multilayered vibrator with increasing stiffness from the cover to the body. Thus, the cover is responsible for most of the vibratory action of the vocal folds and the body for the stiffness, depending on the degree of vocalis muscle contraction.

The vocalis muscle has "multimotor end-plates" and a diffuse distribution, although there have been neuromuscular junctions described which are scattered over an area occupying about two-thirds of the entire muscular mass of the muscle. However, our studies [5] showed that the motor end-plates of the thyroarytenoid muscle were more diffusely distributed with a preferential area of higher concentration at the middle third of the vocal folds (Fig. 3).

It is also important to refer an additional layer on the surface of the vocal fold, a layer of mucus or a mucus blanket, because without this layer the vocal fold would stay dry most of the time and the vibratory movement would be more difficult. The vocal folds do not have glandular elements and the mucous and serous glands which provide lubrication and protection are mainly located within the saccule of the ventricle, along the free margins of the false vocal folds, and near the bodies of the arytenoid cartilages and posterior commissure. The presence of the mucus blanket together with the fine arrangements of the different anatomic structures of the vocal folds are essential to the "flowing" movement of the epithelium over the underlying ligament and musculature which is necessary for normal vibratory mechanisms of voice production.

The vocal fold is generally homogeneous along its length with some changes at the anterior and posterior ends. The lamina propria is thickened anteriorly as it approaches its attachment to the posterior surface of the thyroid cartilage which is called the anterior macula flava. In the region of the vocal process, the thickening of the lamina propria is denominated posterior macula flava. The anterior macula flava is attached to the thyroid cartilage anteriorly through another mass of collagenous fibers, known as the anterior commissure tendon or Broyles tendon. The posterior macula flava is connected to the vocal process of the arytenoid cartilage through a transitional structure consisting mainly of chondrocytes and fibroblasts. The anterior

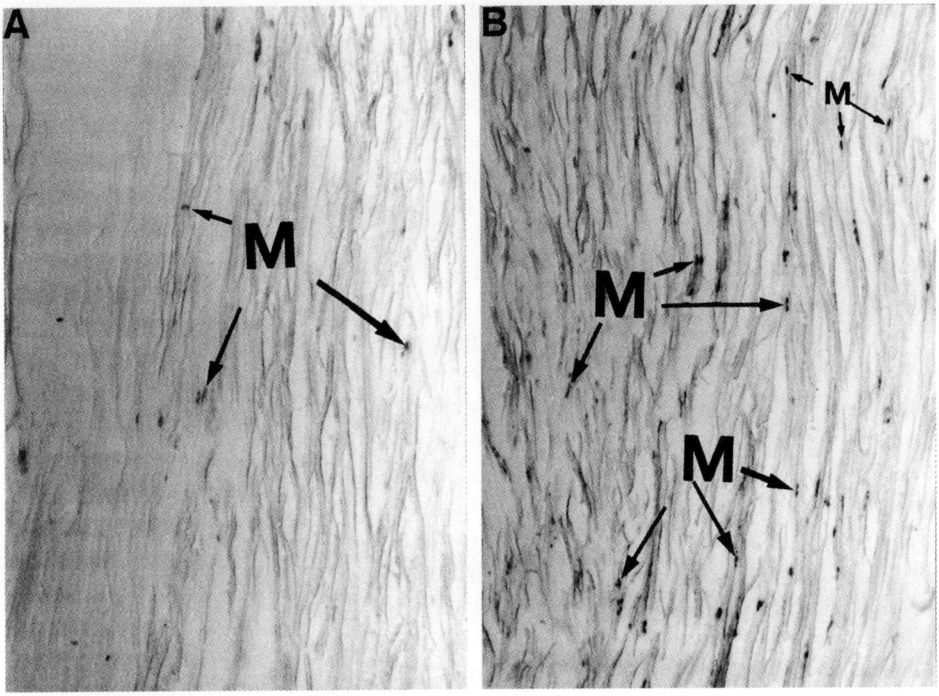

Fig. 3. Motor end-plates (darkly staining dots) of the thyroarytenoid muscle (25×). **A**: Longitudinal section of the anterior third of the muscle. **B**: Longitudinal section of the middle third of the muscle with higher concentration of motor end-plates.

and posterior macula flavas are composed of elastic fibers, fibroblasts and stroma and they are thought to function as "cushions" protecting the ends of the vocal cords from vibratory changes.

The same cover-body concept does not apply to the larynx of children because of the more homogeneous nature of the entire lamina propria which resembles the superficial layer of the lamina propria in adults. Differentiation of the other two layers is progressively observed, and near the end of adolescence the lamina propria mature into its adult form. In the senile larynx the cover becomes thickened and edematous, secondary to changes in the superficial layer of the lamina propria, although the epithelium does not change significantly. The transition layer and the vocalis muscle also tend to atrophy and be replaced by a thicker collagenous tissue [6].

Physiologic principles of laryngeal function

Laryngeal physiology is extremely complex and will be briefly described in this section. The larynx may be regarded as a valve that has three major functions: 1) respiration; 2) protection of the lower airway; and 3) phonation.

The larynx ensures a free flow of air into and out of the lungs. During inspiration, the vocal folds abduct moving away from the midline and widening the glottis, and during the expiration they adduct slightly towards the midline, but always maintaining an open glottal tract. The respiratory center of the medulla, the higher central nervous system and peripheral input drives the synchronous opening of the glottis and descent of the diaphragm during inspiration. The opening of the glottis is primarily through the action of the posterior cricoarytenoid but the cricothyroid contracts rhythmically with the posterior cricoarytenoid particularly in hyperpneic situations. The contraction of both these muscles lengthens the glottic opening, thus increasing the cross-sectional area for airflow.

The larynx also moves as a body during respiration, downward during inspiration and upward during expiration. The downward movement increases the airway capacity, admitting a larger volume of inhaled air. The control of respiratory rate primarily occurs through variation of the expiratory phase. The time of expiration depends on the ventilatory resistance produced by the glottis, and the response of the respiratory center to the different physiologic conditions.

A second vital function of the larynx is the closure mechanism. This mechanism is used during intense physical effort, such as pushing and lifting, and other functions like coughing, vomiting, urination, defecation and parturition. The closure of the larynx occurs at three different levels. In the first level, the laryngeal inlet is contracted by collapsing the aryepiglottic folds medially, and the anterior and posterior spaces are filled by the epiglottic tubercle and the arytenoid cartilages which are brought to the midline. At the second level the false vocal folds are brought together by means of slips of thyroarytenoid muscle contraction.

The final and most important level occurs at the true vocal folds. These folds offer the most important protective closure because of the thyroarytenoid and slips from this muscle which contract at each level of closure. This muscle is one of the fastest contracting of all striated muscles in the body. The glottic closure reflex is a polysynaptic reflex that allows the larynx to protect the lower airway from the aspiration of solids or liquids. Consequently, closure of the larynx during swallowing is essential in order to prevent the food from entering the tracheobronchial tree.

During swallowing the larynx rises as the bolus descends into the back of the tongue, the thyroid cartilage elevates towards the hyoid bone and the epiglottis is pushed into the direction of the bolus with its tip against the posterior pharyngeal wall. The larynx remains closed and it continues to rise as the bolus is squeezed downward passing through the mesopharynx towards the cricopharyngeal sphincter into the upper esophagus. As a result, during swallowing a precise coordination of rising pressure in the hypopharynx against the maintenance of subglottic pressure by the contraction of the thoracic musculature tends to force the false and true folds more tightly against each other, thus providing a better glottic closure.

Phylogenetically, the most recent function of the larynx is phonation. The vocal folds are designed for efficient vibration for phonatory activities, which requires an intact valvular function. The progressive stiffness of the five layers of the vocal folds serves to provide a delicate and complex mechanical vibratory system.

In addition to histologic differences, the five layers of the vocal folds have different mechanical properties. The cover (mucosa and the superficial layer of the lamina propria) is the least stiff; the body (vocalis muscle) most stiff; and the transition (intermediate and deep layers of the lamina propria which constitute the vocal ligament) has intermediate stiffness. Consequently, the cover is more mobile than the other portions of the vocal folds. The tissue fibers for most of the layers run in an anteroposterior direction or parallel to the vocal fold margins. Thus, the tissues are most stiff in a longitudinal direction and most pliable in a transverse direction. This particular distribution of the fibers determines that the greatest flexibility for contraction is at the medial portion of the vocal folds. Also, the "cover-body" theory explains some aspects of the vocal fold vibration, by relating it to mechanical properties of the different layers and their interactions.

Another important component of the structure of the vocal fold is the presence of an additional layer of mucus, or mucus blanket, on the surface of the fold. These mucoserous secretions provide lubrication and protection for the vocal folds keeping the mucosa moist and pliant. This mechanism contributes greatly to the mobility of the vocal fold cover during vibration, and prevents vocal fold abrasion resulting from contact during sound production and sphincteric closure.

The physiology of voice production is extraordinarily complex and not yet completely understood. It involves central and peripheral mechanisms.

The larynx must respond to central commands from speech and motor centers. Impulses are relayed to the motor cortex in the precentral gyrus and then to motor nuclei in the brain system and the spinal cord. These signals are transmitted to the respiratory, laryngeal and articulatory muscles responsible for voice production and speech. Additional refinement of motor activity is provided by the extrapyramidal system including the cerebral cortex, cerebellum and basal ganglia. Also, most of the cranial nerves contribute to voice production and speech.

The role of peripheral mechanisms in phonation has been better documented using airflow and pressure studies in the vocal tract, electromyography as well as imaging techniques. Phonation requires interaction among the power source, oscillator and resonator. Power is produced by the chest, abdomen and back musculature generating a high-pressure air stream. The oscillator is represented by the vocal folds and the resonator by the supraglottic region and upper respiratory tract. During phonation rapid and complex vibratory movements of the vocal folds take place because the resistance changes almost continuously as the glottis closes and opens.

The typical vibratory cycle consists of opening, closing and closed phases [4]. The rate and duration of each phase are determined by the pitch and loudness used, and by other physical factors. By convention, the cycle is described as beginning with the vocal folds closed (Fig. 4). This allows subglottic pressure to raise to a level of about 7 cm of water for conversational speech. Viewed cross-sectionally, each vocal fold is a wedge with a fairly flat surface on top and a sloping section below. At this stage the vocal folds are convergent, closing the airway. Contraction of the expiratory muscles produces a rise in subglottic air pressure which acts on the sloping surface of the glottal walls. The pressure tends to push the lower surface of the vocal folds

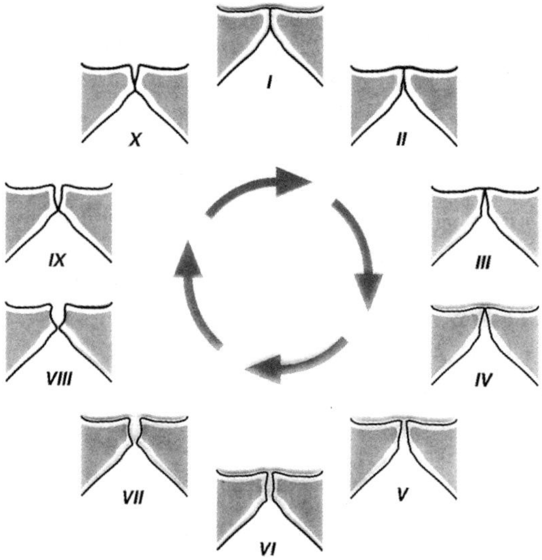

Fig. 4. Cross-sectional illustration of the vibratory changes of the vocal folds during one typical vibratory cycle (modified from [4]).

somewhat apart and the separation grows wider and wider as the pressure continues to build up and air begins to flow. The upper portion of the vocal fold is pushed inward because of the incompressibility of the folds, and the pressure changes within the glottis and the mechanical linkage between upper and lower surfaces of the folds. The difference in timing between the opening of the lower and upper portions of the vocal folds is called vertical phase difference.

This mechanism is very important because it produces a wave-like movement along the mucosa. This movement of the traveling wave depends on a soft and pliant superficial lamina propria and it contributes to the shape and texture of the glottis. The mucosa wave is propagated in the vertical plane by the pressure of subglottic airflow and it extends along the vocal fold. The greatest amplitude of the wave is found in the area closest to the vibrating edge and it becomes significantly reduced further lateral.

During the opening phase a puff of air is released as the vocal folds are being separated. As the cycle proceeds, the lower margins of the folds have begun their return to the midline, resulting primarily from the elastic properties of the tissues, while the upper edges of the vocal folds are still being blown apart. The upper edge of the vocal folds, therefore, begin to snap back towards the midline. As the vocal folds approach each other, narrowing the glottis, a sudden pressure drop caused by the Bernouilli effect sucks the folds into close contact. These events occur during the closing phase and are also mediated by elastic recoil and aerodynamic forces. This phase will remain until subglottic pressure builds up again and the next cycle begins. This interval is called the closed phase. The duration of the closed phase is determined by the compliance of the vocal folds, adductor muscle activity and subglottic pressure. The larynx thus serves as an acoustic wave generator, producing a tone that can be modulated by the supraglottic structures.

The frequency of vibration (number of cycles of openings and closings per second) depends on the air pressure and mechanical characteristics of the vocal folds. The basic frequency of the voice is called fundamental frequency (Fo) and it is measured in hertz (Hz). The time required for one entire vibratory cycle is called the fundamental period (P). Frequency (pitch) increases when the larynx rises in the neck, with increased subglottic pressure, vocal fold length and tension.

The vocal folds normally exhibit some degree of cycle-to-cycle variability in rate (fundamental frequency) which is called jitter or perturbation. Excessive short-term frequency variability has been associated with the perception of hoarse, harsh or rough voice quality in pathologic voices.

Vocal intensity corresponds to our perception of loudness and it increases as subglottic air pressure raises. By increasing the air pressure a greater amplitude of vocal fold vibration is generated and consequently vocal intensity is increased. Cycle-to-cycle variation in vocal amplitude is denominated vocal shimmer. Mean shimmer tends to be higher in voice disorders than in normal voices.

The characteristics of the human voice are owed in great part to this unique laryngeal structure and to the myoelastic – aerodynamic mechanism of phonation. This section could only touch some of the aspects of what is known about laryngeal function. Much still needs to be learned about the vocal folds in health and disease but this work is a challenge for the future.

Treatment strategies

Etiology of organic voice disorders

Before discussing the treatment strategies of benign organically based dysphonias it is important to present a classification of these voice disorders according to their etiology.

A voice disorder is organic if it is caused by structural changes of the larynx or by systemic diseases which alter the normal laryngeal anatomy or function. Table 1 lists the most common causes of organic voice disorders.

Before considering the different treatment strategies we must refer that our patient population with voice disorders has a very careful clinical evaluation with objective measurements of vocal function at our vocal laboratory, and if surgery is indicated, a preoperative counseling is carried out. All our patients have the following preoperative and postoperative voice assessments:

1) subjective judgements of voice quality;
2) laryngovideostroboscopy;
3) acoustic assessment; and
4) aerodynamic testing.

The patients are also informed about our postoperative protocols.

The treatment strategies of benign, organically based dysphonias depend on their etiology, and the causes can be single or multifactorial. Depending on the disease, the treatment can be medical, surgical, vocal rehabilitation, or a combination of any of those treatment modalities. The otolaryngologist may also need the collaboration of other medical and/or surgical specialities which means the multidisciplinary approach of the voice disorders.

Some of these disorders and their treatment will be referred somewhere in this

Table 1. Etiology of organic voice disorders of the larynx.

Congenital disorders	
Laryngomalacia	
Laryngeal webs	
Subglottic stenosis	
Cysts	
Laryngotracheal cleft	
Down's syndrome	
Ageing body	
Inflammatory disorders	
Acute infections:	Viral or bacterial laryngitis
	Supraglottitis (epiglottitis)
	Laryngotracheitis ("croup")
Chronic diseases:	Bacterial diseases
	Tuberculosis
	Mycotic diseases
Inhalation laryngitis	
Environmental pollution	
Tobacco smoking	
Acute thermal injury	
Gastroesophageal (laryngopharyngeal) reflux disease (GERD)	
Benign vocal fold mucosal disorders	
Vocal fold hemorrhage	
Vocal nodules	
Vocal fold polyps	
Polypoid corditis (chronic Reinke's edema)	
Vocal fold cysts	
Contact granulomas and contact ulcers	
Sulcus vocalis	
Postsurgical dysphonia	
Neurological disorders	
Vocal cord paresis/paralysis	
Central	
Peripheral	
Disorders of the neuromuscular junction	

(*continued*)

Table 1. Continued.

Laryngeal motion disorders
Parkinsonism
Dystonia
Vocal tremor
Myoclonus
Stuttering
Tics (Tourette's syndrome)
Choreic disorders
Allergic disorders
Hypersensibility reactions
Angioedema
Endocrine disorders
Hypothyroidism
Hyperthyroidism
Hormonal dysfunction
Systemic diseases
Sarcoidosis
Wegener's granulomatosis
Amyloidosis
Systemic lupus erythematosus
Rheumatoid arthritis
Relapsing polychondritis
Laryngeal trauma
Acute laryngeal injury
Acute laryngeal stenosis
Chronic laryngeal stenosis
Benign tumors
Laryngeal papillomas
Laryngeal hemangiomas
Chondromas
Saccular disorders
Laryngocele
Saccular Cysts
Radiation injury
Radiation laryngitis
Radionecrosis

book. In this chapter we will discuss very briefly our concepts of treatment of some benign vocal fold mucosal disorders such as the vocal fold hemorrhage, vocal fold nodules, vocal fold polyps, polypoid corditis, vocal fold cysts, contact granulomas and contact ulcers, and laryngeal papillomas. We neither present the results nor the complications of these voice disorders because it is out of the scope of this chapter, only relating the different treatment strategies with the knowledge applied to basic sciences.

Surgical treatment

The carbon dioxide laser has been our surgical treatment of choice for benign voice disorders for the past 22 years since we started this surgical technique in 1973, during our Residency Program at Boston University School of Medicine under the direction of Strong, following his pioneer work with the introduction of CO_2 laser in Otolaryngology [7]. It is our conviction that a laser surgeon must have a thorough knowledge of laser biophysics, instrumentation, surgical indications, safety protocols, and technical skills to perform CO_2 laser surgery. Laser technology continues to improve at an increased speed, and it is imperative to keep an update knowledge of current and potential applications of lasers in our speciality.

CO_2 lasers produce light at a wavelength of 10.6 μm in the midinfrared range of the electromagnetic spectrum, and are therefore invisible. The site where the invisible CO_2 laser beam will impact the target tissue is indicated by a built-in coaxial helium-neon laser beam that is red. This aiming beam acts as a guide for delivery of the invisible CO_2 laser beam.

These lasers can be used free-hand, for microscopic surgery attached to the operating microscope, or adapted to a bronchoscopic coupler for rigid bronchoscopy.

We are quite lucky to be familiar with the different generations of CO_2 laser equipments, since the first one developed at the American Optical Corporation (1972), the AO-100 model, until the last model built by Sharplan, the new compact CO_2 30-W system (Fig. 5). This equipment features an extremely accurate laser beam (as fine as 0.1 mm) as well as pulsed and superpulse operation modes. Also, the Sharplan's recent advance — the high precision Acuspot™ micromanipulator can be included in the delivery system.

By using a 400 mm focal length (operating microscope) and varying the spot size, the power output of the laser unit or the time of exposure, the surgeon can adjust the CO_2 laser to incise, coagulate or vaporize the target tissue. Therefore, the treatment of mass lesions is very predictable, and it is possible to remove the lesion very confidently without causing unnecessary additional damage to the cover, transition or the body of the fold.

The wavelength of the CO_2 laser has a high coefficient of absorption for water, and so its energy is well absorbed by all soft tissues with a high water content. The interaction of the CO_2 laser on soft tissues was well studied by Miashi et al. [8], particularly the crater formation and the surrounding structures. Laser energy produces a thermal effect when it is absorbed by the target tissue and converted to heat. When the tissue absorbs a specific amount of radiant energy to raise its temperature to approximately 60—65°C, protein denaturation starts to occur. Blanching of the tissue surface is then visible and when laser light raises the temperature of the tissue to approximately 100°C vaporization of intracellular water occurs with

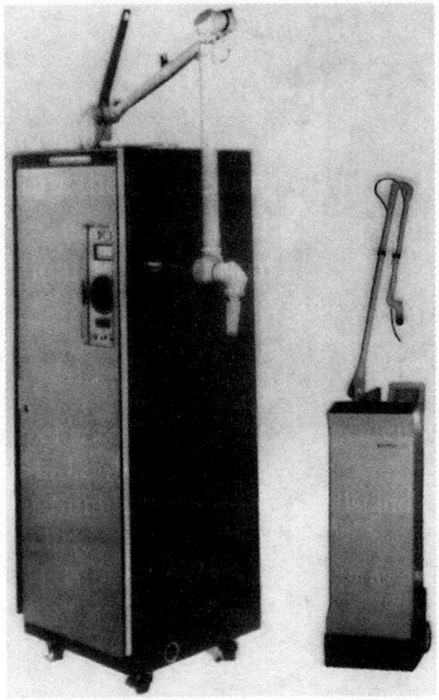

Fig. 5. The evolution of CO_2 laser technology. On the left – the first CO_2 laser equipment, developed at the American Optical Corporation, called the AO-100 model (1972). On the right – the last compact and portable CO_2 laser 30-W system built by Sharplan.

vacuolization, followed by crater formation and tissue shrinkage.

Disintegration, carbonization, smoke and gas formation with destruction of the laser-irradiated tissue occurs at several hundred degrees centigrade. The rapid thermal drops of laser energy in the tissue surrounding the impact, result in shallow and predictable tissue penetration. Consequently, the tissue edema is minimal. However, the hemostatic effect of the CO_2 laser is limited to small blood vessels and with the current CO_2 laser equipment it is possible to defocus the laser beam to produce coagulation of these vessels (approximately 1 mm). The nerves and lymphatics are sealed in the area of thermal necrosis.

The minimal mechanical trauma, the excellent hemostasis achieved with laser beam for small vessels, the sealing of lymphatics and nerves probably accounts for minimal postoperative edema and pain. The combination of these characteristics with other features of the CO_2 laser surgery, such as precise surgery, maximum visibility, preservation of adjacent structures, excellent healing and short hospitalization offers great advantages when compared with other conventional surgical techniques (Fig. 6). This fact represents an extraordinary progress in the field of surgery in general, and in otorhinolaryngology in particular [9].

Benign laryngeal disorders

Benign vocal fold mucosal lesions such as vocal fold hemorrhage, vocal nodules and vocal fold polyps seem to be caused primarily by excessive voice use and misuse. Professional and lifestyle vocal demands are also very important factors. Other

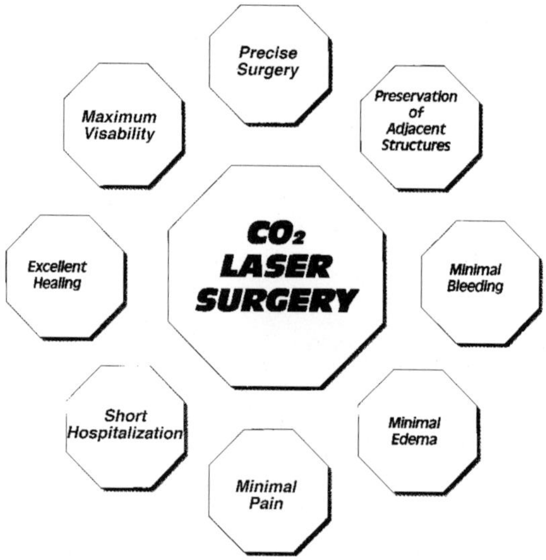

Fig. 6. Advantages of CO_2 laser surgery.

influences such as tobacco smoking, chronic gastroesophageal reflux, laryngeal infections and allergy may contribute to increase the mucosa susceptibility to these disorders during vocal fold vibratory function. Frequent throat clearing may also be responsible for benign vocal fold mucosal lesions [10]. The development of some benign vocal fold mucosal lesions may be explained by the multifactorial theory which includes intrinsic and extrinsic factors (Fig. 7). The intrinsic factors are represented by an individual's susceptibility, anatomic and histologic features of the vocal folds, voice abuse and misuse, laryngeal inflammatory disorders, chronic gastroesophageal reflux, throat clearing and chronic coughing. The extrinsic factors include noisy environments, deficient acoustic conditions, environmental pollution and tobacco smoking.

We believe that these disorders are multifactorial in origin, with one factor being more important than the other(s), depending on the establishment of one or more of the above factors for its development.

Also, the cover-body concept together with our findings on the distribution of the motor end-plates in the vocalis muscle might explain some of the aspects related to the preferential location of those lesions on the middle third of the vocal folds. The peculiar anatomical distribution of the tissue fibers most stiff in a longitudinal direction and most pliable in a transverse direction determines the greatest flexibility for contraction at the medial portion of the vocal folds. Our studies on laryngeal microneuroanatomy [5] showed that the motor end-plates of the vocalis muscle were increased at the middle third of the vocal folds which might contribute to the increased incidence of these lesions at this area, where higher forces of contraction are applied.

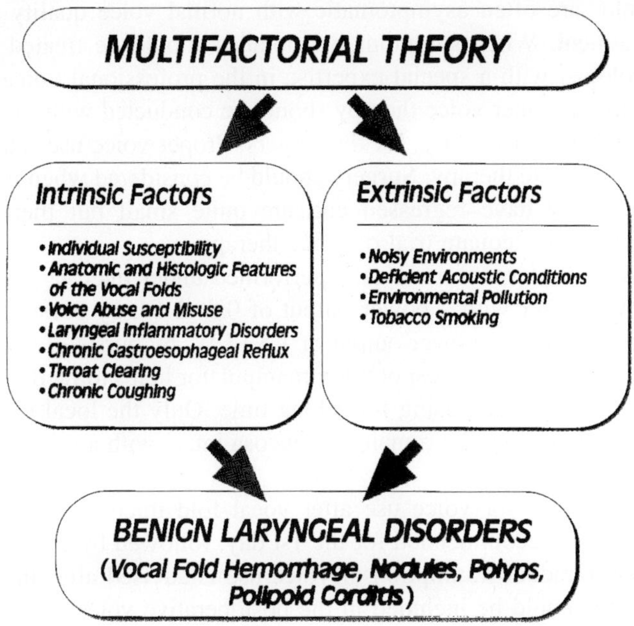

Fig. 7. The multifactorial theory for some benign vocal fold mucosal disorders.

The benign vocal fold mucosal disorders are quite common and account for approximately 30% of our clinical practice between 1978 and 1995.

Vocal fold hemorrhage

Vocal fold hemorrhage can occur with a respiratory infection, laryngitis, acute vocal abuse, particularly with shouting. This disorder may be seen in a few women using aspirin products at the onset of the menstrual period. The singers with a vocal fold hemorrhage should cancel their performances.

Treatment of this disorder is conservative with strict vocal rest, body hydration and aerosol inhalation. Clinical evaluation of the vocal fold hemorrhage should be monitored with videostroboscopy. Recurrent episodes of hemorrhage are usually best treated by vaporization of the bleeding vessel(s) with defocused 1-W CO_2 laser bursts.

Vocal nodules

Vocal nodules typically appear as small bilateral swellings at the junction of the anterior and middle thirds of the phonating margin of the vocal folds. Initially they may be soft and edematous, but become more fibrotic with time and long-term voice abuse. The nodules are usually symmetrical and often impede a complete glottic closure during phonation. The mass and stiffness of the cover are slightly increased, whereas those of the transition and body remain unchanged. The change in mucosal mass interferes with vibratory motion of the focal folds and together with the incomplete glottic closure explains the vocal symptoms referred by the patients.

Vocal nodules are often asymptomatic with normal voice quality and therefore require no treatment. When symptomatic, nodules should be treated by a speech-language pathologist with a special expertise in the professional voice. A minimum of 6 to 12 weeks of proper voice therapy should be conducted with the collaboration of a singing teacher, if necessary, for the singers. Proper voice use rather than voice rest is the most adequate therapy. Surgery should be considered when nodules persist, and even when they have regressed and are quite small but there is no vocal improvement after an adequate trial of voice therapy.

Surgical excision of vocal nodules is performed under microlaryngoscopy using the microspot CO_2 laser with a power output of 0.8–2 W, by bursts of 0.05 s, in a superpulse mode, or with a power output of 1.5–2 W, by bursts of 0.1 s, in a pulser mode. The new generation microspot micromanipulator helps to facilitate the shaving technique that we have been using for a long time. Only the local tissue elevations should be removed, leaving the remaining mucosa intact with a minimal raw surface area to heal.

We have a protocol for voice use after vocal fold microsurgery. Postoperative absolute voice rest is recommended for the 1st day, followed by a period of 2 weeks using soft voice. Gradual resumption of voice use is advised after the beginning of the 3rd week and should be included in the postoperative voice therapy protocol to prevent recurrence of nodules. Also, the vocal folds are monitored with videostroboscopy to evaluate when the mucosal wave is returning to normal.

Vocal fold polyps

Vocal fold polyps frequently arise on the phonating edge of the vocal folds at the junction of the anterior and middle thirds of the folds. The majority of vocal polyps are solitary (90%), although they may be bilateral, or even multiple on one fold.

Polyps often have a feeding blood vessel coursing along the superior surface of the vocal fold and entering at the base of the polyp. The etiology of polyps remains unclear, but most can be related to acute vocal trauma such as shouting, intermittent severe voice abuse or a prolonged period of vocal effort in those who work in noisy environments. Tobacco smoking may contribute to the development of vocal polyps and some of the other factors described in the multifactorial theory.

It may be possible that the polyp begins with breakage of a capillary in Reinke's space during extreme vocal exertion with flowing of blood and accumulation of edema. At least some polyps start as vocal fold hemorrhage. Consequently, if the voice is not immediately rested, the resulting hematoma can become organized into a polyp. After a long duration, a hemorrhagic polyp may lose its vascular appearance and become pedunculated which may also be seen as the final stage of the polyp.

A short period of conservative management with relative voice rest and 2 weeks of low-dose steroid therapy should be tried for small polyps. However, most of them require surgical excision because if the polyps are not treated they may produce contact injury to the opposite vocal fold.

Microlaryngoscopy with microspot CO_2 laser is our treatment of choice because of the already described advantages of this surgical technique. We are not afraid to use laser surgery along the vibratory margins of the vocal folds and we never had any of the potential complications described with this technique, like the formation of an adynamic segment along the vocal fold.

Voice therapy should also be used after surgery for a better vocal rehabilitation and to avoid recurrences.

Polypoid corditis

Polypoid corditis is a bilateral, diffuse swelling of the free edge of the vocal fold within the Reinke's space. There have been a number of terms used to denote this voice disorder. These terms include: chronic Reinke's edema, polypoid laryngitis, polypoid degeneration, chronic hypertrophic laryngitis, and bilateral diffuse polyposis.

We believe the name polypoid corditis is more appropriate, when compared with other terms. It is a chronic inflammatory process of the vocal cord (corditis) with edema and vascular congestion containing a mixoid stroma with a few structural proteins such as collagen and elastin (polypoid-like material). Patients are frequently vocal abusers and overusers, they have typically high subglottic aerodynamic pressures (vocal hyperfunction) and rarely may suffer from hypothyroidism.

Polypoid corditis can also be explained by the multifactorial theory for these benign vocal fold mucosal disorders due to intrinsic and extrinsic factors.

We have already described the Reinke's space as a potential space made possible by the lost of adherence of the vocal epithelium to the underlying vocal ligament. This loose attachment contributes to the vocal fold vibrations. However, owing to the poor lymphatic drainage of this area, it is prone to the accumulation of edema in the loose submucosal layers known as Reinke's space. We believe that vocal fold hemorrhage, vocal fold nodules, vocal fold polyps and polypoid corditis are different stages of the basic inflammatory process of exudation, organization and fibrosis.

Like other authors [11], we found that most individuals with polypoid corditis have persistent hyperfunctional vocal behaviours and chronic glottal mucositis secondary to tobacco smoking and gastroesophageal reflux associated with throat clearing and/or coughing. Interestingly, these patients have elevated subglottal pressures. An explanation for this condition is that the chronic mucosal irritation due to the factors described above change the mechanical properties of vocal fold tissues by increasing the stiffness of the vocal fold cover, which in turn generates higher subglottal pressures to drive the vocal folds into vibration. The mass and stiffness of the transition and body remain unaffected. The lesion also interferes with the vibratory motion of the opposite vocal fold. However, it may also be possible that vocal hyperfunction presented by these patients causes the vocal folds to be abnormally stiff and tense, increasing the force of adduction and consequently requiring higher subglottal pressures for phonation. Trying to find out which one is the first event originating from the sequential mechanisms is a vicious circle that is difficult to interpret.

The treatment consists of a short-term preoperative voice therapy in order to lead the patient to a correct vocal behaviour. The patient is also advised to stop smoking and the gastroesophageal reflux is treated with omeprazole. The surgical technique is performed under microlaryngoscopy with a microspot CO_2 laser for incision on the superior surface of both vocal folds, raising a superior microflap. The mixoid stroma in the superficial lamina propria is then suctioned, reducing its volume to the desired contour without traumatizing the remaining superficial lamina propria and vocal ligament. It is very important not to remove too much stroma of the superficial lamina propria, which avoids adherence of the mucosa basement membrane to the vocal ligament. This adherence decreases the vibratory motion of the vocal folds by making an iatrogenic scar and by increasing its stiffness which has a deleterious effect on sound production.

After the superficial lamina has been reduced to the desired contour, the redundant mucosa is then redraped to determine the extent of epithelial resection for adequate opposition of the mucosal edges. Any suspicious epithelium for atypia and/or microinvasion is removed for biopsy. However, in some cases it is necessary to complete this "cosmetic" vocal procedure with a minimal superficial microcauterization of the remaining superior surface of the vocal fold using the microspot CO_2 laser, 1–2 W, of 0.05 s, in a superpulse mode.

Classically, the common practice of "vocal cord stripping" often results in scarring and dysphonia for a postoperative period of many weeks and the final result could be even worse than before surgery. This more precise "mucosa-sparing" and polypoid-reducing surgical technique is the current management of polypoid corditis for an earlier and optimal return of voice.

The patients are also advised to have postoperative voice therapy to control vocal hyperfunction and avoiding recurrences, to give up smoking and to continue the treatment for gastroesophageal reflux as long as necessary.

When treating this disorder in professional voice users great caution should be taken with the surgical indication in those patients. These performers with polypoid corditis are well recognized and accepted for their abnormal voices and improving their voice quality can be the end of their career [12].

Vocal fold cysts

Vocal fold cysts are submucosal cysts that are probably the consequence of vocal overuse. These cysts can be classified as mucus-retention and epidermoid cysts. The mucus-retention cysts occur when the duct of the mucus gland become obstructed by glandular secretions. The epidermoid cysts contain accumulated keratin. The mucus-retention cysts are usually unilateral but they may cause contact swelling on the opposite side and are frequently misdiagnosed as vocal nodules. However, with the use of videostroboscopy the correct diagnosis can easily be made.

The recommended treatment is the surgical removal of the cyst under microlaryngoscopy with microspot CO_2 laser. A small and superficial incision with CO_2 laser is performed on the fold's superior surface, followed by a careful dissection with delicate microlaryngeal surgical instruments. The cyst is completely removed and care is taken to avoid any injury to the mucosa and vocal ligament. The mucosa is then reapproximated and the wound is closed with the opposed edges. The opposite fold should be examined carefully because of the possibility of bilateral cyst formation.

Although the surgical results are not as good as for nodules and polyps, excellent results can be obtained with proper microsurgery technique. Postoperative voice therapy contributes for vocal rehabilitation.

Contact granulomas and contact ulcers

Contact granulomas and contact ulcers usually appear at/or around the vocal process of the arytenoid cartilage. The lesions may be unilateral or bilateral. They are often seen in individuals who suffer from vocal abuse, gastroesophageal reflux, throat clearing, chronic coughing, and patients who have undergone endotracheal intubation or rigid bronchoscopy.

Voice therapy is the first modality of treatment to change the persistent hyperfunctional behaviour, eliminate throat clearing and nervous coughing. Treatment for gastroesophageal reflux with omeprazole is also indicated. Microlaryngoscopy with microspot CO_2 laser for the removal of the contact granulomas is justified, if with the above-described conservative treatment the lesion(s) do not disappear. Postoperative voice therapy is also recommended.

Benign tumors of the larynx

Benign tumors of the larynx are rare compared to the benign vocal fold mucosal disorders, inflammatory disorders, neurologic diseases and malignant tumors of the larynx. However, laryngeal papillomas are the most common benign tumors of the larynx. The correct terminology for this disease is "recurrent respiratory papillomatosis" (RRP) [13]. It should be regarded as a specific clinical entity, involving the respiratory tract, histologically benign, although with a malignant behaviour, because of its tendency to become recurrent.

The agent responsible for human respiratory papillomas is a human papilloma virus (HPV). Human papillomas virus typing further identifies the involved virus, which in the larynx is most often HPV types 6 and 11. We were able to demonstrate the presence of virus-like particles in three out of 17 surgical specimens (18%) examined by electronmicroscopy and to document the existence of an inflammatory reaction around papilloma cells [14].

The reservoir of RRP seems to be the condyloma accuminatum. In a group of 150 patients, the incidence of genital lesions among their mothers is statistically higher (34.4%) than the one found in the patients (10.0%), and even higher than the overall incidence of this disease in women of the same population groups as ours (1.5%) [15]. Another source for RRP could be the skin warts. Like other authors [16,17] we found an increased incidence of skin warts in patients with this disease (28.7%), which is higher than the incidence attributed to a general hospital population (13.0%) [15].

RRP have a worldwide distribution. According to a national survey in the USA (1976), nearly 1,500 new cases are examined each year, which corresponds to one case per 142,000 inhabitants, particularly prevalent in Southern States such as the States of Florida, Georgia, Alabama, Louisiana and New Mexico [18]. This study permits to conclude that this clinical entity is not as rare as many authors seek to imply [19,20].

The larynx occupies a preferential location for the RRP, followed by the tracheobronchial tree, oropharynx and nasal vestibule. The glottic region is more frequently involved than the supra and subglottic areas. The mass and stiffness of the cover are increased, which interferes with the normal vibratory mechanisms of the vocal folds.

Microlaryngoscopy with the CO_2 laser is the most widely accepted method for treatment of laryngeal papillomas because of the known characteristics of this surgical technique. Many other treatments have been tried in the past, such as cryotherapy, ultrasound, radiation, vaccines, chemotherapy, and most recently interferon. However, the current management would seem to be serial CO_2 laser excisions of the papillomas, waiting hopefully for a remission.

Conclusions

1. Complete knowledge of basic sciences is the master key to a more rational and adequate treatment of benign organically based dysphonias.
2. A team approach including an otolaryngologist with a special differentiation in voice disorders, a speech-language pathologist, a voice teacher, a psychologist and/or a psychiatrist is recommended when treating patients with voice disorders.
3. Great clinical skills and experience with the different objective measurements of vocal function are needed for a correct planned treatment of voice disorders.
4. The treatment strategies for benign organic disorders are multidisciplinary, comprehending medical, surgical, voice rehabilitation or a combination of these different treatment modalities.
5. The preferred phonosurgical technique is microlaryngoscopy using the microspot CO_2 laser, although excellent voice results could also be achieved with other conventional techniques throughout the world.
6. Microdissection limited to the mucosa and the superficial layer of the lamina propria of the vocal fold is the current surgical management of benign voice disorders when indicated.

References

1. Hollinshead WH. Anatomy for Surgeons, vol 1. The Head and Neck. 3rd edn. Philadelphia: J.B. Lippincott, 1982.
2. Sasaki CT, Discol BP, Gracco C. Anatomy and physiology of the larynx. In: Ballenger JJ, Snow JB Jr (eds) Otorhinolaryngology Head and Neck Surgery. Baltimore: Williams & Wilkins, 1996.
3. Pais Clemente M, Pratas R, Cardoso V. Recent findings on laryngeal microneuroanatomy. In: M. Pais Clemente (ed) Voice Update. Amsterdam: Elsevier Science B.V., 1996.
4. Hirano M, Bless DM. Vocal fold vibration. Videostroboscopic Examination of the Larynx. San Diego: Singular Publishing Group, Inc., 1993.
5. Pais Clemente M, Lima Rodrigues M. Distribution of motor end-plates in intrinsic laryngeal muscles of the rat. A comparative study with man. In: M. Pais Clemente (ed) Voice Update. Amsterdam: Elsevier Science B.V., 1996.
6. Hirano M, Kurita S, Sakaguchi S. Ageing of the vibratory tissue of human vocal folds. Acta

Otolaryngol (Stockh) 1989;107:428–433.

7. Strong MS, Jako GJ. Laser surgery in the larynx. Ann Otol Rhinol Laryngol 1972;81:781–789.
8. Mihashi S, Jako GJ, Incze J, Strong MS, Vaughan CW. Laser surgery in otolaryngology: interaction of CO_2 laser and soft tissue. Ann NY Acad Sci 1976;267:263–294.
9. Pais Clemente M. Lasers in otorhinolaryngology. In: Soares OD, Scheggi AM (eds) Bioptics. Bellingham: SPIE – The International Society for Optical Engineering, 1992.
10. Benninger MS. Medical disorders in the vocal artist. In: Benninger MS, Jacobson BH, Johnson AF (eds) Vocal Arts Medicine The Care and Prevention of Professional Voice Disorders. New York: Thieme Medical Publishers, Inc, 1994.
11. Zeitels SM. Personal Communication.
12. Sataloff RT. Structural and neurological disorders and surgery of the voice. In: Sataloff RT (ed) Professional Voice The Science and Art of Clinical Care. New York: Raven Press Ltd., 1991.
13. Strong MS, Vaughan CV, Healy GB, Cooperband SR, Clemente MAC P. Recurrent respiratory papillomatosis – management with the CO_2 laser. Ann Otol Rhinol Laryngol 1976;85:508–516.
14. Incze JS, Lui PS, Strong MS, Vaughan CW, Pais Clemente M. The morphology of human papillomas of the upper respiratory tract. Cancer 1977;39:1634–1646.
15. Pais Clemente MAC. Microcirurgia com laser na papilomatose respiratória recorrente – estudo clínico e experimental. Ph.D. Thesis. Oporto, 1978.
16. Bjork H, Weber C. Papilloma of the larynx. Acta Otolaryngol (Stockl) 1956;46:499–516.
17. Majoros M, Parkhill EM, Devine KD. Papilloma of the larynx in children. A clinicopathologic study. Am J Surg 1964;108:470–475.
18. Strong MS, Pais Clemente MAC. Incidence of recurrent respiratory papillomatosis in the United States. In: Microcirurgia com laser na papilomatose respiratória recorrente – estudo clínico e experimental. Ph.D. Thesis, Oporto, 1978.
19. Dekelboum AM. Papillomas of the larynx. Arch Otolaryngol 1965;81:390–397.
20. Marres Ehma, Wentges RTR, Brinkman WFB. Cryosurgical treatment of juvenile laryngeal papillomatosis. Laryngoscope 1966;76:1976–1983.

Voice Update.
M. Pais Clemente, editor.

Conservative phonomicrosurgery in the treatment of premalignant vocal fold lesions

Oskar Kleinsasser
ENT-Department, Marburg, Germany

Key words: carcinoma in situ, endolaryngeal surgery, precancerosis.

Speaking on premalignant, preinvasive or precancerous lesions we first have to find an acceptable definition of precancerosis. In general pathology a precancerosis is called an epithelial lesion from which a carcinoma will arise. In laryngological practise, unfortunately, no uniform terminology has become generally accepted, so that a multitude of terms are applied to lesions that are sometimes the same and sometimes different, e.g., dysplasia, severe dysplasia, leucoplakia, erythroplakia, keratosis, keratoma, verruca and papilloma. A correct diagnosis can only be made by a meticulous histopathologic examination of the whole lesion, preferably using paraffin step serial sections. In practise this means we must remove the whole lesion first before we can say that we have treated a true premalignant lesion at all, excluding a benign lesion as well as microinvasive cancer.

Histopathologically, a premalignant lesion consists usually of a thickened hyperplastic squamous epithelium with nuclear atypias of varying degrees and disturbances of the regular differentiations. In respect to prognosis there is no difference in between the so-called severe dysplasia with more mature cells and carcinoma in situ consisting of immature atypical cells through the whole thickness of the epithelium.

Nobody knows when these premalignant lesions proceed to true invasive cancer. The preinvasive state certainly can be a short episode of a continually developing carcinoma, but we also know of carcinomata in situ staying as preinvasive small tumors even for several years.

In practice that means that we have to treat each suspicious lesion to be a premalignant one and immediately remove it completely as if it were a true small cancer. A classical punch-biopsy from such a lesion is insufficient as many cancers are surrounded by preinvasive malignant epithelium. The minimal procedure has to be an excisional biopsy enabling us to investigate the whole specimen. If we find benign keratoma or a benign reactive lesion the excisional biopsy has been the correct

Address for correspondence: Prof Dr O. Kleinsasser, ENT-Department, 3 Deutschhausstraße, 35037 Marburg, Germany.

procedure. If it is a premalignant lesion or even a small cancer a well performed excision also constitutes the final therapy.

The treatment of premalignant lesions should be a surgical one, preferably performed endoscopically by endolaryngeal microsurgery. This is the minimum procedure with the lowest morbidity and costs, results usually in an excellent voice and a nearly 100% cure rate and can be done on an outpatient basis. If the tumor cannot be brought well into endoscopic vision I prefer open surgery performing a so-called decortication of the cord. Irradiation, lasting 6 weeks and affording an average of 60 Gy, I consider to be an overtreatment in small tumors. Only in extensive superficially spreading bilateral lesions do we recommend radiotherapy.

The technique of endolaryngeal microsurgery in premalignant lesions is demonstrated by a video tape. We use classical "cold" instruments only and no laser.

Results in 66 carcinomata in situ treated by endolaryngeal microsurgery from 1977 to 1994 are good: no patient has lost his life from a tumor. We saw five recurrences, three of them on the contralateral vocal fold independent from the primary tumor. Two were true recurrences obviously arising from residual tumors. In four of the five cases with a second endoscopical resection the recurrences were treated successfully. One patient lost her larynx after resection of a bilateral carcinoma in situ. She did not come to the regular follow-up for 4 years until an extensive cancer growing far subglottically had developed. Additionally, we had similar good results in 63 pT1 carcinomas resected endoscopically with no recurrence up to this time, no lost larynx and no death by tumor.

Open surgery in premalignant lesions by decortication of the vocal cord epithelium was performed only in some larynges that were difficult to access mainly before 1976. In 36 cases within 22 years there were two local recurrences successfully treated, no larynx was lost, no death by tumor occured.

Voice Update.
M. Pais Clemente, editor.

Voice preservation by CO_2 laser surgery for early and advanced laryngeal cancer

Wolfgang Steiner and Petra Ambrosch
Department of Otorhinolaryngology, Georg August University, Gottingen, Germany

Key words: advanced, early, laryngeal cancer, transoral laser microsurgery.

Introduction

Since 1979 we have preferred laser microsurgery for the treatment of laryngeal cancer as an alternative to conventional surgery or radiotherapy. The therapeutic concept and the advantages of transoral laser microsurgery compared to standard therapy are described below.

Laser microsurgery has similar oncological results (1% secondary laryngectomy as salvage surgery and no tumor-related death) to conventional surgery, but functionally, laser microsurgery achieves better results. In comparison to radiotherapy, laser microsurgery is clearly superior with respect to oncology, while the functional results are similarly favourable.

In the treatment of advanced tumors, there is no therapeutic concept as favourable as that of transoral laser microsurgical partial laryngectomy: organ and function can be preserved in 90% of the cases with the survival rates being comparable to those after total laryngectomy.

The oncological results of 466 previously untreated patients who had transoral laser microsurgery (± neck dissection, ± radiotherapy) with curative intention (pTis–pT4, (p) N0–N2 M0, UICC 1987) between 1979 and 1991 are presented and discussed.

The first report on successful treatment of a carcinoma in situ using CO_2 laser surgery was given by Strong and Jako [1], the pioneers of endolaryngeal laser microsurgery.

Evaluating 23 reports (published between 1984 and 1993) there were 1,230 patients with early glottic cancer (mainly T1a) treated primarily by laser microsurgery. In 12% there were local recurrences, 5% needed total laryngectomy as a salvage treatment.

Our laser surgical experience is based on more than 900 patients treated since 1979 [1] for primary or recurrent cancer of the larynx with curative or palliative intention.

Our presentation deals with the oncological results after laser microsurgery of the early stages of glottic cancer, and also with the results of advanced tumor stages. While in the first group (early stages) the functional goal is to achieve a good quality of voice, in the second group (advanced stages) the functional goal is to preserve the natural voice and to avoid permanent tracheotomy.

This report concerns 466 previously untreated patients who had CO_2 laser microsurgery with curative intention (pTis–4 (p) N0–2, M0, UICC 1987/1992) between 1979 and 1991. Patients with simultaneous second primaries were excluded.

Glottic cancer (pTis – 2a, N0, M0)

The results concern 271 patients with early glottic cancer treated exclusively by laser microsurgery between 1979 and 1991.

There were 39 patients with a vocal cord carcinona in situ, 151 had a T1 and 81 a T2a glottic carcinoma. The median age was 61 years. In 83% of the patients the tumor covered more than one-third of the vocal cord.

Of the 271 patients 112 (42%) had lesions involving the anterior commissure, 78 (69%) of them had unilateral and 34 (31%) bilateral vocal cord carcinoma. No patient needed a tracheotomy, and some of the surgery was performed on an outpatient basis. Only one patient had postoperative hemorrhage, which needed coagulation under general anesthesia. The voice quality was satisfactory in 92% of the cases with slight or no dysphonia.

In our material 8% of the 271 patients with early glottic cancer (pTis, pT1a, pT1b, pT2a) had local recurrences (or new cancers) until 1994. Only in three cases was total laryngectomy as salvage procedure necessary, two of which only after 6 years. So the voice could be preserved in 99% of the patients. What is more, no patient died due to his primary tumor. The 5-year overall survival rate was 85%, which corresponds to the survival curve of age- and sex-matched controls, 28% of the patients were over 70 years old and 9% over 80 years.

Under these circumstances, it is understandable that we consider laser microsurgical primary resection as the treatment of choice. The (almost) bloodless preparation with the CO_2 laser under microscopic magnification allows a precise and safe resection of the tumor, the surgery is individually adapted to the size of the tumor and is thus efficient. The smaller the lesion the better the resectability with preservation of function.

Laser surgery is superior to conventional open surgery for several reasons. First of all, the surgery is comparatively short and often possible as an outpatient procedure. Moreover, the morbidity is minimal because tracheotomy and nasogastric feeding can be avoided. For all this, the stress on the patient is minimalized. Apart from that, also the postoperative quality of voice is remarkable. All in all, there is a trend to overtreat in conventional surgery as we can see from several surgical manuals and papers worldwide.

Laser microsurgery is definitely superior to radiotherapy. In our opinion, radiotherapy is an absolute overtreatment for small lesions, which are often already entirely removed by diagnostic biopsy. The three most important arguments by radiotherapists (avoiding major surgery, better voice quality and lower costs) lose importance in the face of laser microsurgery. In larger tumors better voice quality after radiotherapy does not counterbalance the higher recurrence rate with the possible necessity of a salvage laryngectomy. Furthermore, tumor-related deaths are seen more often in primarily irradiated patients than in surgically treated patients.

While laser microsurgery of early glottic cancer has become more common in the 80s, and its application has been extended beyond purely T1a vocal cord cancer, the supraglottic tumors, which are rarely recognized in their early stages, have been operated transorally by laser microsurgery in some ENT centres only. However, to date no paper has been published reporting a routine laser surgical treatment of the more advanced stages of glottic and supraglottic tumors, especially the T3 and T4 categories.

The conventional partial resections – vertical, horizontal as well as near total laryngectomies – are performed very rarely in very advanced cancer stages. Unfortunately, the treatment of choice is mostly total laryngectomy even for T2-stages. Furthermore, even when partial resections are performed, it is evident that there is a trend to surgical overtreatment.

Recent studies in the USA showed that with sequential chemo-radiotherapy it was possible to avoid total laryngectomy in some of the patients with advanced tumor stages. But we have to remember that in these trials (e.g., T2-supraglottic tumors were considered as advanced stages requiring total laryngectomy) this is not acceptable.

Glottic cancer (pT2b–4 (p)N0–2 M0)

Between 1979 and 1991, 116 previously untreated patients with more advanced glottic cancer (pT2b vocal cord mobility impaired: 79, pT3: 28, pT4: 9/37% belonged to stage III and IV) were treated by CO_2 laser microsurgery for the primary tumor with curative intention. A selective neck dissection was performed in one-third; one in four patients needed postoperative radiotherapy. Twenty-two percent of the patients (n = 26) had local recurrences. Salvage laryngectomy was carried out in 9% of the patients (n = 10). Thirteen percent of the patients (n = 15) died from tumor-related causes. The 5-year overall survival rate (Kaplan Meier) was 61%.

Supraglottic cancer (pT1–4 (p)N0–M0)

Between 1979 and 1991, 79 previously untreated patients with supraglottic cancer (pT1: 12, pT2: 42, pT3: 13, pT4: 12/50% belonged to stage III and IV) were treated by CO_2 laser microsurgery for the primary tumor. Three in four patients underwent a selective neck dissection but only one in four needed postoperative radiotherapy.

Of the 54 patients with T1 and T2 supraglottic cancer, 13% had local recurrences needing salvage laryngectomy in 4% of the cases. Five and a half percent of the patients died from tumor-related causes. The 5-year overall survival rate (Kaplan Meier) was 67%.

In the group of 25 patients with advanced supraglottic cancer 32% of the patients had local recurrences. Salvage laryngectomy was carried out in 12% and 12% of the patients died from tumor-related causes. The 5-year overall survival rate (Kaplan Meier) was 53%.

Laser microsurgery enables part of the larynx to be preserved in about 90% of the patients, even in advanced tumor stages. The oncological results are comparable to those after radical surgery.

Concerning the possibilities of voice therapy and rehabilitation after laser microsurgery, especially after very large resections, and also of the patient's professional and social reintegration, I would like to refer to the contributions of Petra Zwirner MD and Hans Heinrich Niehaus MD, collaborators of Professor Kruse, Chairman of the Department for Voice Rehabilitation (Phoniatry) in Gottingen, with whom we closely cooperate.

The patients with laryngeal lesions are generally analyzed and documented before and after laser microsurgery in the phoniatric department.

Let me briefly explain our therapeutic concept: every laryngeal tumor, which can be resected with preservation of functionally important structures of the larynx (at least one mobile arytenoid) is treated primarily by transoral laser microsurgery.

If neck surgery is indicated, we perform a selective neck dissection only of the levels II and III if there is no advanced neck disease. We prefer a delayed neck dissection.

Postoperative radiotherapy is mainly indicated when advanced neck disease is found. Adjuvant radiotherapy can start early, which means as early as 2 weeks after laser microsurgery with the important advantage of biologically favourable conditions because of optimal blood supply and no scar formation.

Regardless of our intention to preserve as much organ integrity and function as possible we recognize that complete – oncologically radical – removal of the tumor is essential.

The surgical strategy is not only based on and determined according to the preoperative findings, but the transoral resection rather follows the individual spread of the tumor as seen under the microscope as a "custom-tailored surgery".

In the case of early lesions, which are excised en bloc, the specimen is histologically analyzed by step serial sections. Using modern CO_2 lasers the line of carbonization is usually about 25 m. By leaving a sufficient safety margin when circumcising the tumor, the complete removal can be verified by negative margins.

Resection of advanced tumors is done blockwise. Through vertical incisions we identify the infiltration into the depth and then determine an adequate security margin. In nontreated tumors the experienced surgeon is able to distinguish between healthy and diseased tissue with the help of a highly magnifying microscope. In cases of an infiltration of the pre- and/or paraglottic space or the thyroid or cricoid cartilage the infiltrated tissue can be removed together with the tumor and histologically analyzed.

If very advanced tumors are removed in several sections, it is impossible to examine all margins. This, however, also applies to conventional extended partial or complete resections of the larynx.

Limits

Insufficient exposure during microlaryngoscopy and extensive tumor spreading to the neck are the technical limits of the transoral approach, depending on the surgeon's experience. In these rare cases we continue by the external approach but always with the aim of organ preservation. Our experience shows that the most limiting factor is severe postoperative swallowing disorder after very extensive resections.

According to our experience, the long-term results published so far, and respecting certain precautions, the laser microsurgical resection is the best treatment for many cases of laryngeal cancer regarding oncology, function and economy.

Reference

1. Strong M St, Jako GJ. Laser surgery in the larynx. Early clinical experience with continuous CO_2 laser. J Ann Otol 1979;81:791–798.

Voice Update.
M. Pais Clemente, editor.

Treatment of laryngeal cancer: implications for voice conservation and restoration

J.J. Alvarez Vicent
Otolaryngology Department, Hospital 12 de Octubre, Madrid, Spain

Key words: implications for voice, laryngeal cancer.

In the study of voice aspects related to treatment of laryngeal cancer, we should consider the following parameters of the laryngeal tumor sites: supraglottis, glottis, subglottis and mixed. Each of these sites of origin requires a different surgical treatment; in some cases the changes in voice are minimal (standard supraglottic laryngectomy).

Voice production is mainly altered when the tumor arises on the glottic segment of the larynx:

- anterior, midcord and posterior vocal cord lesions (T1, T2);
- total vocal cord lesion;
- bilateral cord lesions;
- anterior commissure lesions; and
- fixed cord lesion.

Surgical procedures are different for the distinct lesions as they affect speech production to a different degree. This ranges from a moderate dysphonia in cordectomy, noticeable dysphonia in subperichondrial cordectomy, to severe dysphonia in bilateral vocal cord resection.

Therapeutic tools

First, we ought to consider radiation therapy. Its main advantage is the avoidance of the surgical morbidity, an important disadvantage is edema with the possibility of persistent dyspnea and dysphonia. Nevertheless, early localized tumors are well managed either with radiation or with surgery.

Surgery is the treatment with better long-term results in the management of laryngeal cancer.

Different authors have published many surgical procedures taking into account tumor origin and pathways of spreading. The goal in the functional management of

---

Address for correspondence: Prof J.J. Alvarez Vicent MD, Chairman of the Otolaryngology Department, Hospital 12 de Octubre, Crtra. de Andalucía, Km. 5400, 28041 Madrid, Spain.

carcinoma of the larynx is control of the primary tumor with preservation of functions including swallowing, respiration and voice, in this order.

Basic principles of oncologic surgery are en bloc resection of tumor, and a pathological confirmation that the whole tumor is included in the specimen.

Related to preservation of voice, surgical techniques are:

1. Functional surgery which aims to preserve the three, already named, laryngeal functions. The best example is standard supraglottic laryngectomy, the indications of this approach are lesions confined to the supraglottis. This technique represents the only one that preserves the voice.
2. Glottic-site tumors require resection of the whole or part of the phonatory segment. These surgical effects will change laryngeal phonatory behavior. Tumors arising on the membranous portion of the true cord, anterior, midcord or posterior vocal cord lesions are treated by cordectomy.
3. Cordectomy is performed through laryngofissure or by endoscopic removal (Kleinsasser); transoral laser excision has also been successfully employed by experienced hands.
4. Dysphonia depends on what type of cordectomy has been employed; sub-perichodrial cordectomy affects voice production more seriously than muscular cordectomy does.

Different techniques have been described with an aim to preserve phonatory laryngeal function (voice, the third vital function):

- Three-quarters laryngectomy.
- Vertical hemilaryngectomy preserving thyroid ala.
- Hemilaryngectomy.
- Crico-ariteno-epigloto-hyoido-pexy.
- With autograft or homograft: thyroid cartilage transposition reconstruction, or with epiglottic flap reconstruction.
- Frontolateral, anterior frontal partial laryngectomy, etc.

All these procedures cause dysphonia. Voice can then be improved with other surgical treatment. It is important to consider that cordectomy increases the glottic gap and the remaining vocal fold is sometimes not mobile.

After treatment of laryngeal cancer for voice restoration, there are the following options:

Phonatory surgery

When total laryngectomy or near-total laryngectomy has been performed, the surgical establishment of a tracheoesophageal fistula is one choice: it allows an acceptable phonation.

No phonatory surgery

In some patients who have undergone total laryngectomy, esophageal voice constitutes the only means of speech production.

Techniques for reconstruction

Vocal cords: when partial surgery has resected one or both vocal cords, they can be reconstructed. The reconstruction is done during the same operation or later. The reconstruction consists of transposing the strap muscles. The sternohyoid and omohyoid (Hirano) muscles are most commonly used.

Other repairing methods rotate the thyroid cartilage inwards, which is then joined to the external perichondrium (Brocca). These techniques allow better swallowing and better phonation.

There are methods for voice reconstruction using a deferred approach. These are laryngeal injection techniques. Different materials have been used for this purpose (cartilage particles, silicone, Teflon, etc.). The results are not homogeneous.

Other techniques for reconstruction

These include procedures in which:

1. The epiglottis is mobilized downwards to cover the resected cartilage in extended frontal anterior laryngectomy or in vertical hemilaryngectomy. Torrents, a Spanish author in the 50s, published a technique that used a skin flap to cover the laryngeal defect.
2. After the hemilaryngectomy or near total laryngectomy has been performed, we cover the cartilage defect with thyroid cartilage homograft, so the results are satisfactory.

The functional surgery has its complications. Those that affect the voice are:

- postsurgical stenosis,
- granulomata,
- anterior commissure stenosis,
- muscle atrophy, and
- cartilage absorption.

Related to this surgery we must remember that it is important to attend to the three vital laryngeal functions:

- deglutition,
- respiration, and
- phonation.

If we do so we keep in mind the laryngeal physiological studies of Presmann.

Voice Update.
M. Pais Clemente, editor.

Common etiologies of vocal fold scarring: clinical and objective assessment

Paulo Pontes
Escola Paulista de Medicina, Instituto da Laringe, São Paulo, Brazil

The concept of scar includes the presence of a previous lesion that has been repaired by fibrous tissue. Specifically a vocal fold scar is a mark in the structure which involves a modification into the connective tissue.

So, we can consider the existence of three groups of scars according to their etiologies:
- from intrinsic factors,
- from extrinsic factors, and
- from phonotrauma.

Intrinsic factors

To this first group belong all the scars derived from a constitutional predisposition.

The majority of these alterations have an hereditary character. Clinically, the manifestations of a scar are deviations introduced in the quality of voice according to the extension of the scar, age of the individual and vocal demand.

Two important situations are:
- minor structural changes of vocal fold cover, and
- geriatric stiffness and atrophy.

Extrinsic factor

The scars in this group represent the ultimate and definitive result of a repetitive and aggressive action of an external agent. Those external aggressive agents can be of a mechanical, chemical or biological nature.

Phonotrauma

Faulty vocal behavior can generate laryngeal inflammatory processes with secondary reparation by scar formation. Usually, a phonotrauma by itself is not enough to produce these intense reactions but predisponent factors — of an external or internal

Address for correspondence: Prof Paulo Pontes, Escola Paulista de Medicina, Instituto da Laringe, Rua Diogo de Faria, 171, CEP 04037-000, São Paulo, Brazil.

nature can trigger the tissue alteration.

There are several causes in each etiological group. For the first group the causes are named according to their visual appearance and the so-called minor structural changes are the causes of a scar. They are:

- striae, } "sulculus vocalis"
- vocal fold pocket, } "sulculus vocalis"
- vocal fold stiffness, and
- microdiaphragm.

Several extrinsic factors can produce a scar, such as:

- hematoma and tissue disruption,
- ulcera and intubation granuloma,
- surgical scarring (intentionals and accidentals),
- gastroesophageal reflux,
- aspiration of irritative agents,
- laryngitis, and
- actinic alterations.

All these causes belong to the second group of scar formation.

The deviations introduced in the vocal quality from the presence of a scar can be evaluated through several procedures.

The laryngeal and vocal semiology are based on two parameters common to almost all scars, regardless of its nature in different degrees and combinations:

- glottic closure alterations, and
- vibratory cycle alterations.

Auditory perceptual evaluation

There are five main parameters to be considered for an auditory perceptual evaluation:

- hoarseness,
- breathiness,
- asteny,
- strain,
- diplophonia.

Hoarseness is the noise component produced by irregularities in the successive vibratory cycles.

Breathiness is the air leak component. It represents the quantity of air non-modulated by the glottic source. The degree of breathiness depends upon the relation between the area of the glottic chink and the quality of the mucosal wave.

Asteny is the weakness of the voice translated into a lack of projection due to a reduced subglottic pressure and glottic resistance.

Diplophonia is a bimodal sensation of two concomitant or consecutive tones. This sensation is produced by a phase or period difference in the mucosal vibration.

Laryngoscopy

The most common finding in this evaluation is the presence of spindle-shaped glottic chinks or irregular glottic chinks, with hyperfunctional gestures such as medial vestibule constriction of the vestibular folds.

Laryngostroboscopy

The most frequent alterations under strobe light are:
- asymmetry of vibration,
- vibration amplitude reduction,
- mucosal wave impairment, and
- adynamic segment.

Maximum phonation time

The duration of a sustained voiced emission is reduced by the association of three factors:
- glottic chink,
- reduction of mucosal wave, and
- lower subglottic pressure.

An associated increase of the airflow rate can be observed.

Acoustic analysis

From the clinical point of view there are four major parameters to consider when performing an acoustic analysis. They are:
- fundamental frequency,
- jitter and shimmer,
- harmonic-to-noise ratio, and
- spectrographic trace.

Fundamental frequency — higher due to tissue rigidity and compensatory effort.

Jitter and shimmer — higher values due to the irregularity of the successive vibratory cycles.

Harmonic-to-noise ratio — lower proportion due to a stronger noise component and large formant bands.

Spectrographic trace:
- irregularities,
- higher energy at the upper level of the spectra,
- turbulence at the lower frequency, and
- bimodal fundamental frequency distribution.

Conclusion

We believe that this classification of vocal fold scars can help in the treatment planning and can be related to prognosis.

Voice Update.
M. Pais Clemente, editor.

Vocal fold scarring: current concepts in management

Robert Thayer Sataloff
Department of Otolaryngology, Thomas Jefferson University, Philadelphia, Pennsylvania, USA

Abstract. New insights into the anatomy and physiology of phonation, along with technological advances in voice assessment and quantification, have led to dramatic improvements in medical voice care. Techniques to prevent vocal fold scar have been among the most important, especially scarring and hoarseness associated with voice surgery. Nevertheless, dysphonia due to vocal fold scar is still encountered all too frequently. Although it is not generally possible to restore such injured voices to normal, patients with scar-induced dysphonia can usually be helped. Voice improvement is optimized through a team approach. Treatment may include sophisticated voice therapy, and vocal fold surgery. Recent experience with collagen injection and autologous fat implantation is particularly encouraging.

Key words: dysphonia, hoarseness, vocal fold scar.

Introduction

Vocal fold scar poses great therapeutic challenges for medical voice professionals. Familiarity with the latest concepts in vocal fold anatomy and physiology is essential in understanding the consequences of vocal fold scar.

Anatomy and physiology of phonation

Extensive review of the anatomy and physiology of phonation is beyond the scope of this brief chapter. Reviews are readily available in the literature [1–4]. However, when considering vocal fold scar, certain aspects of anatomy and physiology are worthy of emphasis. The larynx is essential to normal voice production, but the anatomy of the voice is not limited to the larynx. The vocal mechanism includes the abdominal and back musculature, rib cage, lungs, pharynx, oral cavity, nose, and many other parts of the body. Each component performs an important function in voice production, although it is possible to produce voice even without a larynx, for example in patients who have undergone laryngectomy. In addition, virtually all parts of the body play some role in voice production and may be responsible for voice dysfunction. Even something as remote as a sprained ankle may alter posture, thereby impairing abdominal, back, and thoracic muscle function and resulting in voice inefficiency, weakness, and hoarseness. Conveniently, various parts of the body outside of the larynx may also be used to enhance phonation therapeutically, helping

---

Address for correspondence: Robert Thayer Sataloff MD, DMA, 1721 Pine Street, Philadelphia, PA 19103, USA.

to compensate for such problems as vocal fold scar.

The soft tissues comprising the vocal folds are much more complex than originally thought. The mucosa forms the thin, lubricated surface of the vocal folds that makes contact when the two vocal folds are closed. It consists of five layers. The thin, lubricated epithelium covering the vocal folds forms the area of contact between the vibrating vocal folds and acts somewhat like a capsule, helping to maintain vocal fold shape. The epithelium lining most of the vocal tract is pseudostratified ciliated columnar epithelium, typical respiratory epithelium involved in handling mucous secretions. The vibratory margin of the vocal fold is covered with stratified squamous epithelium, better suited to withstand the trauma of vocal fold contact. The superficial layer of the lamina propria, also known as Reinke's space, is made up of loose fibrous components and matrix. It contains very few fibroblasts, the cells primarily responsible for scar formation. The intermediate layer of the lamina propria contains more fibroblasts and consists primarily of elastic fibers. The deep layer of the lamina propria is composed primarily of collagenous fibers and is rich in fibroblasts. The thyroarytenoid or vocalis muscle makes up the body of the vocal fold and is one of the intrinsic laryngeal muscles. The region of the intermediate and deep layers of the lamina propria is called the vocal ligament and lies immediately below Reinke's space. Mechanically, the vocal fold structures actually act more like three layers consisting of the cover (epithelium and Reinke's space), transition (intermediate and deep layers of the lamina propria), and the body (the vocalis muscle) [5]. The epithelium is connected to the superficial layer of the lamina propria by a complex basement membrane structure [6]. The attachments involve an intricate series of type VII collagen loops which emanate from and return to basement membrane cells. Type III collagen fibers of the superficial layer of the lamina propria pass through them. Basement membrane structures and the integrity of their attachments are probably related to numerous vocal fold functions, including wound healing, if we can extrapolate from basement membrane behavior elsewhere in the body. It is essential for surgeons to understand this anatomy, and the importance of preserving it during surgical intervention. The vocal folds act as the oscillator of the vocal tract.

The supraglottic larynx, tongue, lips, palate, pharynx, nasal cavity, and possibly the sinuses, shape the sound quality produced at the level of the vocal folds by acting as a series of complex interconnected resonators. Minor alterations in the configuration of these structures may produce substantial changes in voice quality. Such alterations may be due to illness, injury, technique, or other causes. During the course of vocal training for singing, acting, or healthy speaking, changes occur not only in the larynx, but also in the muscle motion, control, and shape of the supraglottic vocal tract.

The infraglottic vocal tract serves as the power source for the voice. Singers and actors refer to the entire power source complex as their "support" or "diaphragm". Actually, the anatomy of support for phonation is especially complicated and not completely understood. Yet it is quite important because deficiencies in support are frequently responsible for voice dysfunction that may lead to injury and subsequent scar. Similar voice dysfunction may limit one's ability to compensate for vocal fold scar; hence, making voice worse than it actually needs to be in the presence of a specific vocal fold injury.

Vocal fold scar

Symptomatic vocal fold scarring alters phonation by interfering with the mucosal wave. This may be due to obliteration of the layered structure of the vibratory margin, as seen commonly after vocal fold stripping or, to a limited extent, after other vocal fold surgery or trauma. Similar disruption of the layered structure and mucosal wave function may also occur congenitally, such as in some cases of sulcus vocalis. Scarring may also cause dysphonia by mechanical restriction of vibration or glottic closure, as seen in some cases of dense vocal fold web, or fibrotic masses on the membranous vocal fold such as may form subsequent to vocal fold hemorrhage. Scar involving the posterior, subglottic, and arytenoid regions may also be troublesome, but this discussion will be limited to scar involving the membranous portion of the vocal folds.

Diagnosis of vocal fold scar

Reliable, valid, repeatable, objective voice assessment is essential in diagnosing vocal fold scar, as well as in the assessment of other voice disorders. Familiarity with some of the measures currently available and in clinical use is extremely helpful [7–9]. A fully equipped voice laboratory measures phonatory ability, aerodynamic function, acoustic output, vibration, electromyographic signals, and includes psychoacoustic evaluation. Accurate assessment of vibration is critical, and strobovideolaryngoscopy is virtually indispensable to proper diagnosis and management of vocal fold scar [10,11].

Integrity of the vibratory margin of the vocal fold is essential for the complex motion required to produce good vocal quality. Under continuous light, the vocal folds vibrate approximately 250 times/s while phonating at middle C. Naturally, the human eye cannot discern necessary details during such rapid motion. Assessment of the vibratory margin may be performed through high-speed photography, strobovideolaryngoscopy, electroglottography, or photoglottography. Only strobovideolaryngoscopy provides the necessary clinical information in a practical fashion.

Strobovideolaryngoscopy is the single most important technological advance in diagnostic laryngology with the possible exception of the fiberoptic laryngoscope. Stroboscopic light allows routine, slow-motion evaluation of the mucosal cover layer of the leading edge of the vocal fold. This improved physical examination permits detection of vibratory asymmetries, structural abnormalities, small masses, submucosal scars, and other conditions that are invisible under ordinary light [10,11]. For example, in a patient with a poor voice following laryngeal surgery and a "normal-looking larynx", stroboscopic light reveals adynamic segments (scar) that explains the problem even to an untrained observer (such as the patient). In addition, it often permits differentiation between cysts and nodules, allowing better treatment and outcome predictions.

Therapy for vocal fold scar

Therapy for vocal fold scar depends upon the size, location, and severity of the scar, the vocal needs of the individual patient, the patient's motivation, and the skill of the voice team. In general, once the vibratory margin of the vocal fold has been scarred (the layered structure obliterated), it is not possible to return the voice to normal. However, several options are available to improve the voice.

Voice therapy is essential for anyone interested in obtaining optimal results. Most patients do not use their vocal mechanisms optimally. Consequently, even in the presence of vocal fold scar, teaching the individual to make effective use of the support and resonator systems generally improves vocal intensity and ease, and helps diminish fatigue. Nearly everyone with significant vocal fold injury develops compensatory gestures in an effort to decrease breathiness and hoarseness. These gestures are usually hyperfunctional, counterproductive, and in some cases they are dangerous. Such subconscious adjustments are seen even in the most skilled voice professionals following vocal fold injury and scar. Expert voice therapy eliminates this compensatory muscular tension dysphonia, further decreasing fatigue and allowing a more accurate assessment of vibratory margin function. After voice technique has been optimized, and the vocal fold scar has matured (usually about 6–12 months), judgements can be made about the acceptability of the final voice result. If voice function is not satisfactory to the patient, then surgery may be considered. However, it is essential for the laryngologist to be sure that the patient's expectations are reasonable. These do not include restoration to normalcy. However, in some cases, it is possible to decrease hoarseness and breathiness substantially.

Surgery for vocal fold scar

Vocal fold scar causes dysphonia by disrupting or obliterating the mucosal wave, and by interfering with glottic closure. Clear understanding of these facts is essential to rational surgical intervention. At present, there is no generally accepted, highly successful surgical treatment for vocal fold scar. However, numerous procedures have been tried, and some are useful in selected cases. Although there is very little information published on older attempts at surgical procedures to correct vocal fold scar, anecdotally, many busy voice surgeons admit to having attempted surgery in very small numbers of patients. Procedures to restore the mucosal wave have included injection of steroids into the vibratory margin, elevation of a microflap to "lyse adhesions", followed by simply replacing the microflap, elevation of a microflap with placement of steroids under the flap, and other procedures. Although none of these procedures produces consistently excellent results, they may help somewhat. Bouchayer, for example, uses microflap elevation and steroid injection and obtains at least some improvement in a majority of patients (personal communication). Recently, Pontes suggested a unique approach to the treatment of sulcus vocalis which essentially involves multiple releasing incisions [12]. The voice results have been surprisingly good, considering the limited success achieved by previous procedures for this condition. Recently, these principles have been applied to iatrogenic vocal fold scar and may prove useful for patients with extensive severe adynamic areas (P. Pontes, personal communication).

The problem of glottic incompetence is generally addressed through medialization surgery. Most medialization procedures in the past have involved injection of Teflon. Because this substance can itself cause profound scarring, many of us have abandoned its use in most cases since the mid-to-late 1980s. At present, the medialization techniques of choice are generally thyroplasty, or injection of a substance other than Teflon. Medialization techniques have been discussed widely in the literature and will not be reviewed here [13,14]. For extensive failure of glottic closure, the author has found type I thyroplasty to be most effective. For limited medialization, lateral injection of autologous fat (in the same place where Teflon used to be injected) has proven quite successful [14]. However, approximately 30% overinjection is necessary to account for resorption. Techniques to manage vibratory margin scar are worthy of more complete discussion.

Collagen injection was investigated most extensively by Ford and co-workers [15–17]. Collagen is clearly useful in selected cases. It is injected into the region of the vocal ligament and appears particularly appropriate for limited vocal scarring. Such cases are common, e.g., following laser resection of vocal nodules. For more extensive scarring, as may be seen following stripping of an entire vocal fold, collagen appears less effective.

During the last 2 years, the author has treated a small number of severely scarred vocal folds with autologous fat implantation [18]. The technique involves creating a tunnel along the vibratory margin and filling the tunnel with autologous fat. Preliminary results have been extremely encouraging. In some cases, this technique has resulted in restoration of a fairly normal-looking mucosal wave in vocal folds that were entirely adynamic. Further research into the use of collagen and autologous fat is needed.

Occasionally, surgeons are faced with extreme cases of vibratory margin scar. These are especially common following major trauma or extensive cancer surgery. When a nonvibrating scarred vocal fold is lateralized so that glottic closure is impossible, and when the involved hemilarynx is so densely scarred that the vocal fold cannot be adequately medialized even with thyroplasty, occasionally more extensive surgery for vocal fold scar may be appropriate. For example, some such cases may be improved through resection of the scarred hemilarynx, and creation of a pseudovocal fold using modifications of strap muscle techniques employed routinely following cordectomy or vertical hemilaryngectomy [19]. Certainly, this is an unusual and extreme approach for the treatment of vocal fold scar, but it is an option that should be in the surgeon's armamentarium for the rare, appropriate patient.

Conclusions

Vocal fold scar may produce profound dysphonia. Accurate diagnosis based on understanding of anatomy and physiology, and utilizing the latest technology, generally leads to a rational treatment program. Combinations of expert therapy and surgery offer improvement for most patients with vocal fold scar. However, extensive additional research is needed into current surgical techniques, especially collagen injection and autologous fat implantation, and into the development of new and better approaches for the treatment of vocal fold scar.

Acknowledgements

Published with permission of The Voice Foundation, Philadelphia, Pennsylvania.

References

1. Sataloff RT. The human voice. Sci Am 1992;267(6):108–115.
2. Sataloff RT. Professional Voice: The Science and Art of Clinical Care. New York: Raven Press, Ltd., 1991;7–18.
3. Hirano M. Surgical anatomy and physiology of the vocal folds. In: Gould WJ, Sataloff RT, Spiegel JR (eds) Voice Surgery. St. Louis: C.V. Mosby Co., 1993;135–158.
4. Sataloff RT. Functional anatomy and physiology of the voice. In: Gould WJ, Sataloff RT, Spiegel JR (eds) Voice Surgery. St. Louis: C.V. Mosby Co., 1993;159–172.
5. Sataloff RT. Professional Voice: The Science and Art of Clinical Care. New York: Raven Press, Ltd., 1991;7–9.
6. Gray S. Basement membrane zone injury in vocal nodules. In: Gauffin J, Hammarberg B (ed) Vocal Fold Physiology. San Diego: Singular Press, 1991.
7. Sataloff RT, Heuer RJ, Hoover C, Baroody M. Laboratory assessment of voice. In: Gould WJ, Sataloff RT, Spiegel JR (eds) Voice Surgery. St. Louis: C.V. Mosby Co., 1993;203–216.
8. Martin GF. The contribution of the speech sciences to the development of phonosurgery. In: Gould WJ, Sataloff RT, Spiegel JR (eds) Voice Surgery. St. Louis: C.V. Mosby Co., 1993;97–122.
9. Baken RJ. Clinical Measurement of Speech and Voice. Boston: College Hill Press, Little, Brown, 1987.
10. Sataloff RT, Spiegel JR, Carroll LM, Schiebel BR, Darby KS, Rulnick R. Strobovideolaryngoscopy in professional voice users: Results and clinical value. J Voice 1988;1:359–364.
11. Sataloff RT, Spiegel JR, Hawkshaw MJ. Strobovideolaryngoscopy: Results and clinical value. Ann Otol Rhinol Laryngol 1991;100:725–757.
12. Pontes P, Behlau M. Treatment of sulcus vocalis: auditory perceptual and acoustic analysis of the slicing mucosa surgical technique. J Voice 1993;7(4):365–376.
13. Gould WJ, Sataloff RT, Spiegel JR. Voice Surgery. St. Louis: C.V. Mosby Co., 1993.
14. Mikaelian D, Lowry LD, Sataloff RT. Lipoinjection for unilateral vocal cord paralysis. Laryngoscope 1991;101:465–468.
15. Ford CN, Bless DM, Loftus JM. The role of injectable collagen in the treatment of glottic insufficiency: A study of 119 patients. Ann Otol Rhinol Laryngol 1973;101(3):237–247.
16. Ford CN, Bless DM. Collagen injected in the scarred vocal fold. J Voice 1988;1:116–118.
17. Ford CN, Bless DM. Selected problems treated by vocal fold injection of collagen. Am J Otolaryngol 1993;14(4):257–261.
18. Sataloff RT, Spiegel JR, Hawkshaw MJ, Rosen D, Heuer RJ. Autologous Fat Implantation for Vocal Fold Scar: A Preliminary Report. Presented at The Voice Foundation's 24th Annual Symposium: Care of the Professional Voice, Philadelphia, PA, June 11, 1994.
19. Spiegel JR, Sataloff RT. Surgery for carcinoma of the larynx. In: Gould WJ, Sataloff RT, Spiegel JR (eds) Voice Surgery. St. Louis: C.V. Mosby Co., 1993;307–338.

Voice Update.
M. Pais Clemente, editor.

Acquired vocal fold web prevention and management

Michael S. Benninger
Department of Otolaryngology — Head and Neck Surgery, Henry Ford Health System, Detroit, Michigan, USA

Key words: laryngeal webs, microwebs, treatment.

Vocal fold webs occur congenitally or can be acquired following laryngeal injury. The most common causes of acquired laryngeal webs are noted in Table 1. Although caustic or burn injuries and radiation therapy for small glottic cancers can result in webbing, these are relatively infrequent. Webs which result from prolonged intubation, laryngeal trauma or as a sequelae of iatrogenic injury during vocal fold surgery, are the conditions which account for the majority for webs which require management. This paper will describe the pathophysiology of web formation, will discuss methods to prevent webbing during intubation, trauma or laryngeal surgery and will describe methods of nonsurgical and surgical treatment.

Vocal fold histology and pathophysiology of laryngeal web formation

The vocal folds histologically are composed of three major layers: a superficial mucosal layer, a middle lamina propria, and a deep muscular layer. The mucosa is stratified squamous epithelium on the free margins of the vocal folds and a pseudostratified ciliated columnar (respiratory) epithelium in the supraglottis and subglottis. The middle layer is composed of three layers of lamina propria; superficial, transitional and deep layers. The superficial layer of the lamina propria (Reinke's space) is just beneath the basement membrane, contains few fibroblasts, elastic or collagen fibers but a relatively high concentration of reticulum fibers. The transitional or middle layer of the lamina propria is sometimes poorly recognized histologically but has somewhat more collagen fibers and extracellular matrix with moderate fibroblasts and elastic fibers. The deep layer of the lamina propria (vocalis ligament) has many collagen and elastic fibers, a moderate number of fibroblasts and a dense concentration of extracellular matrix. The deep layer of the lamina propria merges with the muscular layer (vocalis muscle).

The greater the concentration of fibroblasts and collagen, as occurs in the deeper

Address for correspondence: Michael S. Benninger MD, Chairman, Department of Otolaryngology – HNS, Henry Ford Hospital, 2799 West Grand Boulevard, Detroit, MI 48202, USA. Tel.: +1-313-876-3275. Fax: +1-313-876-7263.

Table 1. Etiology of acquired laryngeal webs.

Iatrogenic
— laryngeal surgery
— intubation
Traumatic
— blunt trauma
— penetrating trauma
Caustic ingestion
Laryngeal burns
Inflammatory
Radiation therapy

layers of the lamina propria, the greater the risk of scarring. Although injury to the superficial layer of the lamina propria can result in scarring, it has been shown that laryngeal surgery confined to this layer has little functional consequence [1–3]. Injury to the mucosa of one vocal fold generally heals without sequelae, however, when de-epithelialization occurs on two opposing surfaces such as near the anterior commissure, scarring can occur across the defect with web formation. Such opposing de-epithelialized areas can follow sharp or blunt laryngeal trauma after aggressive or prolonged intubation, or with laryngeal surgery for bilateral vocal fold disease, particularly if vocal fold stripping or injudicious laser surgery is performed [1]. One of the most common sequelae of surgical treatment of benign laryngeal papillomas is vocal fold webbing [4]. Webs can occur either anteriorly or posteriorly or can be at the glottic, supraglottic or subglottic levels. Given the closer approximation of the vocal fold and the comparatively less motion to the posterior commissure, anterior webs at the glottic level are the most common site of web formation.

Evaluation of the patient with a vocal web

The symptoms of laryngeal webs are largely dependent on the size and site of the webbing. Small anterior commissure webs may have little or no symptoms. This is particularly true in individuals who have little voice demands. However, in individuals who require their voices either for their occupation or avocation such as public speakers or singers, even small webs may be detrimental. Recent evaluations have identified small anterior commissure microwebs. These have been found to be associated with an increased likelihood of vocal nodules or other laryngeal pathologies such as granulomas [5–7]. The cause of these relationships has not been identified but it is speculated that nodules may form due to alterations in the vibration of the vocal folds, due to the slight foreshortening caused by the microweb [7]. Many of these patients have resolution of the nodules with voice therapy alone [5], although failure of voice therapy for nodules may be greater for those that have a microweb.

Larger webs or posterior commissure webs always present with some degree of dysphonia. Many have developed voice behaviors such as elevated pitch either to compensate or as a result of the shortened vocal fold. Airway compromise tends to occur primarily in patients with large webs. This is typically exertional dyspnea but can occasionally be dyspnea at rest.

The evaluation of a patient with a vocal fold web should be based on a thorough evaluation of the cause of web formation. Once this is established, an assessment of the degree and site of webbing should be undertaken by indirect, flexible, or rigid laryngoscopy. Videostroboscopic evaluation will help to assess the effect on the vocal fold waveform and will help to determine if there are other areas of scarring other than the web. This is particularly important following trauma, intubation, or iatrogenic surgical injury. A voice assessment by a skilled voice-language pathologist will help to evaluate the level of dysfunction, and will help to determine the patient's need and desire for treatment. The voice pathologist will help to establish a healthy voice technique and eliminate adverse compensatory behaviors, and will also assist in postsurgical voice instruction.

The treatment of vocal webs

The best treatment for vocal webs is prevention. Appropriate assessment of patients who have sustained blunt or penetrating trauma should take into consideration the possibility of subsequent web formation. In patients who have bilateral mucosal disruption, those who have sustained massive laryngeal injury or those where significant laryngeal edema occurs and where there are mucosal tears, should be considered for laryngeal stenting once the airway is secure, and during the surgical treatment of the laryngeal trauma or fracture [8].

Patients who require prolonged intubation should be monitored carefully to assure that as small a tube as necessary is used and that tube movement is minimized. Furthermore, if it is clear that the patient is not going to be weaned in the near future, then a tracheostomy should be recommended.

Care with laryngeal surgery for benign laryngeal lesions is an area where there is significant opportunity for prevention of web formation. Microinstruments should be used wherever possible and avoidance of disruption of the middle and deep layers of the lamina propria should be a priority. As little of the normal vocal fold should be removed as possible and stripping, which has poor control of resected margins, should not be performed under most circumstances. Attention should be payed to the avoidance of bilateral mucosal resection near the anterior commissure. If necessary, such as in the excision of papilloma, staged procedures should be performed to allow regeneration of the mucosa on one side prior to resection on the other. Injudicious laser use should be avoided even in the case of large lesions or papilloma. Heat spread from the laser may result in injury a distance from the primary focus. The use of microdissection instruments and the microspot CO_2 laser will aid the surgeon in avoidance of vocal scars and webs. Close attention to postoperative care with humidification, hydration, and voice hygiene should be recommended in all patients. Antireflux measures or medications should always be considered and anti-inflammatory agents, steroids, and antibiotics may be of benefit for some.

Surgical management of webs are dictated by the severity of the airway compromise, the patient's occupational and social voice requirements and their desire for improvement. Once a decision has been made to proceed, the specific treatment depends on the location and the size of the web. Anterior commissure microwebs generally do not require any treatment. If surgical treatment of associated vocal nodules is necessary, the microweb can be lysed [5]. Small, thin mucosal bridges may be able to be managed by lysis alone. Thicker webs or those extending more than 5 mm usually require either mucosal coverage or placement of a stent or keel.

In order to prevent web recurrence without a stent, one, if not both vocal folds need to have a mucosal cover. This can be accomplished by mucosal rotation or advancement flaps, or possibly by a free mucosal graft. After lysis of small webs, the mucosa on the ventricular surface of the vocal fold can be elevated and undermined to the level of the ventricle, and advanced on both sides to attempt to cover the free margin of the vocal fold. This may be held in position with fibrin glue, 8-0 chromic sutures, or spot-welded with a microspot CO_2 laser. These cases are infrequent. In 1984, McGuirt and his colleagues described an endoscopic microflap technique for the management of anterior commissure webs [9]. The mucosa over the web is elevated and retracted, the web and any scar is excised, and the elevated mucosa is then draped over the vocal fold and spot-welded with a laser to provide mucosal coverage to one vocal fold. They reported excellent control of the webbing and good voice outcomes.

I have found it difficult to hold the flap on the undersurface with spot-welding and therefore have developed a variation of McGuirt's technique (Figs. 1–3) which adheres to the same principles, but I find simpler to perform. The mucosa and scar on the upper surface is removed with defocused laser or microdissection leaving the undersurface mucosa intact (Fig. 1). The remaining scar is excised and the

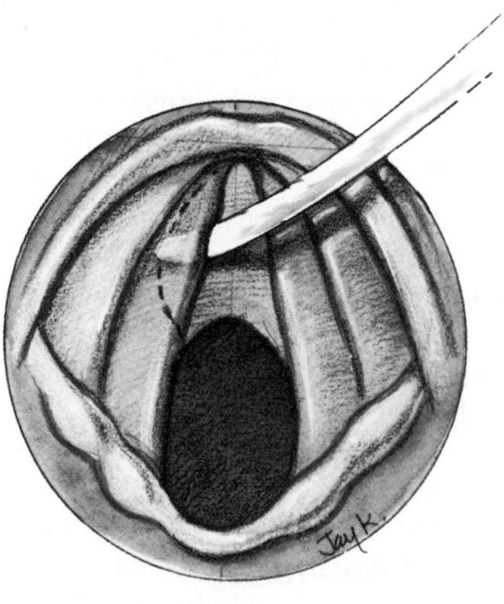

Fig. 1. Mucosa on upper surface removed by defocused laser or microdissection.

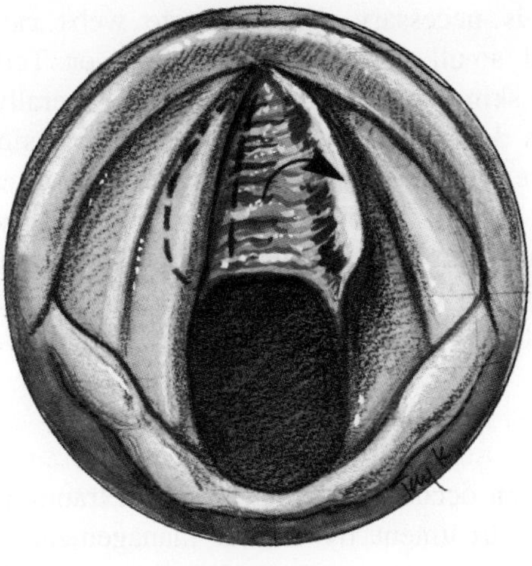

Fig. 2. Scar excised and undersurface mucosa cut.

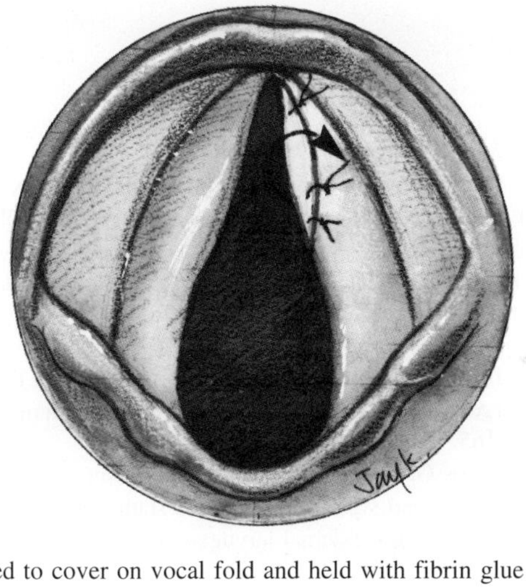

Fig. 3. Mucosal flap rotated to cover on vocal fold and held with fibrin glue or 8-0 chromic sutures.

undersurface mucosa is cut either on the margin of the opposite vocal fold or under the opposite fold depending on the size of the defect and amount of mucosal coverage that is necessary (Fig. 2). The mucosal flap is then rotated to cover the free margin of one fold and sutured into position with two 8-0 chromic sutures. If a small microweb persists due to the angle of rotation, the voice is usually not affected but can be treated with simple lysis at another time. This provides for ample coverage and preserves good voice quality. It also obviates the need for an open laryngeal procedure or stenting. Free mucosal grafts can also be performed usually through a thyrotomy with good results [10].

Large and thick webs do not respond well to microsurgery and mucosal flaps. In such cases, stenting is necessary. Medium size webs can be stented with an endoscopically placed small catheter, silastic [11] or Teflon keel and sutured anteriorly through the skin over a button. These are generally left in place for 2 to no more than 4 weeks depending on the size and thickness of the web. Still larger webs generally require an open procedure with anterior thyrotomy, web and scar excision and stenting. This is usually necessary only with large scars which have required a tracheotomy for airway management. With involvement of excessive areas with laryngeal stenosis, an epiglottoplasty has been described to provide anterior mucosal and structural support [12].

Summary

Laryngeal webbing often occurs following laryngeal trauma, surgery or intubation. Prevention is the best treatment by careful management of traumatic laryngeal injuries, microsurgical laryngeal surgery and endotracheal tube care. Webs can be treated surgically with lysis, microflaps or stenting with good results and satisfactory voice.

References

1. Hirano M, Hirade J, Yoshida T, Sanada T. Improved surgical technique for epidermoid cysts of the vocal fold. Ann Otol Rhinol Laryngol 1989;98:791–795.
2. Bastian R. Treatment of benign mucosal disorders of the larynx. Ear Nose Throat J 1988;67:408–410.
3. Alessi D, von Leden H. Stroboscopy and phonosurgery. Arch Otolaryngol Head Neck Surg 1992;118:1003–1005.
4. Ossoff RH, Werkhaven JA, Dere H. Soft-tissue complications of laser surgery for recurrent respiratory papillomatosis. Laryngoscope 1991;101:1162–1166.
5. Benninger MS, Jacobson B. Vocal nodules, microwebs and surgery. J Voice (In press).
6. Bouchier M, Cornut G. Instrumental microscopy of benign lesions of the vocal folds. In: Ford CN, Bless DM (eds) Phonosurgery: Assessment and Surgical Management of Voice Disorders. New York: Raven Press, 1991;143–165.
7. Ford CN, Bless DM, Campos G, Leddy M. Anterior commissure microwebs associated with vocal nodules: Detection, prevalence and significance. NCVS status and Progress Report 1993;85–92.
8. Schaefer SD. The treatment of acute external laryngeal injuries ‘state of the art’. Arch Otolaryngol Head Neck Surg 1991;117:35–39.
9. McGuirt WF, Salman J, Blalock D. Normal speech for patients with laryngeal webs: an achievable goal. Laryngoscope 1984;95:1176–1179.
10. Isshiki N, Nose K, Taira T, Kojima H. Surgical treatment of laryngeal web with mucosa graft. Ann Otol Rhinol Laryngol 1991;100:95–100.
11. Parker DA, Das Gupta AR. An endoscopic silastic keel for anterior glottic webs. J Laryngol Otol 1987;101:1055–1061.
12. Delaere PR, Ostyn F, Segers A, Vandyck W. Epiglottoplasty for reconstruction of posttraumatic laryngeal stenosis. Ann Otol Rhinol Laryngol 1991;100:447–450.

Voice Update.
M. Pais Clemente, editor.

Glottic physiology after Botox treatment of adductor spasmodic dysphonia, abductor spasmodic dysphonia and vocal tremor

Krzysztof Izdebski[1,2] and Ronald R. Ward[1,2,3]

[1]*Pacific Voice and Speech Foundation, San Francisco;* [2]*Department of Otolaryngology – Head and Neck Surgery, University of California at Davis, Sacramento; and* [3]*Department of Otolaryngology – Head and Neck Surgery, Kaiser Permanente Medical Center, San Francisco, California, USA*

Abstract. The action of botulinum toxin type A (Botox) on glottic phonatory biomechanics was studied stroboscopically, acoustically, and aerodynamically in a series of adductor spasmodic dysphonia (ADD SD) patients, abductor spasmodic dysphonia (ABD SD) patients, patients who had vocal tremor (VT) and ADD SD, and patients who had VT only. After chemodenervation, glottic gap size, which narrowed from its initial maximum as a function of delayed reinnervation/recovery, was a primary physiologic element responsible for symptom elimination in ADD SD. Breathiness as well as pitch and loudness control were reflected by glottic gap size. Mucosal vibratory wave (MVW) asymmetry accounted for aperiodicity (hoarseness). Symptoms were eliminated for a mean of 4 months in ADD SD. Drug dosage criteria did not correlate well with physiologic and acoustic findings. Voice therapy appeared to prolong interinjection interval. Shifting of the vocal fold toward the midline after denervation of the posterior cricoarytenoid (PCA) muscle to reduce the posterior glottic gap produced variable results in ABD SD. Although glottic physiology in VT was similar to that in ADD SD, results in VT were also variable. Resultant data are used to construct a typical phonatory profile after Botox treatment, which can be used to explain the results of this treatment method for all patients.

Key words: botulinum toxin, dystonia, electromyography, laryngeal muscles, phonoscopy, recurrent laryngeal nerve, spasmodic dysphonia, vocal tremor, voice analysis, voice disorders.

Introduction

Intramuscular injection of botulinum toxin type A (Botox, Allergan Pharmaceuticals, Irvine, CA, USA) causes transient chemical paralysis followed by delayed (≤6 months) recovery of the injected muscle [1–3]. This technique has recently become popular for treating various phonatory movement disorders [4–14] and is used especially as an alternative to unilateral surgical resection of the recurrent laryngeal nerve (RLN) in treating adductor spasmodic dysphonia (ADD SD) [15–17]. As a result, researchers generally agree that Botox injection is effective in short-term elimination of ADD SD symptoms [4–10,14] and that RLN resection produces long-term (up to 16 years) results [18–21].

In general, authors [4–10] who have described phonatory results after Botox treatment have concentrated on short-term acoustic changes in ADD SD symptoms, including clinically significant reduction in spasmodic symptoms (i.e., strained or

Address for correspondence: Dr Krzysztof Izdebski, 350 Parnassus Ave, Suite 501, San Francisco, CA 94117, USA. Fax: +1-510-444-7179.

strangled voice) but higher mean values of nonnormal phonation (breathy-aperiodic-weak voice) immediately after Botox treatment than in control patients. Similarly, sequential clinical assessments of laryngeal function after Botox treatment by using phonatory airflow and stroboscopic measurements, showed increased airflow (breathiness) and incomplete vocal fold adduction with an asymmetric vibratory pattern [8]. The authors concluded that bilateral Botox injection, which causes bilateral denervation of the true vocal folds (TVFs), appeared to produce better glottic approximation and better vibratory symmetry than unilateral RLN chemical blocks [8,11–14,21]. However, others are less conclusive regarding the effect of unilateral vs. bilateral injections on glottic closure and postinjection phonatory quality [11], although some research suggests that a cumulative toxin dose can be decreased and spasmodic voice quality eliminated when both vocal folds are injected. By using a flexible fiberoptic scope to study glottic hyperfunction (including excessive activation of intrinsic laryngeal musculature, extrinsic muscular hyperfunction, dystonic glottic and supraglottic motion, and tremor), Woodson et al. [10] showed that Botox reduces unwanted laryngeal muscle activation, except in tremor. In one study [12], ADD SD patients' self-ratings of voice course and phonatory effort after three consecutive Botox injections indicated that voice change after toxin injection is not predictable, equal, or uniform, although improved phonation after Botox treatment has been reported in almost all patients studied by other investigators.

However, the underlying physiologic glottic changes caused by chemical denervation and their effect on phonation have rarely been systematically detailed. In particular, studies which have evaluated glottic physiology in relation to phonatory consequences and have included observation of induced longitudinal change in phonatory biomechanics, are scarce. However, such systematically detailed description of glottic phonatory biomechanics after Botox treatment is important because it explains the variability of clinically assessed phonatory results, aids discussion of the long-term efficacy of Botox compared with other current treatment methods, and assists in predicting the long-term effect of Botox on symptom elimination and in establishing a pattern of phonatory quality after injection. Moreover, such a description can aid clinicians in choosing injection site(s), can guide drug dosage and reinjection timing, can help document recurrence, and can help explain and substantiate the role of voice therapy in prolonging interinjection interval. Understanding glottic physiology after Botox treatment may also help explain failures in treating abductor spasmodic dysphonia (ABD SD), ADD SD and vocal tremor (VT) combined (ADD SD/VT), or VT alone. Moreover, assessment of glottic physiology after Botox treatment can support the currently proposed physiologic model of ADD SD [22].

In this investigation, we searched for the elements of Botox-induced glottic physiologic change which were most capable of explaining and predicting symptom reduction after treatment, and the mechanisms which generate breathiness and aperiodicity, which maintain a symptom-free voice, and which are responsible for symptom recurrence. Our search for these crucial elements was guided by a physiologic model of ADD SD symptom generation [22]. This model explains ADD

SD symptoms as a misprocessing of sensory information from the glottis by the brainstem and basal ganglia affecting fine neuromotor control of the TVFs during phonation. In this phonotopic model of symptom generation, the presence or absence of symptoms is systematically predictable, and symptom severity depends on the nature of the phonatory task executed. The physiologic factors responsible for symptom generation in this model include vocal fold contact area, vocal fold collision force, and glottic compression. Therefore, eliminating or reducing these factors will eliminate or reduce symptoms.

In addition, our data are compared with other results of Botox treatment of various forms of phonatory dystonias and are used as a foundation for further discussion of the effectiveness of all current treatment of forms of spasmodic dysphonias caused by abnormal laryngeal movements. Our data are also used to construct a profile of phonation after Botox treatment which can be universally applied to explain the results of treatment.

Materials and Methods

The various types of spasmodic dysphonia and their physiologic correlates are briefly reviewed here because discrepancies in their description in the biomedical literature may aid in the explanation of discrepancies regarding treatment outcomes.

Patient selection

ADD SD

Patients selected for this study were diagnosed as having ADD SD on the basis of the criteria proposed in the biomedical literature [10,14,22–24]. Consequently, they all exhibited characteristic overpressure (strained or strangled voice) with or without vocal arrests. Symptoms were organized phonotopically: they were more severe at the habitual voice fundamental frequency levels than in the higher vocal ranges and were absent during whispering, falsetto phonation, and vegetative tasks as predicted by the model [11]. When auditory or phonoscopic examination was difficult, diagnostic unilateral RLN block was administered according to the protocol described in our previous study [25].

ADD SD/VT and VT

The physiologic mechanism of ADD SD/VT and VT is thought to include some additional symptom-generating site(s) (the cerebellum) [26,27]. Vocal oscillations were judged as tremorous in nature rather than of the ADD SD vocal arrest type on the basis of the criteria established in our previous study [26]. According to those criteria, VT may coexist with ADD SD, and VT oscillations are more regular than the vocal arrest patterns of ADD SD, although both occur at a frequency of about 5.5 Hz. In contrast to vocal arrests, VT indiscriminately affects all vocal intensity and frequency ranges, including whispering and falsetto phonation, and is present during vegetative tasks [22,26]. Further, tremor rate was not affected by chemical RLN blocks (including co-block of ipsilateral or contralateral superior laryngeal nerve).

although these blocks reduced tremor magnitude [25]. As demonstrated, RLN block eliminated vocal arrest [25].

ABD SD

This rare condition was diagnosed when patients displayed sudden increases in transglottic phonatory airflow during speech (i.e., after a voiceless consonant) which resulted in involuntary devoicing or unvoicing of the voiced speech segments to follow. The speech pattern of these patients was characterized clinically by a sudden severe breathiness during phonation which made completing a word, phrase, or sentence laborious or impossible. Excessive compensatory straining of facial muscles was accompanied by intermittent breathy spasms. Although sometimes associated with ADD SD, VT was not noted as a co-symptom in any ABD SD cases.

ABD SD treatment has been clinically unsatisfactory, although some clinicians have reported reasonable success after Botox injection [28]. Moreover, ABD SD symptoms have been less thoroughly modeled than ADD SD symptoms. Therefore, ABD SD has been most commonly explained as a clinical antipode of ADD SD which causes a dysfunction (spasm) of the abductor musculature [28,29]. Our evidence suggests that ABD SD patients may either relax the PCA too slowly or may not activate the adductors quickly enough to counteract the action of the PCA, which belies the assumption that ABD SD mirrors ADD SD. RLN resection has not been advocated for ABD SD, and our results after chemical RLN block have been inconsistent.

Since we started Botox treatment 3 years ago, 86 consecutive patients have participated in this study. Of these, 55 patients had ADD SD (16 men, 39 women); 11 had ADD SD/VT (two men, nine women); three had ABD SD (three women); and seven had VT only (two men, five women). All patients had a thorough medical history assessment and a complete head and neck examination. They also had extensive voice pathology assessment both before and after treatment. This assessment included phonatory function studies comprised of acoustic recording and analysis, and 90°, rigid, transoral laryngovideostroboscopy (phonoscopy) with Rhino-Larynx Stroboscope Type 4914 (Bruel and Kjaer, Marlborough, MA, USA) [30–32]. Transnasal flexible phonoscopy was done when appropriate. No topical anesthesia was required for either type of phonoscopy. These studies were repeated after each initial injection and when clinically indicated after consecutive injections.

Before we administered the toxin, potential risks were explained to the patient, who completed a consent form. All patients were told that Botox injection neither cures SD nor guarantees a good speaking voice. Voice therapy after Botox treatment was considered an integral part of the treatment regimen. Therapy after Botox treatment was outlined according to previously published protocols [17,33]. Possible complications after Botox treatment were outlined.

Injection protocol

The patient was positioned supine on a mechanized examining table with a pillow placed under the shoulders to achieve comfortable neck extension. Only one patient requested and later received oral sedative medication (i.e., diazepam) before treatment. The needle injection site on the anterior neck was cleaned with alcohol, and 0.4 ml, 1% Xylocaine (lidocaine hydrochloride, Astra Pharmaceutical Products, Inc, Westboro, MA, USA) with 1:100,000 epinephrine was injected subcutaneously. For increased patient comfort, topical anesthetic (Hurricane (20% benzocaine, Beutlich L.P., Niles Ill), or 10% Xylocaine) was applied transorally to diminish the gag and coughing reflexes.

The Nicolet Viking IIe multichannel electromyographic (EMG) monitoring system (Nicolet Instrument Corporation, Madison, WI, USA) was used to monitor EMG discharge patterns recorded above a simultaneous display of an acoustic signal (voice). A recording microphone was positioned 3 inches away from the patient's mouth to obtain acoustic information. Both visual and auditory monitoring were performed simultaneously to verify laryngeal muscle activities. All relevant signals were retrieved in a hard-copy format. The EMG reference lead was positioned on the sternocleidomastoid muscle on the same side as the injection site. All leads were grounded either on biceps or on the forehead. A standard monopolar, 25-gauge, Teflon-coated needle (Oculinum, Inc., Berkeley, CA, USA) with an exposed tip was used to inject the toxin. A 1-ml tuberculin syringe containing a single dose of toxin which had been appropriately stored and which was mixed immediately before injection was attached to the injection electrode.

This injection protocol was used for all but four patients, who received direct perioral TVF injection via standard laryngoscopic techniques [34].

Target sites and tasks

ADD SD

The left thyroarytenoid (TA) muscle complex was targeted in most ADD SD cases. Injection was aimed at the middle of the TA complex. Intramuscular needle placement was verified by utilizing simultaneous voice signals during phonation, the Valsalva maneuver, grunting, swallowing, and pitch/loudness increments. The Botox dose ranged from 5 to 15 units. Depending on the results, the dose was increased or decreased in future injections.

ADD SD/VT

The cricothyroid (CT) was also (unilaterally) ipsilaterally or contralaterally targeted for injection in addition to the TA in ADD SD/VT. The monitoring method was similar to that described under *"Injection protocol"* and included pitch raising, respiration, and swallowing. Doses ranged from 15 to 25 units.

VT

VT was treated by injecting the TA and ipsilateral or contralateral CT. The CT was identified and its location verified during respiration, swallowing, and production of the fundamental frequency (Fo) from the lowest to the highest pitch. The CT usually responds at about half an octave above the base Fo [35].

ABD SD

The PCA was injected unilaterally in all ABD SD cases. The dose did not exceed 10 units so as to avoid unwanted spread of toxin to the opposite PCA muscle [36]. The larynx was rotated contralaterally to allow the EMG needle to pass behind the thyroid cartilage and through the inferior constrictor muscle. The midposterior aspect of the cricoid cartilage was targeted for correct identification and later injection of the PCA. Simultaneous voice and EMG monitoring is imperative to verify placement. Tasks activating the PCA included inspiration as well as production of alternating voiced and voiceless speech segments.

Follow-up

All patients received a telephone evaluation beginning the day after injection. A short course (48 h) of modified voice rest was advised for TA-injected patients because of injection-related vocal fold trauma. Complete initial reassessment of vocal functions was done within 14 days of injection and then at intervals determined by telephone evaluation until symptoms recurred. This intensive approach was used for all patients after the initial injection, and patients were re-evaluated as needed after later injections.

Measurements

Pitch

Voice pitch and intensity ranges were measured after Botox treatment. Pitch was measured either directly with the Rhino-Larynx Stroboscope Type 4914 by reading the Fo values on the face of the instrument, or by feeding the acoustic signal through a Kay Elemetrics computer processing unit (VISI-Pitch, Kay Elemetrics Corp, Pine Brook, NY, USA). Resultant sustained and connected speech was assessed for overpressure, aperiodicity, and breathiness according to previously published criteria [37]. Standardized voice recordings were made by using a constant mouth-to-microphone distance. Recordings were made either by using a C60 audio cassette analog system or, once it became available, a DAT audio cassette system. Recordings were made for archival and clinical purposes [38]. Voice quality judgments were made on line.

Loudness

Maximum and minimum vocal loudness was measured directly with an SPL meter (Bruel and Kjaer, Model 4814) set to C scale and positioned 12 inches away from the mouth. All acoustic recordings and measurements were made either in an IAC booth or in a sound-insulated room.

Aerodynamics

Air consumption was estimated indirectly on the basis of maximum phonation time (MPhT) measured in milliseconds and averaged over three consecutive phonatory episodes, each made during maximum inhalatory effort and executed as close to similar Fo and intensity targets as possible.

Measurement of stroboscopic (phonoscopic) findings
All phonoscopic images were recorded on video tape and played back from a Sony SLV 900HF VCR (Sony Corp of America, Park Ridge, NJ, USA) on a 21-inch, flat video display terminal screen for later analysis. Factors of interest were studied subjectively according to recommendations [8,32] and included level of closure, smoothness of glottic edge, supraglottic compensation, and bilateral characteristics of the mucosal wave. Size of the glottic gap (degree of lateral shifting) of the injected vocal fold was estimated in relative units as the length of each vocal fold in relation to anterior glottic angle. This method is similar to a recently proposed method used to estimate the position of the paralyzed vocal fold by measuring anterior glottic and vocal fold angles [39,40].

These subjective observations and relative numeric measurements were carried out on images of consecutive phonoscopic examinations. Maximum care was taken to obtain images compatible across settings by fitting the new image recorded during live phonoscopy to an old image represented by a tracing on translucent gel placed on the video monitor, a technique recommended to increase accuracy of comparison [41].

Results

General clinical observations, complications, and interinjection interval

We completed 228 unilateral injections in our patient population. The interinjection interval ranged from 3 to 10 months (mean, 4 months). Injection produced minimal complications including minor intracordal hematoma, which resolved spontaneously, in three patients. One of these hematomas occurred in a patient who failed to report taking anticoagulants; the other two were due to repeated intramuscular needle manipulation.

Several times we encountered needle patency problems which presumably resulted when fatty, areolar, cartilaginous, or muscular tissue clogged the needle tip during neck penetration. Other complications included brief coughing while swallowing liquids and overall cervical ache and discomfort, including referred otalgia on the injected side. In general, however, the TA-targeted patients showed only minor dysmotility of the injected vocal fold in adductory or abductory directions. This degree of dysmotility contrasts sharply with that of PCA-targeted patients. Decreased adductor or abductor motility was also observed in TA/CT-targeted cases. Motility decrease lasted a mean of <30 days except in PCA-targeted patients.

For ADD SD, the longest interinjection interval (10 months) was achieved in patients who previously had unilateral RLN resection and whose symptoms had recurred. Our results also showed that the mean 4-month interinjection interval could be increased to 5.5 months for patients in whom improved vocal fold control developed through voice therapy.

For ADD SD/VT, the interinjection interval was similar to that for ADD SD only. Tremor was only slightly diminished, and although patients subjectively reported improved phonatory control, we were unable to correlate their subjective impressions with any objective measurement done in this study.

Similarly, no objective verification of patient self-ratings of VT symptom reduction was generally obtained. However, more chaotic MVW characteristics were associated with increased aperiodicity (hoarseness), and decreased glottic closure (glottic gap) was associated with increased breathiness and decreased total vocal loudness. However, this combination of factors reduced the magnitude of tremor without affecting its rate. Consequently, tremor symptoms were slightly diminished but not eliminated. This finding may account for the substantial subjective symptom reduction reported by our patients.

Of the three ABD SD patients studied, one showed considerable symptom reduction which lasted a mean of 8 months between injections. This patient received extensive voice therapy both before and after Botox injection. Another patient showed no clinically significant symptom relief after two consecutive injections and declined further treatment. A third patient, who had a >25-year history of the most severe ABD SD we have ever encountered, showed no symptom elimination despite successful unilateral shifting toward the midline of the left TVF, after PCA injection with 10 units of Botox; she also declined further treatment.

Stroboscopic findings

Level of closure

This observation relates to relative vertical alignment of the vocal folds during closure. No differences in level of closure were observed in any of the Botox-treated dysphonic conditions studied as a function of any muscle or combination of muscles injected.

Smoothness of glottic edge

Because TA injection may result in convexity and displacement of the mucosal edge of the TVF, we observed smoothness of the phonatory glottic edge after Botox injection. Neither transitory nor chronic changes were noted in the phonatory edge between either the upper or the lower phonatory lips, regardless of injection site or size of dose. PCA and CT injection resulted in similar findings.

Supraglottic compensation

The supraglottic compensatory behavior occasionally seen before Botox treatment in ADD SD patients was generally absent after Botox treatment. However, just after Botox injection and in relation to degree of the glottic gap created by the injection, some patients showed more prominent ventricular fold contraction on the side contralateral or ipsilateral to the injection.

Glottic gap

According to the physiologic model of ADD SD, widening the glottic gap is crucial for eliminating overpressure. This widening was achieved in all TA-injected patients and reduced or eliminated symptoms in most patients within the first 24–36 h. The glottic gap was widest – about 2 mm – immediately after injection. The phonatory glottic configuration seen during laryngovideostroboscopy was fusiform or spindle and skewed to the injected side. The gap narrowed rapidly in the first 2–3 weeks after injection (Fig. 1) and then remained constant (±1–1.5 mm) until minor symptoms recurred, usually in 3–3.5 months. In the last stage, the glottic gap appeared to be eliminated or to be of the same size as it was before injection. This gap reduction occurred despite continuous asymptomatic or barely symptomatic phonation, and distinguishing between its size before injection and its size at the last stage or after the recurrence of symptoms was difficult. Within each patient, glottic gap assessment after consecutive injections showed a similar pattern: no substantial differences in glottic gap size were noted as a function of 5-unit increases or decreases in dose. Moreover, at this stage of our research, we could not correlate the dose injected with the size of glottic gap or angulation characteristics. Therefore, we are determining dosage empirically, primarily on the basis of symptom severity before injection. A dose of 10 units injected unilaterally and properly targeted is sufficient to achieve a maximal gap. We are of the opinion that exceeding this dose in patients who have not received trial treatment may result in prolonged breathiness and possible aspiration.

Bilateral characteristics of the MVW

Observing the MVW is critical when interpreting voice quality – specifically, aperiodicity and breathiness – after Botox treatment. All TA-targeted patients showed increased MVW asymmetry between the left and right TVFs as a function of Botox

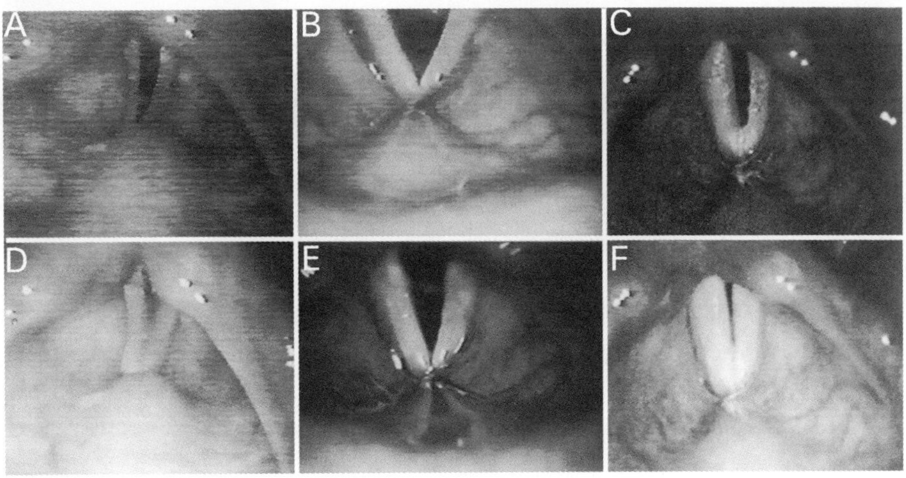

Fig. 1. Glottic configuration in a male adductor spasmodic dysphonia patient observed during a 90° laryngovideostroboscopy (**A**, **B**, **D**) 1 week after and (**C**, **E**, **F**) 4 weeks after an injection of 10 units of Botox into the left thyroarytenoid muscle complex. Note the narrowed glottic gap and reduced bowing of affected left true vocal fold as a function of time.

injection. Dosage-to-asymmetry correlation was low. Asymmetry and MVW amplitude on the injected side was more pronounced immediately after injection (Figs. 2 and 3). With time, both MVW asymmetry and amplitude variability diminished. MVW eventually became quasisymmetric as early as 2 weeks after injection, but asymmetry persisted for as long as 2.5 months in some cases and rendered the voice hoarse and subject to sudden, uncontrollable pitch breaks, particularly during loudness increases. Voice therapy aimed at controlling intensity appeared useful for improving this condition.

Acoustics

Pitch (Fo) and loudness (dB) measurements obtained at various intervals after Botox injection showed initial reduction in high-voice Fo production and limited loudness characterized by breathiness. Restoration of normal phonatory function was generally observed as early as 2 weeks after injection in most TA-targeted ADD SD patients (Fig. 4), a period which correlated well with glottic gap reduction. Initial increase in Fo aperiodicity (hoarseness) correlated well with restoration of a more symmetric MVW, a pattern which also occurred within 3 weeks after injection. The most normal phonation occurred between the first 3 and the last 4 recorded weeks after injection (Fig. 4). Aggressive voice therapy eliminated or reduced aperiodicity and pitch or

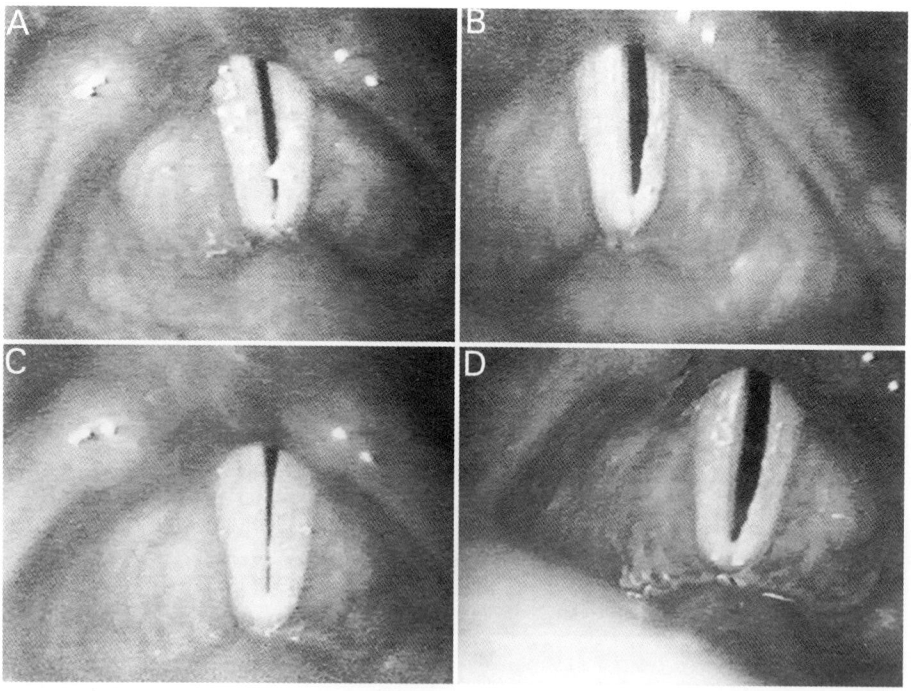

Fig. 2. Post-Botox glottic configuration showing aperiodic vibratory mucosal wave observed stroboscopically at a 90° angle. Note that aperiodicity, representing consecutive vibratory frames, is more pronounced on the injected (**A**, **C**) side.

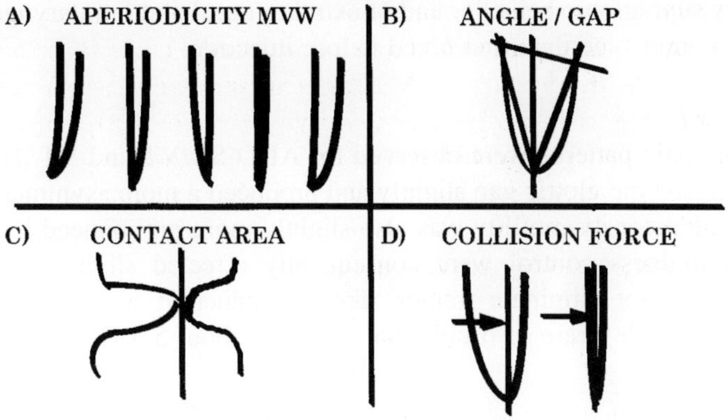

Fig. 3. Idealized and computer-enhanced glottic configuration in adductor spasmodic dysphonia patients after an injection of 10 units of Botox into the left thyroarytenoid complex. **A**: Aperiodicity of vibratory mucosal wave, which accounted for hoarseness and in part for breathiness. **B**: Glottic gap size as a function of time. **C**: Estimated reduction in glottic contact area. **D**: Estimated reduction in collision forces.

loudness control problems and appeared to prolong the symptom-free interval.

Maximum air consumption (<5 s of MphT per full inhalation) predominated in the first 2–3 weeks after injection and correlated well with glottic gap size in a pattern similar to that for pitch restoration. MphT improved rapidly from 2 to 3 weeks after Botox injection (Fig. 4). This improvement allowed normal breath group management for proper linguistic phasing and sentence construction and eliminated the need to reinhale frequently to complete a sentence sequence which typifies the first stage after injection. Improved air consumption apparently coincided with elimination of

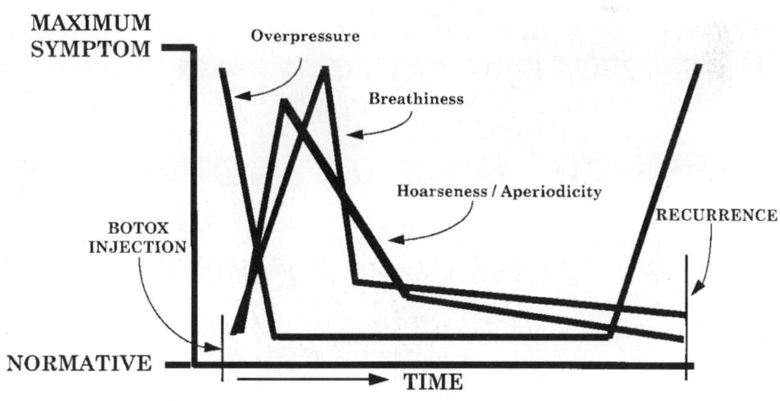

Fig. 4. Simplified profile of relevant phonatory changes as a function of time in adductor spasmodic dysphonia patients treated with Botox injection of the thyroarytenoid. Maximum breathiness and aperiodicity, as well as reduced overpressure and loudness and increased air consumption (short maximum phonation time), occur within the first 2 weeks after injection. Voice quality improves after this period. Voice therapy is routinely provided toward the end of the symptom-free period. Note the relatively short period before symptom recurrence.

compensatory supraglottic behavior and of extralaryngeal and intralaryngeal struggle, albeit of a different type than that noted before injection.

ADD SD/VT, VT

Similar physiologic patterns were observed for ADD SD/VT and VT. However, CT injection increased the glottic gap slightly and produced a more asymmetrical MVW. Abductor or adductor dysmotility was also slightly more pronounced in these cases, and Fo and loudness control were consequently affected slightly longer, which reduced, but did not eliminate tremor. Tremor reduction was mainly limited to magnitude (amplitude); rate of oscillation remained about 5.5 Hz.

ABD SD

PCA injection resulted in time-dependent ipsilateral medialization and dysmotility of the injected vocal fold (Fig. 5). This shifting toward the midline followed by gradual lateralization and increased motility was observed for up to 4 months. Normal abductory motility was observed at the 4-month interval (Fig. 6). Asymptomatic phonation paradoxically persisted for the next 4 months. In the remaining two cases, a shift toward the midline (medialization) of shorter duration and abductory dysmotility were achieved but failed to eliminate symptoms.

Discussion

The glottic physiologic factor most responsible for symptom elimination and symptom recurrence after Botox injection was the glottic gap-angulation factor. This finding is consistent with the proposed physiologic model of ADD SD. Changes induced by muscle paresis, weakening, and gradual recovery are reflected acoustically

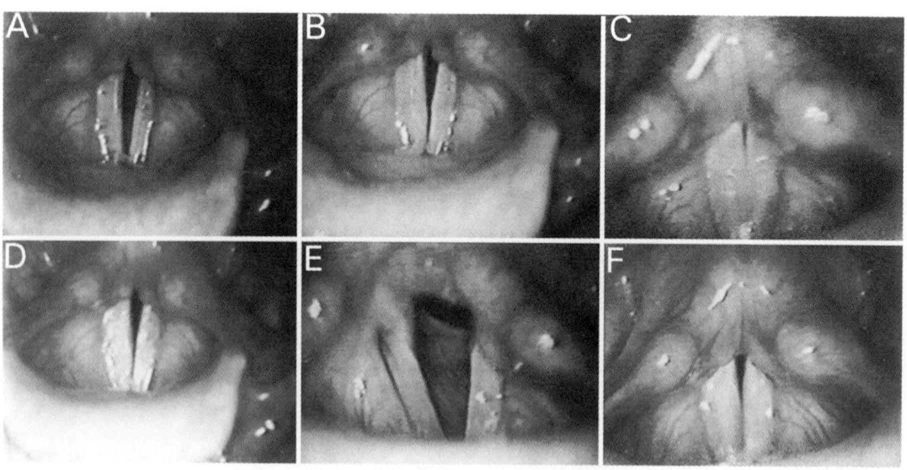

Fig. 5. Glottic configuration in a female abductor spasmodic dysphonia patient observed with a 90° laryngovideostroboscope: (**A**, **B**, **D**) before and (**C**, **E**, **F**) after an injection of 12.5 units of Botox into the left posterior cricoarytenoid muscle. Note the narrowed glottic gap and reduced abductor motility immediately after injection. Also note the gradual increase in abductor motility as a function of time.

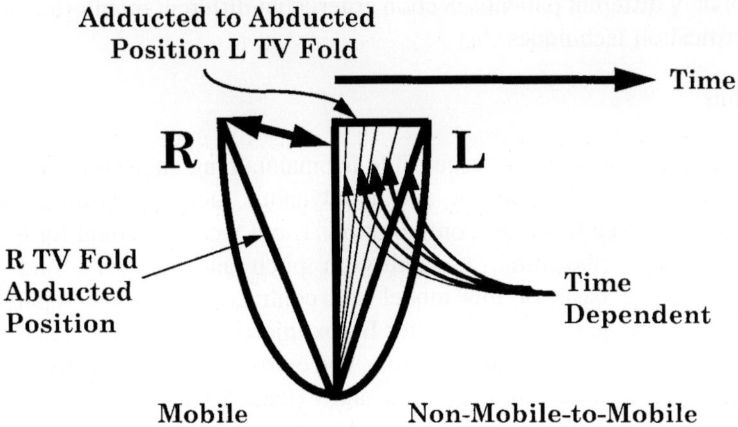

Fig. 6. Computer-enhanced glottic configuration in an abductor spasmodic dysphonia patient after an injection of 12.5 units of Botox into the left posterior cricoarytenoid muscle. Note the time-dependent reduction in glottic gap and increased motility (shifting to the side) of the affected left true vocal fold.

by time-dependent aperiodicity [42], changes in loudness and pitch, and phonatory air consumption [42,43]. Our Botox injection technique did not eliminate pure or associated vocal tremor, which substantiates theories postulating a more central (cerebellar) tremor-generation site. The variable effects of PCA denervation in ABD SD described here are difficult to explain in view of the consistently achieved medialization of the ipsilateral TVF and abductory dysmotility. Our data indicate a need to re-examine the concept that the physiology of ABD SD mirrors that of ADD SD. In addition, the efficacy of either unilateral or bilateral Botox injection for PCA denervation remains untested.

Although variable among patients and between consecutive reinjections, the physiologic elements described here form a solid basis for predicting voice quality after Botox injection in most cases. However, more detailed study of these changes is needed to establish better criteria for drug dosage in response to symptom severity. This need is especially urgent because our data did not show any clinically relevant changes in symptom elimination as a function of cumulative effects of consecutive injections.

Because symptoms were affected (improved) in all our ADD SD patients, administering this toxin bilaterally appears unnecessary, a finding consistent with the proposed ADD SD model and with data obtained from more than 400 RLN resections. These findings are of particular importance because duration of symptom relief achieved appears to be similar to or better than that in patients treated bilaterally at equivalent doses. Finally, glottic physiology after Botox injection differs considerably from that which results after unilateral RLN resection. These two techniques consequently produce considerably different durations of relief.

Our findings regarding voice quality variability and complications after Botox injection in ABD SD patients also differ from those of others. This difference may reflect not only different patient selection criteria but different monitoring and muscle action verification techniques.

Conclusion

The physiologic element most responsible for maintaining an asymptomatic voice is the glottic gap-angle. All acoustic and aerodynamic factors measured after Botox injection were derived from this configuration. These factors account for breathiness, aperiodicity, weak phonation, variability in pitch and loudness, and symptom recurrence. On the basis of this model and contrary to a recent report [12], no worsening of voice quality resulted after Botox injection. Moreover, contrary to that report [12], we did not find that phonatory voice profiles varied greatly from patient to patient. Uniform injection techniques and extended therapeutic voice care after injection may account for these differences. Duration of each voice quality phase after Botox injection appears to depend on symptom severity before injection, compensation after injection, and use of voice therapy to control glottic gap configuration after injection. On the basis of our model, the time-limited efficacy of Botox injection is best for pure ADD SD and is worst for pure VT. Our data are insufficient to meaningfully address ABD SD treatment but contrast sharply with reports of successful treatment of ABD SD by injecting Botox into the PCA [28].

Our results can be used to explain recovery course and voice-production capability to patients. The utility of our results in instructing patients contrasts with recent skepticism regarding this issue [12]. In addition, our results agree with other research on the symptom relief and recurrence cycle after Botox injection. Therefore, ADD SD treatment efficacy clearly relates to the capacity of a denervation technique to create, sustain, and maintain a minimal glottic gap. After chemodenervation using Botox, this effect may last 6 months at best in de novo cases. Therefore, reinjection is required to recreate these conditions after inevitable reinnervation. Treatment which prolongs the denervation pattern and maintains a minimal glottic gap should thus be more effective, and we believe that RLN resection produces such results as it can eliminate symptoms for up to 16 years [18–21,44,45]. Symptom recurrence after RLN resection correlates with a shift toward the midline of the paralyzed vocal fold and with reinnervation. Recurrence after RLN resection is treated by thinning the paralyzed vocal fold with a CO_2 laser to recreate the critical glottic gap. When recurrence after these treatments is then managed with Botox, almost 12 months of symptom relief can be achieved. Such prolonged symptom-free periods compare favorably with the 4–6-month symptom elimination typical after treatment with Botox alone.

Finally, although our data support the efficacy of combined RLN resection and voice therapy for treating ADD SD, we believe that combined Botox injection and voice therapy has been firmly established as an option in managing ADD SD because it enables patients to make an informed choice about treatment and its consequences.

Acknowledgements

The research was supported in part by the Pacific Voice and Speech Foundation, San

Francisco, California.

The Medical Editing Department, Kaiser Foundation Research Institute, provided editorial assistance, and the Audiovisual Department, Kaiser Permanente Medical Care Program, assisted with graphics production.

References

1. Scott AB. Clostridial toxins as therapeutic agents. In: Simpson L (ed) Clostridial Neurotoxins. San Diego: Academic Press, 1989:399–412.
2. Jankovic J, Brin MF. Therapeutic uses of botulinum toxin. N Engl J Med 1991;324:1186–1194.
3. Simpson LL. Clinically relevant aspects of the mechanism of action of botulinum neurotoxin. J Voice 1992;6:358–364.
4. Blitzer A, Brin HF, Fahn S, Lange D, Lovelace RE. Botulinum toxin (BOTOX) for the treatment of spastic dysphonia as part of a trial of toxin injections for the treatment of other cranial dystonias (letter). Laryngoscope 1986;96:1300–1301.
5. Blitzer A, Brin MF. Laryngeal dystonia: a series treated with botulinum toxin therapy. Ann Otol Rhinol Laryngol 1991;100:85–89.
6. Ludlow CL. Treatment of speech and voice disorders with botulinum toxin. JAMA 1990;264: 2671–2675.
7. Ludlow CL, Naunton RF, Sedory SE, Schulz GM, Hallett M. Effects of botulinum toxin injections on speech in adductor spasmodic dysphonia. Neurology 1988;38:1220–1225.
8. Woo P, Colton R, Casper J, Brewer D. Analysis of spasmodic dysphonia by aerodynamic and laryngostroboscopic measurements. J Voice 1992;6:344–351.
9. Zwirner P, Murry T, Swenson K, Woodson GE. Acoustic changes in spasmodic dysphonia after botulinum toxin injection. J Voice 1991;5:78–84.
10. Woodson GE, Zwirner P, Murry T, Swenson M. Use of flexible fiberoptic laryngoscopy to assess patients with spasmodic dysphonia. J Voice 1991;5:85–91.
11. Brin MF, Blitzer A, Fahn S, Gould W, Lovelace RE. Adductor laryngeal dystonia (spastic dysphonia): treatment with local injections of botulinum toxin (BOTOX). Mov Disord 1989;4: 287–296.
12. Aronson AE, McCaffrey TV, Litchy WJ, Lipton RJ. Botulinum toxin injection for adductor spastic dysphonia: patient self-ratings of voice and phonatory effort after three successive injections. Laryngoscope 1993;103:683–692.
13. Ludlow CL, Hallett M, Sedory SF, Fujita M, Nauton RF. The pathophysiology of spasmodic dysphonia and its modification by botulinum toxin. In: Berardelli A, Benecke R, Manfredi M, Marsden CD (eds) Motor Disturbances II: A Selection of Papers Delivered at the 2nd Congress of the International Medical Society of Motor Disturbances held at Rome, Italy, 2–4 June, 1988. San Diego: Academic Press, 1990:274–288.
14. Ludlow CL, Naunton RF, Fujita M, Sedory SE. Spasmodic dysphonia: botulinum toxin injection after recurrent nerve surgery. Otolaryngol Head Neck Surg 1990;102:122–131.
15. Dedo HH. Recurrent laryngeal nerve section for spastic dysphonia. Ann Otol Rhinol Laryngol 1976;85(4 Pt 1) 451–459.
16. Dedo HH, Izdebski K. Surgical treatment of spastic dysphonia. Contemp Surg 1981;18:75–90.
17. Dedo HH, Shipp T. Spastic Dysphonia: a Surgical and Voice Therapy Treatment Program. Houston, TX: College-Hill Press, 1980.
18. Izdebski K, Dedo HH, Shipp T, Flower RM. Postoperative and follow-up studies of spastic dysphonia patients treated by recurrent laryngeal nerve section. Otolaryngol Head Neck Surg 1981;89:96–101.
19. Dedo HH, Izdebski K. Intermediate results of 306 recurrent laryngeal nerve sections for spastic dysphonia. Laryngoscope 1983;93:9–16.
20. Dedo HH, Izdebski K. Problems with surgical (RLN) section for spastic dysphonia. Laryngoscope 1983;93:268–271.

21. Dedo HH, Behlau MS. Recurrent laryngeal nerve section for spastic dysphonia: 5- to 14-year preliminary results in the first 300 patients. Ann Otol Rhinol Laryngol 1991;100(4 Pt 1):274–279.
22. Izdebski K. Symptomatology of adductor spasmodic dysphonia: a physiologic model. J Voice 1992;6:306–319.
23. Izdebski K, Dedo HH. Spastic dysphonia. In: Darby JK Jr (ed) Speech Evaluation in Medicine. New York: Grune & Stratton, Inc., 1981;ii:105–127.
24. Izdebski K, Dedo HH, Boles L. Spastic dysphonia: a patient profile of 200 cases. Am J Otolaryngol 1984;5:7–14.
25. Izdebski K, Dedo HH. Selecting the side of recurrent laryngeal nerve section for spastic dysphonia. Otolaryngol Head Neck Surg 1980;89(3 Pt 1):423–426.
26. Izdebski K, Dedo HH. Characteristics of voice tremor in spastic dysphonia: a preliminary study. In: Lawrence VL (ed) Spastic Dysphonia: State of the Art 1979. New York: Voice Foundation, 1979:17–23.
27. Ludlow CL, Bassich CJ, Connor NP, Coulter DC. Phonatory characteristics of vocal fold tremor. J Phonetics 1986;14:509–516.
28. Blitzer A, Brin MF, Stewart C, Aviv JE, Fahn S. Abductor laryngeal dystonia: a series treated with botulinum toxin. Laryngoscope 1992;102:163–167.
29. Aronson AE, Brown JR, Litin EM, Pearson JS. Spastic dysphonia. II. Comparison with essential (voice) tremor and other neurologic and psychogenic dysphonias. J Speech Hear Dis 1968;33: 219–231.
30. Izdebski K, Ross JC, Klein JC. Transoral rigid laryngovideostroboscopy (phonoscopy). Speech Lang 1990;11:16–26.
31. Hirano M. Clinical Examination of Voice. New York: Springer-Verlag, 1981.
32. Hirano M, Bless DM. Videostroboscopic Examination of the Larynx. San Diego, CA: Singular Publishing Group, 1993.
33. Izdebski K. Surgical and medical treatment of spasmodic dysphonia. In: Stemple JC (ed) Voice Therapy: Clinical Studies. St. Louis: Mosby Year Book, 1993:131–147.
34. Ward R, Izdebski K, Fross R, Glass A. Laryngeal muscle verification during percutaneous Botox injection for spasmodic dysphonia. Paper presented at ASHA Annual Convention, Anaheim, CA, November 19–22, 1993. ASHA 1993;35:195 (abstract).
35. Shipp T, Doherty ET, Morrissey P. Predicting vocal frequencies from selected physiologic measures. J Acoust Soc Am 1979;66:678–684.
36. Shaari CM, George E, Wu B-L, Biller HF, Sanders I. Quantifying the spread of botulinum toxin through muscle fascia. Laryngoscope 1991;101:960–964.
37. Izdebski K, Shipp T, Dedo HH. Predicting postoperative voice characteristics of spastic dysphonia patients. Otolaryngol Head Neck Surg 1979;87:428–434.
38. Izdebski K. Practical techniques of office voice recording. Otolaryngol Head Neck Surg 1983;91: 638–642.
39. Woodson GE. Configuration of the glottis in laryngeal paralysis. I: Clinical study. Laryngoscope 1993;103:1227–1234.
40. Woodson GE. Configuration of the glottis in laryngeal paralysis. II: Animal experiments. Laryngoscope 1993;103(11 Pt 1):1235–1241.
41. Peppard RC, Bless DM. A method for improving measurement reliability in laryngeal videostroboscopy. J Voice 1990;4:1280–1285.
42. Woo P, Colton R, Casper J, Brewer D. Diagnostic value of stroboscopic examination of hoarse patients. J Voice 1991;5:231–238.
43. Izdebski K. Overpressure and breathiness in spastic dysphonia: an acoustical LTAS and perceptual study. Acta Otolaryngol (Stockholm) 1984;97(3–4):373–378.
44. Fritzell B, Feuer E, Haglund S, Knutsson E, Schiratzki H. Experiences with recurrent laryngeal nerve section for spastic dysphonia. Folia Phoniatr (Basel) 1982;34:160–167.
45. Schiratzki H, Fritzell B. Treatment of spasmodic dysphonia by means of resection of the recurrent laryngeal nerve. Acta Otolaryngol Suppl (Stockholm) 1988;449:115–117.

Voice Update.
M. Pais Clemente, editor.

Laryngeal framework surgery — a tailored approach to voice improvement

Hans F. Mahieu
Department of Otorhinolaryngology — Head and Neck Surgery, Academisch Ziekenhuis Vrije Universiteit, Amsterdam, The Netherlands

Abstract. *Background.* Laryngeal framework surgery is gaining popularity as a phonosurgical procedure. Two different categories of laryngeal framework surgeries can be distinguished:
1. With the objective to correct incomplete glottis closure by medialization.
2. With the objective to adjust the tension of the vocal folds.
Both categories are performed under local anaesthesia to allow fine-tuning of the voice.

Methods. 100 patients who underwent laryngeal framework surgery have been evaluated. In 70, the primary aim was correction of incomplete glottis closure and in 30, the correction of vocal fold tension, mostly to raise the vocal pitch. The voice parameters used for assessment were maximal phonation time, maximal dynamic intensity range, dynamic intensity range at the mean pitch of the speaking voice, maximal vocal intensity, melodic range and mean habitual pitch of the voice.

Results. Good results, short-term as well as long-term results have been obtained in the correction of incomplete glottis closure. Most of the patients requesting a raise of the vocal pitch have obtained a mean pitch within the normal female range. Complications were few and not serious.

Conclusions. Laryngeal framework surgery offers a safe and effective method to improve certain dysphonias, and it enables a tailored approach to the individual dysphonic patient's need.

Key words: medialization laryngeal framework surgery, phonosurgery, pitch-raising surgery, surgical correction of vocal fold tension.

Introduction

Dysphonias resulting from incomplete glottis closure or inadequate vocal fold tension are eligible for phonosurgical correction, and laryngeal framework surgery is rapidly gaining popularity as the treatment of first choice for these conditions. Not only because of the physiological approach but also because of the possibility to monitor the voice during this type of surgery. Although some types of laryngeal framework surgery had already been suggested decades ago [1,2], the concept remained fragmentary until Isshiki [3—7] modified some of these procedures, introduced some others and integrated them all into the functionally oriented set of phonosurgical techniques which is available to us today.

Two different categories of laryngeal framework surgeries can be distinguished:

Address for correspondence: Prof Hans F. Mahieu MD, PhD, Department of Otorhinolaryngology — Head and Neck Surgery, Academisch Ziekenhuis Vrije Universiteit, Postbus 7057, 1007 MB Amsterdam, The Netherlands.

1. With the objective to correct incomplete glottis closure by medialization of one or both vocal folds.
2. With the objective to adjust the tension of one or both vocal folds.

Sometimes a single modality laryngeal framework surgical technique sufficiently improves the voice, but often a better voice can be obtained by combining different techniques in one stage. This is not always predictable preoperatively, so that voice and functional fiberoptic endolaryngeal monitoring are essential during the procedure, not only to determine the required degree of medialization or change of vocal fold tension, but also to decide whether or not to continue with a combination of laryngeal framework surgical procedures. To enable this monitoring, the laryngeal framework surgical techniques are performed under local anaesthesia. After a premedication of 10 mg of morphine and 0.5 mg of atropine, local anaesthesia is obtained by infiltration of xylocaine 1% and epinephrine 0.001% solution, 5–8 cc. Brief descriptions of the surgical procedures are outlined below, for a more elaborate description see Isshiki [7] and Mahieu et al. [8].

Correction of incomplete glottis closure

The surgical treatment strategy in dysphonia resulting from incomplete glottis closure is generally based on trying to medialize the affected vocal fold(s). This can be achieved by two laryngeal framework surgical techniques:

1. Thyroplasty type 1, which consists of a window cut in the ala of the thyroid cartilage at the level of the vocal fold. The window can then be impressed, thus medializing the vocal fold. The window is secured in the optimal medialized position by a silicon wedge, a silicon plug or by sutures. If necessary, a posterior extension can be added to the silicon wedge to medialize the vocal process of the arytenoid as well. Contrary to the recently advocated procedure of removing the cartilage window in order to more directly influence the shape and position of the vocal fold by using differently shaped silicon implants [9–11], the author personally prefers to leave the cartilage window in situ, as a buttress against endolaryngeal extrusion of the silicon implant. Such extrusions have only been reported following removal of the cartilage window and incision of the inner perichondrium [12]. Because thyroplasty type 1 does not interfere with vocal fold mobility, it can be used bilaterally if necessary in cases with incomplete glottis closure and mobile vocal folds.
2. Arytenoid adduction, which consists of sutures being tied around the muscular process of the arytenoid. Traction on these sutures in the anterolateral direction (mimicking the activity of the thyroarytenoid muscle, pars lateralis, and the lateral cricoarytenoid muscle), will result in rotation of the vocal process medially, thus medializing the vocal fold. Because arytenoid adduction restricts laryngeal mobility it can only be used unilaterally.

In cases with a unilateral vocal fold immobility and incomplete glottis closure, usually a thyroplasty type 1 is performed first, because it is the most simple technique. Only if the glottal gap is extremely large or if there is a marked vertical level difference between both vocal folds, is the procedure started with an arytenoid adduction. If this "single modality" framework surgery results in a satisfying per-operative voice and adequate glottis closure, the procedure is concluded. If the per-operative voice improvement is not satisfactory, then the procedure is extended with the addition of another medializing or tension-adjusting framework technique.

The most frequently used combination in medialization laryngeal framework surgery is thyroplasty type 1 and arytenoid adduction (almost 50% of the cases). The effect of a manual cricothyroid approximation (see adjustment of vocal fold tension) is always tested after the required degree of medialization has been achieved to hear whether increased tension results in a further improvement of voice. If indicated, surgical cricothyroid approximation can then be performed (approximately in 10% of the cases).

Adjustment of vocal fold tension

Indications for adjustments of vocal fold tensions are various. Too lax vocal folds may result in a weak, hoarse, and usually low-pitched voice. Too tense vocal folds may result in a strained, breathy, and usually high-pitched voice. Diminished and asymmetrical vocal fold tension, as may accompany vocal fold palsy, may contribute to the breathy voice quality and can result in diplophonia. These and certain other pitch-related dysphonias may be eligible for surgical correction of vocal fold tension.

Normally the tension of the vocal folds and consequently the vocal pitch are largely determined by the action of the cricothyroid muscles and the vocalis muscles, which act more or less as antagonists. This mechanism is supported by the other intrinsic laryngeal muscles which counterbalance the forces applied to the arytenoid and assist in increasing the tension of the vocal folds. Contraction of the cricothyroid muscles results in an anterior approximation of the cricoid and thyroid cartilages and consequently the anterior commissure is displaced anteriorly and caudally. As a result of this displacement the vocal folds are stretched, thinned and stiffened (body as well as cover), a situation which leads to a rise in vocal pitch. Contraction of the vocalis muscle results in a shortening, thickening and slackening (cover only) of the vocal folds, leading to a lower vocal pitch. Vocal pitch is thus largely controlled by the tension, which influences stiffness, mass and length of the vocal folds.

By and large there are five categories of patients who may benefit from laryngeal framework surgical correction of vocal fold tension:

1. Patients who are undergoing correction of incomplete glottis closure by means of medialization laryngeal framework surgery and in whom additional correction of vocal fold tension may contribute to a further improvement of the voice.
2. Patients who request an elevation of the vocal pitch. The major indications for raising the vocal pitch are androphonia following hormonal medication and gender dysphonia in male-to-female transsexual patients. Voice therapy is the mainstay for gender dysphonia, but additional phonosurgical intervention can be required to raise the habitual vocal pitch. Although vocal pitch is not the only factor in identifying the gender of a speaker, it is generally regarded as the predominant

one. Other factors include patterns of intonation, quality of resonance, articulation characteristics, conversational topics and type of vocabulary [13,14].

3. Patients with slackened vocal folds as may be the result of superior laryngeal nerve palsy, extreme flaccid vocal folds in elderly patients and some cases following laryngeal trauma.
4. Patients with stiff vocal fold(s) due to congenital vocal fold disorders, some cases of sulcus vocalis (after unsatisfactory microlaryngeal surgery) and exceptional cases following laryngeal trauma. In such cases a combination of surgical reduction of vocal fold tension and slight medialization can improve the voice.
5. Patients requesting a lowering of the vocal pitch. Although rare, cases of voice therapy-resistant mutational dysphonia and some cases of congenital vocal fold hypoplasia can benefit from surgical reduction of vocal fold tension.

The two mostly used methods to increase the vocal fold tension (and the vocal fold pitch) are:

1. Cricothyroid approximation, which seems to be the most physiological way to increase the vocal fold tension, because this procedure mimics the activity of the cricothyroid muscles and imitates the situation during falsetto phonation. Sutures are tied around the cricoid cartilage and are fixed to the anterior part of the thyroid cartilage. This can be performed both unilaterally (usually in addition to medialization laryngeal framework surgery) or bilaterally (for example in pitch elevation surgery).
2. Displacement of the anterior commissure anteriorly by making a midline thyroid cartilage flap at the level of the anterior commissure as described by Tucker [15]. This flap is pulled anteriorly, thus displacing the anterior commissure anteriorly as well. The flap can be held in this anterior position with a small plate or shim. This technique was originally developed to tighten flaccid vocal folds, but is also successful in pitch elevation surgery as an adjunct to cricothyroid approximation. Isshiki [7] prefers to displace the anterior commissure anteriorly by using a thyroplasty type 3 with lengthening of the anterior-posterior dimension of the thyroid ala. For this purpose a vertical incision is made through the thyroid ala cartilage (unilaterally or bilaterally) at one-third from the front of the thyroid cartilage. Interposition of a vertical strip of silicone will increase the anterior-posterior dimension of the thyroid ala, resulting in an anterior displacement of the anterior commissure and thus a stretching of the vocal folds.

Reduction of vocal fold tension is rarely required, but can be achieved with a thyroplasty type 3 with shortening of the anterior-posterior dimension of the thyroid ala. The vertical incision through the thyroid ala is performed, just as is described above, but instead of interpositioning of a strip of silicon, a vertical strip of ala cartilage is excised, resulting in a shortening of the anterior-posterior dimension of the thyroid ala, resulting in a posterior displacement of the anterior commissure and thus a slackening of the vocal folds. This procedure can be performed unilaterally or bilaterally and can be used in combination with anterior medialization.

Materials and Methods

The first 100 patients who underwent laryngeal framework surgery in our department between 1987 and 1994 have been evaluated. For 70 of these patients the primary aim was to correct a dysphonia due to incomplete glottis closure. In 30 patients the indication for the surgery was primarily correction of vocal fold tension, 27 of whom requested a raise in pitch.

Voice evaluation was performed by means of a phonetogram (Fig. 1) preoperatively, between 2 and 4 months postoperatively (short-term results) and more than 1 year postoperatively (long-term results). In addition, the maximal phonation time of the sustained vowel /a/ was recorded in the patients undergoing medialization laryngeal framework surgery. Furthermore, the mean pitch of the voice during normal speech was determined by means of a glottal frequency analyser (Teltec type GFA 06, Sweden) in both patient categories. This resulted in the following objective voice parameters:

1. Maximal phonation time (Phon. Time) in seconds of a sustained vowel /a/ (best of three efforts).
2. Maximal dynamic intensity range (Dyn. Range) in dB obtained from the phonetogram (30 cm microphone-mouth distance).
3. Dynamic intensity range at the mean habitual pitch of the speaking voice (Dyn. Range MVP) in dB obtained from the phonetogram.

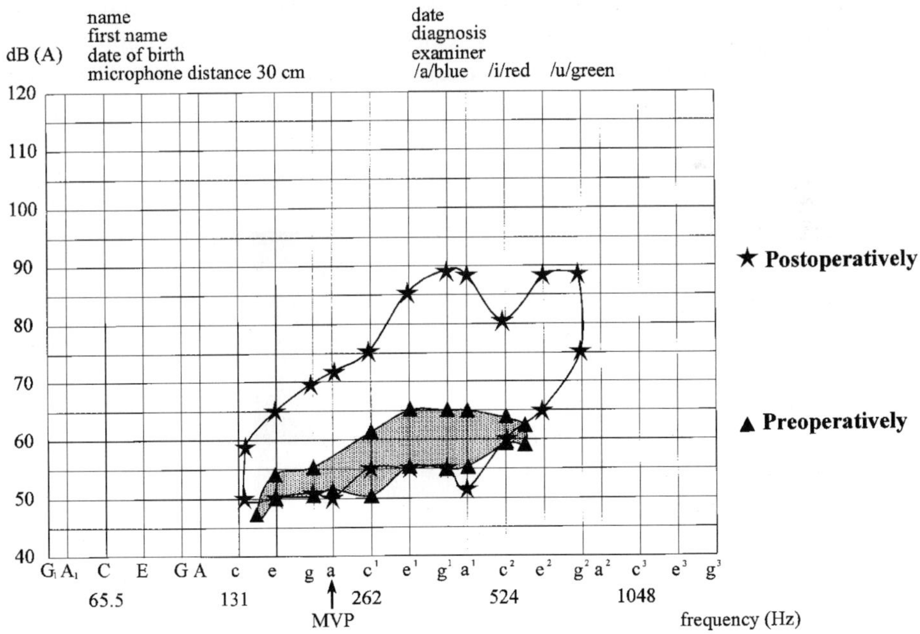

Fig. 1. Example of preoperative and a 3-month postoperative phonetogram following thyroplasty type 1 in a 47-year-old female patient 6 years after thyroid surgery and left-sided vocal fold paralysis: near normal phonetogram postoperatively, mean pitch of speaking voice MVP = 220 Hz.

4. Maximal vocal intensity (Max. Int) in dB obtained from the phonetogram.
5. Melodic range (Mel. Range) in semitones obtained from the phonetogram.
6. Mean habitual pitch of the voice during speech (MVP).

Results

Of 70 patients who had undergone medialization laryngeal framework surgery, none showed a deterioration of the voice. Three patients considered their voice to be unchanged or only marginally improved following the procedure. All three had undergone extensive previous phonosurgical procedures, two of them including teflon injections. All patients with a dysphonia based on vagus or recurrent nerve paralysis who had not previously undergone any phonosurgical procedure obtained a markedly improved voice and were highly satisfied with the result. About one-third of all patients considered their postoperative voice to be absolutely normal, even in demanding circumstances. More than half of the remaining patients considered their voice to be "functionally adequate".

Short-term objective postoperative voice evaluation was obtained in 54 patients following medialization laryngeal framework surgery (Fig. 2). Sixteen patients were excluded from voice evaluation; seven patients because they were from abroad and the voice assessment performed in the respective referring centers was not consistent; nine patients because they had terminal disease (malignant involvement of mediastinum). In 26 patients long-term voice evaluation was also obtained (Fig. 3).

All voice parameters except the melodic range show a postoperative improvement. It is interesting to notice that some of the voice parameters have still improved after 1 year as compared to the voice evaluation a few months postoperatively. This proves

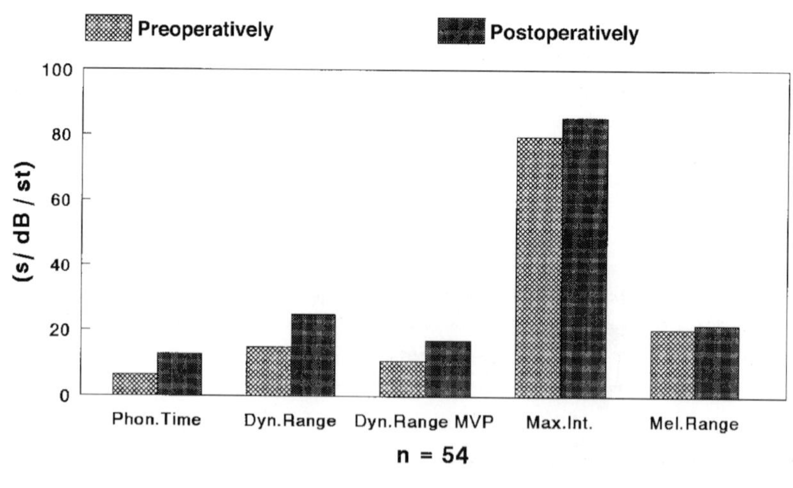

Fig. 2. Short-term (2–4 months postoperatively) results following medialization laryngeal framework surgery: maximal phonation time (Phon. Time) doubled to 13 s. Dynamic vocal intensity range (Dyn. Range): improvement of 10 dB. Dynamic vocal intensity range at the level of the habitual speaking pitch (Dyn. Range MVP): improvement of 6.5 dB. Maximal vocal intensity (Max. Int.); improvement of 6 dB. Melodic range (Mel. Range): improvement of 1.5 semitones.

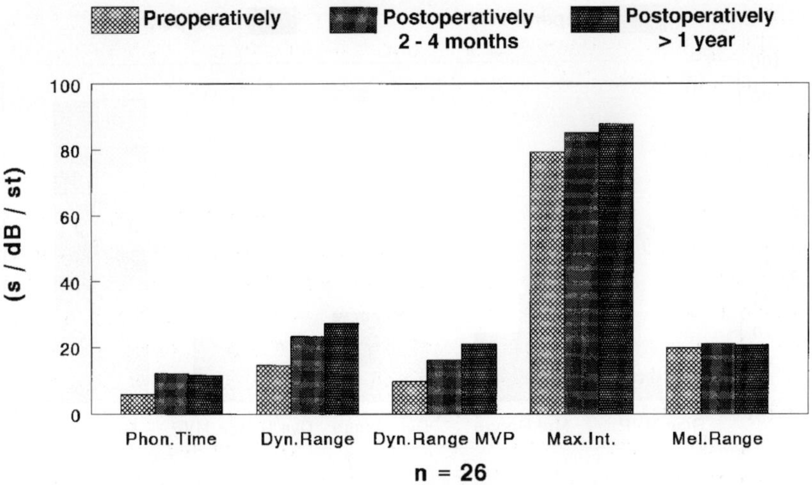

Fig. 3. Comparison of short-term (2–4 months) and long-term (1 year) results after medialization laryngeal framework surgery: phonation time (Phon. Time) and melodic range (Mel. Range) remained stable. Dynamic vocal intensity range (Dyn. Range), dynamic vocal intensity range at the level of the habitual speaking pitch (Dyn. Range MVP) and the maximal vocal intensity (Max. Int.) showed further voice improvement one year following surgery of respectively 4, 4.5 and 2.5 dB.

that the voice improvement obtained by medialization laryngeal framework surgery remains stable.

Generally, the best results were obtained in patients with dysphonia and or aspiration caused by recurrent or vagus nerve paralysis. Worst results were obtained in patients who had previously undergone intracordal teflon injections and patients with laryngeal fibrosis following laryngeal trauma. Complications observed as a result of medializing laryngeal framework surgical procedures were minor (two local infections, successfully treated with antibiotics; one transient stridor because of edema, successfully treated with steroid medication; and one slight dyspnea on exertion because of overcorrection, which was corrected secondarily with preservation of the achieved voice improvement). One patient required a second thyroplasty type 1 when her initially satisfactory postoperative voice deteriorated following an intubation for a gynecological procedure 2 years following the first thyroplasty. The second thyroplasty again resulted in a good postoperative voice.

Laryngeal framework surgery with the objective to raise the vocal pitch has been performed in 27 patients (one androphonia; 26 male-to-female transsexuals). All of these patients underwent a cricothyroid approximation and three of them also underwent anterior commissure advancement according to Tucker [15] (two as a second stage procedure). One patient later also underwent additional scarification and mass reduction of the vocal folds. Six patients had already undergone anterior web creation elsewhere prior to laryngeal framework surgery.

There is a tendency among transsexual patients not to show up for postoperative voice assessment. Seventeen patients could be assessed objectively between 2 and 6

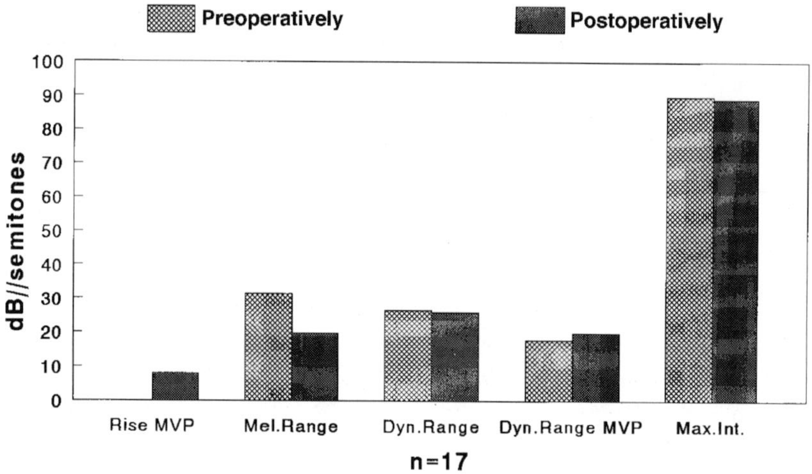

Fig. 4. Results of pitch-raising surgery: rise in the mean habitual pitch of speaking voice of 8 semitones (Rise MVP). Loss of melodic range (Mel. Range) of almost 11 semitones. Other voice parameters were unaltered by pitch-raising surgery.

months postoperatively (Fig. 4). Six of the other 10 patients have communicated by telephone that they were satisfied with the voice result, but were unable or unwilling to come for postoperative voice assessment. Breathiness and diplophonia were often present during the first few weeks postoperatively, but normalized spontaneously within 2 months.

Preoperatively, all voices had a mean pitch of the speaking voice within the male range (98–131 Hz). Postoperatively 14 of the 17 patients had achieved a mean pitch within the normal female range (174–262 Hz). One patient had no pitch rise after cricothyroid approximation but refused further treatment. Two patients demonstrated a drop of pitch after initial successful rise following cricothyroid approximation; both underwent an anterior commissure advancement reintervention resulting in a pitch rise, which again dropped to the preoperative pitch level in one.

The overall mean pitch rise of the speaking voice was 8 semitones. Although the melodic range was almost invariably diminished postoperatively (overall 11 semitones mean loss of melodic range), there were no complaints of monotonous voices. Other voice parameters such as maximal dynamic intensity range, dynamic intensity range at the mean pitch of the speaking voice and the maximal vocal intensity did not change due to the surgery, signifying no loss of overall voice quality.

Most patients were satisfied with the result and considered their voices as "normal female voices". Three patients were not satisfied with the result. One had a rise of 5 semitones on postoperative voice assessment and was almost within the range of the normal female speaking pitch, but did not appreciate this voice as a "normal female voice". In two patients a cricothyroid approximation was performed to correct a superior laryngeal nerve paralysis (one unilaterally, one bilaterally). Both demonstrated a slightly higher pitch and a stronger voice postoperatively.

The indication for lowering the vocal pitch is very rare and has been performed only once using a unilateral thyroplasty type 3 with shortening of the anterior-posterior dimension of the thyroid ala in combination with slight anterior medialization on the same side, and a thyroplasty type 1 on the other side in a case of severe dysphonia with a strained, weak, high-pitched voice, due to congenital hypoplasia of the vocal folds, with incomplete glottis closure. The mean pitch dropped 5 semitones and the glottis closure improved, resulting in a slightly stronger and less strained voice.

Complications of laryngeal framework surgery to correct vocal fold tension included one anterior fracture of the cricoid cartilage and one anterior fracture of the thyroid cartilage, both as a result of sutures pulling through the cartilage in cricothyroid approximation. Both were young transsexual patients with noncalcified cartilage. Both fractures were repaired at the time of initial surgery, without further sequelae. One of these patients had a good vocal pitch rise, the other voice result was unsatisfactory. No other complications were observed.

Discussion

A still frequently applied method other than laryngeal framework surgery to achieve medialization is the endolaryngeal injection of soluble substances, such as teflon, silicone, or collagen and more recently autologous fat. Such treatments with injectable substances are quick and apparently simple procedures, however, they are associated with considerable disadvantages and risks:

1. The mass, volume, and stiffness of the injected vocal fold is influenced by the injected substances. Such changes in vocal fold mass, volume, and stiffness negatively influence the vibratory properties of the vocal fold, which can result in a poor voice.
2. Distribution of the injected substance is difficult to control. The substance will spread according to the path of least resistance, rather than to the area requiring augmentation.
3. The treatment is irreversible. Overinjection is difficult to correct and generally requires partial resection of the vocal fold resulting in severe dysphonia.
4. If performed under general anaesthesia, as many endolaryngeal injection procedures are, voice monitoring during the procedure is not possible. Consequently it is difficult to estimate the proper amount of substance to be injected.
5. Some materials (collagen, fat) are subject to partial absorption so that initial overcorrection is required and repeated injections may be necessary. Other materials (silicone, teflon) are known to have a tendency towards migration, which may also require repeated injections [16].
6. Often vocal fold palsy is associated with a level difference of both vocal folds (vertical shift), which may be difficult to detect (special attention required to asymmetry in the video-laryngostroboscopic image and the position of the vocal processes). Such a level difference usually cannot be corrected by vocal fold

injection.

7. Last but not least, a considerable number of complications and local tissue reactions attributable to the injected substances have been published [17–20]. The injection of autologous fat seems to present less complications [16].

The advantages of the laryngeal framework medialization techniques are:

1. The affected vocal fold is not negatively influenced by mass, volume, or stiffness changes.
2. Direct control can be obtained over the degree, area and level of medialization, also enabling correction for a vertical shift of the vocal fold.
3. The procedure is reversible in the unlikely event of overcorrection.
4. The procedure is performed under local anaesthesia, so that fine-tuning of the voice is possible during the operation and several combinations of techniques can be tested during the operation to achieve the best voice result.
5. The voice results have proved to remain stable with only very few exceptions, so that the need for repeated procedures is rare.
6. Very few complications have been reported following this type of laryngeal framework surgery and those that have been reported were not serious or detrimental to ultimate voice improvement [9].

The only disadvantages of laryngeal framework surgery are the elaborateness of the procedures and the fact that clinical observation of 1 day is advised in all but the most simple procedures. Tucker [9] has suggested a reinnervation procedure (nerve-muscle pedicle) in addition to medialization laryngeal framework surgery. Preoperative laryngeal EMG-studies have, however, taught us that most of the "unilateral laryngeal palsy" patients do not have a lack of innervation of the laryngeal musculature, but they have an inappropriate reinnervation leading to synkinesia, tension dysbalance and sometimes even a tendency towards paradoxal laryngeal mobility. Since hyperinnervation of an, albeit subclinical, innervated muscle is physiologically impossible, the effectiveness of these additional reinnervation procedures is questionable.

Several surgical procedures other than laryngeal framework techniques have been described to elevate the vocal pitch. Some authors [21,22] advocate the creation of a web in the anterior commissure. The general idea of this procedure is that the length over which the vocal fold can vibrate is reduced. By reducing the vibratory length of the vocal fold, the pitch will rise. It, however, proves difficult to control the length over which the vocal folds will form a web. Furthermore, mass reduction of the vocal folds by CO_2 laser evaporization and scarification of the vocal fold mucosa have been described as methods to raise the vocal fold pitch. Clearly all of these procedures will have more or less severe negative consequences on voice quality.

In most cases vocal pitch elevation can safely be achieved by cricothyroid approximation, sometimes in combination with an anterior commissure advancement. Approximately 75% of the patients can thus obtain an habitual vocal pitch within the normal female range. Continuation of voice therapy following pitch elevation surgery is, however, advisable, so that the patient is also trained in other factors which designate the gender of a speaker.

Conclusion

Laryngeal framework surgery offers a safe and usually effective method to improve incomplete glottis closure and adjust vocal fold tension. Local anaesthesia enables fine-tuning of the voice during the procedure. The possibility to combine different laryngeal framework surgeries according to the dysphonic patient's needs illustrates the tailored approach to surgical voice improvement.

References

1. Payr E. Plastik am Schildknorpel zur Behebung der Folgen einseitiger Stimmbandlähmung. Dtsch Med Wochenschr 1915;41:1264–1270.
2. Meurman Y. Mediofixation der Stimmlippe bei ihrer vollständigen Lähmung. Arch Ohren-Nasen-Kehlkopfheilkd 1944;154:296–304.
3. Isshiki N, Morita H, Okamura H, Hiramoto M. Thyroplasty as a new phonosurgical technique. Acta Otolaryngol 1974;78:451–457.
4. Isshiki N, Tanabe M, Sawada M. Arytenoid adduction for unilateral vocal cord paralysis. Arch Otolaryngol 1978;140:555–558.
5. Isshiki N. Recent advances in phonosurgery. Folia Phoniatr 1980;32:119–154.
6. Isshiki N, Taira T, Tanabe M. Surgical alteration of the vocal pitch. J Otolaryngol 1983;12:335–340.
7. Isshiki N. Phonosurgery: Theory and Practice. Tokyo/Berlin/New York: Springer-Verlag, 1989.
8. Mahieu HF, Schutte HK. New surgical techniques for voice improvement. Arch Otorhinolaryngol 1989;246:397–402.
9. Tucker HM. Complications of laryngeal framework surgery for phonation disorders. Operat Tech Otolaryngol Head Neck Surg 1993;4(3):232–235.
10. Montgomery WW, Montgomery SK, Warren MA. Thyroplasty simplified. Operat Tech Otolaryngol Head Neck Surg 1993;4(3):223–231.
11. Wanamaker JR, Netterville JL, Ossoff RH. Phonosurgery: silastic medialization for unilateral vocal fold paralysis. Operat Tech Otolaryngol Head Neck Surg 1993;4(3):207–217.
12. Tucker HM, Wanamaker JR, Trott M et al. Complications of laryngeal framework surgery. Laryngoscope 1993;103:525–528.
13. Brally RC, Bull GL, Gore CH, Edgerton MT. Evaluation of vocal pitch in male transsexuals. J Comm Disord 1978;2:443–449.
14. Oates JM, Dacakis D. Speech pathology considerations in the management of transsexualism; a review. Br J Disord Comm 1983:139–151.
15. Tucker HM. Anterior commissure laryngoplasty for adjustment of vocal fold tension. Ann Otol Rhinol Laryngol 1985;94:547–549.
16. Ford CM. Laryngeal injection techniques. In: Ford CM, Bless DM (eds) Phonosurgery: Assessment and Management of Voice Disorders. New York: Raven Press, 1991:123–141.
17. Rubin HJ. Misadventures with injectable polytef (Teflon). Arch Otolaryngol 1975;101:114–116.
18. Lewy RB. Teflon injection in the vocal cord: complications, errors and precautions. Ann Otol Rhinol Laryngol 1983;92:473–474.
19. Tucker HM. Complications after surgical management of the paralyzed larynx. Laryngoscope 1983;93:295–298.
20. Pohris E, Kleinsasser O. Stenosis of the larynx following Teflon injection. Arch Otorhinolaryngol 1987;244:44–48.
21. Donald PJ. Voice change surgery in the transsexual. Head Neck Surg 1982;4:433–437.
22. Waar CH. Stemveranderingen bij transsexuelen door operatie. Logopedie en Foniatrie 1986;58: 135–137.

Voice restoration and rehabilitation postlaryngectomy

Voice Update.
M. Pais Clemente, editor.

An integrated postlaryngectomy rehabilitation program

Philip C. Doyle
Department of Communicative Disorders, Vocal Production Laboratory, The University of Western Ontario, London, Ontario, Canada

Abstract. The loss of one's larynx due to cancer results in a variety of changes that cross anatomical, physiological, and psychological boundaries. Although oncologic concerns are primary for those undergoing laryngectomy, the loss of verbal communication clearly results in significant challenges to one's wellbeing. According to the World Health Organization (1980) three fundamental areas and their impact on an individual's rehabilitation must be considered: 1) impairment, 2) disability, and 3) handicap. Thus, if rehabilitation is to be successful, professionals who work with individuals who undergo laryngectomy must address the comprehensive effects of such changes on the person. This paper addresses the importance of both primary and collateral concerns encountered by individuals following laryngectomy.

Key words: alaryngeal speech, head and neck cancer, laryngectomy, quality of life, speech rehabilitation.

Introduction

The loss of an individual's larynx due to cancer results in a variety of changes that cross anatomical, physiological, and psychological boundaries. Over the past 40 years, significant changes have been witnessed in the treatment and rehabilitation of individuals with laryngeal cancer [1]. During the past several decades, more refined diagnostic procedures have permitted widespread consideration of additional treatment options such as partial or "conservation" laryngeal surgery [2,3]. Yet despite conservation laryngectomy procedures, many patients with larger tumors of the larynx will require total laryngectomy. Surgical resection associated with tumor removal will always be guided by the need to meet oncologic safety [1,2]. Therefore, more radical surgical procedures such as total laryngectomy are often necessary when a larger laryngeal tumor is identified. When total laryngectomy is undertaken, profound changes in anatomy, physiology, and verbal communication will be noted post-surgically. Because of the breadth of these changes, rehabilitation requires an integrated approach, both from the perspective of the types of professional expertise required, and the domains that will be addressed.

There is no disagreement among professionals who work with patients who are diagnosed with laryngeal cancer, that total laryngectomy has a significant and far-reaching impact on the patient and members of his or her family. This includes the

Address for correspondence: Philip C. Doyle PhD, Department of Communicative Disorders, Vocal Production Laboratory, Elborn College, The University of Western Ontario, London, Ontario, Canada N6G 1H1. E-mail: pdoyle@uwovax.uwo.ca possibility of changes in vocational and avocational interests. Clearly, the patient who undergoes total laryngectomy must confront real and significant changes in a variety of domains. However, the impact of laryngectomy has been viewed in a somewhat narrow manner over the past decades. Although specific areas of change may be noted due to the direct effects of anatomical and physiological alteration, many additional changes are likely to be noted over time. Adaptation and coping with these changes subsequent to laryngectomy is very much a dynamic process, hence, the patient's expectations and experiences in the postoperative period are critical factors that have great potential to influence rehabilitative success. For this reason, it is essential that professionals who work with those individuals who undergo laryngectomy seek to broaden their understanding of some of the issues that may have direct influence on rehabilitation following surgery. That is, although most clinicians are cognizant of many of the changes that will be noted postlaryngectomy, the consideration of other issues that may be less common, and perhaps particular to a given patient, is likely to arise. In order to address some of these concerns in the following sections of this paper, an attempt is made to provide a brief review of issues that many clinicians are fully aware of as it relates to total laryngectomy. Much of this basic information is unchanged from the seminal work offered by Diedrich and Youngstrom [4], Gardner [5], and Snidecor [6]. Thus, an expansion of traditional clinical considerations will be provided. This expansion will hopefully raise clinical awareness of some subtle, but perhaps more important issues that may affect each patient's rehabilitation following total laryngectomy.

Basic components of the postlaryngectomy rehabilitation program

The most comprehensive rehabilitation program for those with laryngeal cancer must integrate both the content of information provided and the appropriate professional expertise so that accurate and complete information is available. Specifically, the provision of adequate information to the patient, both preoperatively and postoperatively, is critical [7–9]. But, professionals from a variety of disciplines and specialties including medicine, speech science, speech-langauge pathology, psychology, nursing, as well as others, must work cooperatively if this goal is to be achieved. Preoperative counseling may provide the single most important dimension of comprehensive patient care following the diagnosis of laryngeal cancer. Such counseling is also likely to form the foundation from which a successful rehabilitation outcome may evolve [7]. Clinicians must recognize that counseling is an integral component of comprehensive patient care in those who will undergo or have undergone surgical treatment for laryngeal cancer. Information provided to the patient and members of his or her family should begin with presentation of general information (i.e., information that all patients will need to know in relation to their surgery). While presentation of specific information as it pertains to each patient's needs must also be undertaken, this is best done in the postoperative period [7–9]. Continued provision of information may be required for many patients into the long-term postlaryngectomy period as specific problems and concerns arise.

Postoperative alaryngeal speech options

An important component of any pre- or early postoperative counseling session should focus on one issue – patients need to know that alaryngeal speech options exist and that in most centers, these methods are available to them. These options include traditional esophageal speech, use of a variety of electronic artificial laryngeal devices (either intraoral or transcervical devices), and tracheoesophageal (TE) speech [10] using a TE puncture voice prosthesis [7,10]. The presentation of information about these alaryngeal options to the patient and possibly members of his or her family, should be conducted in an unbiased fashion. That is, the relative advantages and disadvantages of each potential alaryngeal speech option should be provided to the patient without setting up one method as being superior to another. The rationale behind such an approach is based on a belief that if accurate and complete information is offered, the patient will be better prepared to determine which option may be most suitable to their unique social, vocational, and avocational needs. Ultimately, the patient needs to know that at least one of the three primary alaryngeal options is likely to provide a voice source that will allow them to learn to speak again in the postoperative period. Direct therapeutic intervention that focuses on the acquisition, development, and refinement of vocal and speech skills using one of these three alaryngeal methods should ideally seek to provide a fully functional method of verbal communication that is not restrictive to the patient's communicative needs. However, while many patients are able to acquire highly functional and serviceable alaryngeal voice and speech, additional concerns that often may be considered as collateral issues may have an even more significant influence on the success or failure of their postlaryngectomy rehabilitation. The issues discussed in the following section of this paper should not be interpreted as all-inclusive, but rather, as a thumbnail sketch of some of the concerns that may impact on the patient's well-being following laryngectomy, whether surgical treatment is undertaken using a conservative (partial) or radical (total) laryngectomy procedure.

The influence of laryngectomy on quality of life

Unfortunately, the influence of laryngectomy on the individual in the more intrinsic, personal, qualitative domain is frequently considered in an incomplete manner. Though "quality of life" is by no means a secondary concern of many professionals involved with those with laryngeal cancer, its interpretation or definitional boundaries at times may be incomplete. Professionals must acknowledge that the success of a given treatment procedure cannot be adequately assessed without addressing those qualitative dimensions that are specific and important to each individual patient. According to the definition provided by the World Health Organization [11], quality of life comprises a "...state of complete physical, mental, and social wellbeing, and not merely the absence of disease or infirmity." More simply stated, the removal of malignant tissue via total laryngectomy may result in alterations that will influence the individual for the remainder of his or her life. These changes may result in significant levels of impairment that impact on more that just communicative behavior. The influence of the disease (cancer), its diagnosis and treatment (effects of surgery, etc.), and subsequent outcome (physical disfigurement, loss of normal verbal communication, etc.) also may restrict the patient's quality of life [7].

Clinicians who work with individuals diagnosed and treated for laryngeal cancer clearly realize and typically address the basic domains that are directly affected by conservation or total laryngectomy. These broad domains consist of: 1) anatomical changes, 2) physiologic reductions, and 3) psychological constraints. The details of these three areas must be addressed with all patients in any comprehensive rehabilitation program. As noted, such information will be best provided with input from a variety of professional sources. Using this type of multidisciplinary approach for the provision of information as part of a comprehensive program of patient care would appear to offer the patient the greatest possible opportunity for full understanding of the changes that he or she will experience. Nevertheless, the dramatic and far-reaching effects of laryngectomy on the person cannot be fully appreciated until well into the postoperative period. Although the three broad domains noted permit understanding of the obvious changes that will occur, the range of problems that are likely to be encountered by many patients remains unknown. To better understand the more extensive impact of anatomical, physiological, and psychological changes, these critical and widely acknowledged domains may be best understood if recast from a slightly different perspective.

Expanding the definition of the postsurgical effects of total laryngectomy

Using the World Health Organization's framework for disability [11], conservation or total laryngectomy will result in varying levels of physical impairment, functional disability, and social handicap. These more expansive domains appear better suited for assessing the impact of laryngectomy on the patient's comprehensive wellbeing and their resultant posttreatment quality of life. Questions related to quality of life issues in cancer patients is not a new area of clinical inquiry [12,13]. Quality of life is characterized by a sense that life is worth living and that living has meaning to the patient and others [7]. In this regard, clinicians must consider the effects of a cancer diagnosis, its treatment, and the subsequent residual outcome on the patient's wellbeing. Rehabilitative efforts also must consider the social consequences of the problem. Specifically, the diagnosis and treatment of cancer is often viewed in a rather myopic manner where the treatment itself may be perceived as the "end result" in a patient's care. The contemporary view places increased importance on what occurs in the postdiagnosis and treatment period. Medical treatment is best viewed as the initial stage of the rehabilitation process and the period following treatment may comprise the essential components that ultimately define the true success or failure of treatment (regardless of treatment modality). Treatment success encompasses more than "how long" one lives. A patient who survives for 1 year following cancer diagnosis does not necessarily experience a less complete or fulfilling life than another patient who survives 5 years. It is the quality of what occurs in any given period of time that ultimately defines the "success" of any treatment.

Because of the multidimensional nature of any individual's quality of life, a patient's outcome following treatment for a specific illness is defined along a number of dimensions. For example, while the disease may be eliminated by treatment, the diagnosis itself and/or the primary treatment may result in significant changes that affect the patient's physical, psychological, social, and psychosocial wellbeing. This is certainly evident when treatment results in a noticeable alteration from what is considered to be "normal", whether the changes are physical or otherwise. Though all professionals working with those who are treated for laryngeal cancer are likely to agree that an individual's communicative capacity is of extreme importance, the underlying contribution of communication may be slightly more opaque. Specifically, communication is the essence of a person's personal and social identity [14].

The acknowledgment of illness offers the individual a unique perspective into what qualitative dimensions define health [7]. Because of this, clinicians must consider both quantitative and qualitative aspects of rehabilitation in the hope of optimizing each patient's chance of success. But the astute clinician must also acknowledge the fact that serious illness challenges more than just one's physical health; the patient's emotional and psychological wellbeing is contested and jeopardized. We must not forget that the patient with cancer often confronts stigmata that commonly surround a diagnosis of malignant disease [7].

To briefly expand on this issue, three basic elements are of importance following the diagnosis and treatment of laryngeal cancer: 1) control of malignancy, 2) patient adaptation to anatomical and physiological alterations resulting from treatment, and 3) the patient's long-term psychological and social adjustment. The patient must also cope with the subtle stigma frequently associated with cancer. Thus, the stigma of cancer as a disease, partial or total laryngectomy as the treatment, the disruption of self-concept and body image when disfigurement occurs, as well as postoperative changes in voice and speech production, may significantly impact on recovery and rehabilitation. Therefore, "aesthetic" concerns may emerge for the disease class, the patient's physical appearance, as well as for changes that occur with the new vocal source and subsequent postlaryngectomy verbal (i.e., alaryngeal) communication [7].

The social consequences of laryngectomy

The central feature of the stigmatized individual's situation in life revolves around the question of their "acceptance" by society. This acceptance, when combined with the vocal and communication deficit following either partial or total laryngectomy may present significant challenges to the laryngectomized patient's social competence [14]. Namely, it is society that establishes the criteria defining normality and abnormality [15]. Preconceived standards which define ordinary and natural, permits "society to transform them into normative expectations" [15]. Expectation, therefore, provides a construct from which comparison and evaluation emerges. Individuals "...who do not depart negatively" from the expectation are considered "normal" [15]. In those who undergo partial or total laryngectomy, physical changes, the abnormality in voice/speech quality, and ultimately, why this occurred, may be judged negatively by others. Those who do not conform are "discredited" and one's social identity is threatened. In essence, the individual's social identity is judged relative to the preconceived expectation by others. This expected conformity has been termed a "virtual social identity" [15]. Gender-based concerns relating to expectation must also be considered, particularly with the increasing number of females who will undergo laryngectomy. Such concerns also may be quite independent from what anatomy remains in those who receive less radical surgical methods. That is, in some instances, partial laryngectomy may result in relatively greater levels of disability for a female as opposed to a male patient.

From a voice and speech perspective, data also suggest that the extent of surgery does not always correlate well with postsurgical voice, both in the success of acquisition, and the character and quality of the vocal signal. Preconceived notions of what can be expected following laryngectomy are frequently problematic and these concerns must be addressed relative to each patient's needs and desires [7]. When considered with the concept of "normal expectations" [15], one can see the social importance of achieving acceptable behaviors, both vocally and socially. As stated by Prutting [15], "it is one's social identity that is often affected by having a speech, language, and/or hearing disorder". Although the speech-language pathologist must exhibit a comprehensive understanding of anatomic and physiologic sequelae of laryngectomy, options for speech and voice rehabilitation, and the generalized effects of laryngectomy and alaryngeal communication on the patient, the clinician must also develop an awareness for other factors that ultimately influence the success of rehabilitative efforts [15]. The loss of "normal" verbal communication may isolate some patients from re-entering a variety of activities. However, when coupled with other stigmatizing factors (e.g., cancer, disfigurement, etc.) the collective effects on recovery and rehabilitation may be underestimated.

Conclusion

In summary, rehabilitation following laryngectomy should be guided by one primary goal: to provide the patient with the greatest opportunity for returning to as normal a life as possible. This goal will always be at the core of a successful program of rehabilitation. All patients with laryngeal cancer will endure significant changes and restrictions following either conservative (partial) or radical (total laryngectomy) surgical treatment for laryngeal cancer. Again, we must accept the individualized needs and expectations, as well as the impact of laryngectomy on the patient's total being. This includes comprehensive consideration of factors that influence vocational and avocation interests, social interaction, and family dynamics. As such, the patient is best suited to define the parameters of how truly successful treatment has been. Regardless of specialty, it is incumbent on clinicians who serve these individuals to determine the relative impact of laryngectomy on each patient's postsurgical quality of life. Clearly, we are in a unique position to evaluate and address the multifaceted and complex issues that cut to the core of what makes each patient an individual. If we can begin to consider and acknowledge the importance of these collateral, qualitative issues in clinical practice, we will no doubt be in a position to offer the best and most complete care to our patients. By doing so, the chance of rehabilitative success would appear to be enhanced considerably.

References

1. Bailey BJ. Glottic carcinoma. In: Bailey BJ, Biller HF (eds) Surgery of The Larynx. Philadelphia: W.B. Saunders, 1985;257–278.
2. Biller HF. Conservation surgery of the larynx: Past, present, and future. J Laryngoscope 1987; 97:38–41.
3. Silver CE. Surgery for Cancer of The Larynx and Related Structures. New York: Churchill-Livingstone, 1981.
4. Diedrich WM, Youngstrom KA. Alaryngeal Speech. Springfield: Charles C. Thomas, 1966.
5. Gardner WH. Laryngectomy Speech and Rehabilitation. Springfield: Charles C. Thomas, 1971.
6. Snidecor JC. Speech Rehabilitation of The Laryngectomized. Springfield: Charles C. Thomas, 1978.
7. Doyle PC. Foundations of Voice and Speech Rehabilitation Following Laryngeal Cancer. San Diego: Singular Publishing Group, 1994.
8. Salmon SJ. Pre- and postoperative conferences with the laryngectomized and their spouses. In: Keith RL, Darley FL (eds) Laryngectomee Rehabilitation. San Diego: College-Hill Press, 1986;379–402.
9. Reed CG. Surgical-prosthetic techniques for alaryngeal speech. J Comm Dis 1983;8:109–124.
10. Singer MI, Blom ED. An endoscopic technique for restoration of voice after laryngectomy. J Ann Otol Rhinol Laryngol 1980;89:529–533.
11. World Health Organization – World Health Assembly. International Classification of Impairments, Disabilities, and Handicaps: A Manual of Classification Relating to The Consequences of Disease. Geneva, Switzerland: WHO, 1980.
12. McNeil BJ, Weichselbaum R, Pauker SG. Speech and survival: Tradeoffs between quality and quantity of life in laryngeal cancer. N Engl J Med 1981;305:982–987.
13. Welch-McCaffrey D, Hoffman B, Leigh SA, Loescher LJ, Meyskens FL. Surviving adult cancers. Part 2: Psychosocial implications. J Ann Int Med 1989;111:517–523.
14. Prutting CA. Pragmatics as social competence. J Speech Hear Dis 1982;47:123–134.
15. Goffman E. Stigma: Notes on the Management of a Spoiled Identity. Englewood Cliffs, NJ: Prentice Hall, 1963.

Voice Update.
M. Pais Clemente, editor.

Experience with voice preservation and restoration using shunts

Alberto Staffieri
E.N.T. Clinic, University of Udine, Italy

Abstract. Voice rehabilitation after total laryngectomy is critical to the patient's future. It has become difficult to make the choice of a solely surgical shunt because of the availability of other valid alternatives. Nevertheless, this choice is still frequently made. Recent works have, in fact, demonstrated that a significant percentage of such procedures are used throughout the world. This paper intends to answer some questions regarding experience with voice preservation and restoration using shunts. It will show who uses these techniques, how they are used, when and why. Examination of the results will make it possible to determine what is true and what is false in all that has been said about shunts.

Key words: shunt, speech rehabilitation, total laryngectomy.

Background

The prevailing question which arises whenever one deals with the topic of speech rehabilitation after total laryngectomy is: Is such rehabilitation necessary? The obvious answer to this question is an overwhelming "yes". Of course, this in turn leads to the second question: What type of rehabilitation should be performed? The latter question is much more difficult to answer. Since it is fundamental to the patient's future it requires a wide range of data from all parts of the world.

Some initial insights can be drawn from recent statistical work on voice rehabilitation after total laryngectomy written by Lopez et al. in 1987 [1]. It appears that in the USA shunts are used in approximately 15% of the patients, although it is not particularly clear exactly what type of procedures are used. However, Lopez does make an astute observation when he says that 15% may not reflect the general practice of head and neck surgery in the USA. In fact, the questionnaires used in the study were directed to the relatively select group of society members and thus reflect the work of those who are also involved in research. Almost the same study was performed in Germany by Hagen in 1990 [2] and, in clinical practice, shunts were not even used in 1% of the patients.

Methods

The key word here is obviously research. When does one perform research? When one is unsatisfied with what one has and wants to makes progress; after all "necessity

Address for correspondence: Alberto Staffieri, E.N.T. Clinic, University of Udine, Policlinico Città di Udine, Viale Venezia 410, 33100 Udine, Italy.

is the mother of invention".

Another important factor for comparison emerges from the last three international congresses on the topic (E.G.F.L. Meeting, Grado, Italy, September 1993; Second World Congress on Laryngeal Cancer, Sydney, February 1994; Pacific Voice Conference, San Francisco, October 1994) where an average of one paper was presented on shunts for every three to four papers on prostheses.

The authors who have recently written on purely surgical methods of voice rehabilitation after total laryngectomy are: Brandenburg (USA, 1980), Amatsu (Japan, 1980), Ehrenberger (Austria, 1985), Shu-Ling-Li (China, 1985), Tanabe (Japan, 1985), Strome (USA), Brasnu (France, 1988), Lacau St. Guily (France, 1989), Saito (Japan, 1989), Hagen (Germany, 1990) and Denk (Austria, 1992). The experience of these authors does not involve a large patient population although it does, once more, confirm that purely surgical voice rehabilitation after total laryngectomy is still practiced. However, it must be said that, in daily practice, solely surgical speech rehabilitation after total laryngectomy has fallen out of the limelight. Moreover, new, solely surgical methods for speech rehabilitation after total laryngectomy are being researched in pursuit of an ideal procedure. In all likelihood, given the fact that all the works present nearly analogous data, the ideal procedure has yet to be found.

Discussion

At this point one must take a good look at some of the common misconceptions which have besieged shunts in the past and which still haunt them today.

First of all, from the surgical point of view, it is more difficult to create a purely surgical shunt than, for example, to install a voice button. Moreover, it is not true that shunt surgery is more dangerous for the patient nor does it imply more intra- and postoperative complications. Indeed, any experienced surgeon will realize that even the application of a voice button – a procedure everyone considers "easy" – can still give rise to serious problems.

It is true that the voice achieved with the shunts is analogous to that achieved with the voice button. A comparison of the vocal spectra of two patients – one rehabilitated with a voice button, the other with a shunt – will show them to be identical.

It has been said that the vocal mechanisms are comparable although this has not fully been proven. In a shunt, the vibration of the mucosa takes place much closer to the site of the shunt itself. It may very well be that some shunts vibrate spontaneously.

In addition, the techniques used to create shunts fall into two basic categories: 1) shunts which employ a part of the trachea lying above the tracheostoma; 2) shunts which do not use the trachea but which are created among the muscle tissue between the trachea and the esophagus. Recently Omori published a work entitled "Mechanism of Tracheoesophageal Shunt Phonation" (June 1994) describing the hypothetical formations for the neoglottis [3]. However, his hypotheses are only valid for those shunts which do not use the trachea. Instead, those that do bypass the area of the thyropharyngeal and cricopharyngeal muscles leading to the formation of the voice in the hypopharynx. Moreover, a small portion of the trachea in this hypopharynx might serve as a spontaneous dilator; it could leave the pharynx slightly dilated, just enough to provide some "tone" to the voice. This difference explains why those shunts using the trachea above the tracheostoma do not require selective myotomy. Further confirmation of the above could be the higher site of vibration closer to the air source as mentioned above.

Another factor involved is that while it is true that the shunts give rise to greater problems in terms of inhalation and passage of liquids and saliva through the esophagus into the trachea, it is not true that the percentage of these problems is extremely high. Such complications are linked to the technique used, to the surgeon's ability and to individual patient-related problems.

But there is one other factor which is often overlooked. Should a shunt leak it is always possible to insert a voice button at a later date but it is not possible to create a functional shunt after a hole has been made between the trachea and the esophagus.

References

1. Lopez MJ et al. Voice rehabilitation practices among head and neck surgeons. J Ann Otol Rhinol Laryngol 1987;96:261–263.
2. Hagen R. Voice rehabilitation after total laryngectomy in West Germany (in German). J HNO 1990;38:417–420.
3. Omori K et al. Mechanism of tracheoesophageal shunt phonation. J Arch Otolaryngol Head Neck Surg 1994;120,648–692.

Voice Update.
M. Pais Clemente, editor.

Voice results using the indwelling Provox® voice prosthesis

F.J.M. Hilgers, A.J.M Balm, R.T. Gregor, A.H. Ackerstaff and B.E.G.M. Scholtens
Department of Otolaryngology — Head and Neck Surgery, The Netherlands Cancer Institute, Antoni van Leeuwenhoek Hospital, Amsterdam, The Netherlands

Key words: heat and moisture exchanger, pharyngeal reconstruction, total laryngectomy, voice rehabilitation, voice prosthesis.

Introduction

Vocal rehabilitation after total laryngectomy has been of major concern to head and neck surgeons ever since the first laryngectomy for cancer was performed by Billroth in 1873 [1]. His pupil Gussenbauer described in great detail not only the actual operation, but also the development and use of two "artificial larynges". These "voice prostheses" enabled the patient "to speak loud enough to be well understood at the other end of a large ward". However, due to major clinical and technical problems, the use of such devices was soon abandoned. After many decades, during which vocal rehabilitation after total laryngectomy was achieved mainly with esophageal speech and/or through artificial sound sources, or without consistently successful surgical methods [2], in 1979 Singer and Blom were the first to develop and use a voice prosthesis successfully, enabling lung powered speech [3]. Since then many more voice prostheses have been developed [4—6], commonly containing a one-way valve mechanism to prevent aspiration, being inserted in a tracheoesophageal fistula, and restoring vocalization by diverting the pulmonary air into the pharynx (Fig. 1).

The increasing use of voice prostheses has considerably improved the prospects of vocal rehabilitation after total laryngectomy. Consistently high success rates have been reported during the last 15 years. Compared to esophageal and electrolarynx speech, a higher number of patients achieve an acceptable voice, enabling communication under virtually all social circumstances. Success rates up to 90% are not exceptional any longer [7—10]. These favorable figures can only be achieved if prosthetic voice rehabilitation is approached as a multidisciplinary team effort [11].

It is important to realize that unlike the traditional situation with only esophageal and electrolarynx speech available, the primary responsibility for prosthetic voice restoration again lies with the head and neck surgeon, who should be aware of all the surgical and technical aspects of this rehabilitation method. In most instances, we believe that failure to obtain prosthetic speech can be explained and corrected on the

Address for correspondence: Dr F.J.M. Hilgers, The Netherlands Cancer Institute, Plesmanlaan 121, 1066 CX Amsterdam, The Netherlands. Tel.: +31-20-5122550. Fax: +31-20-5122554.

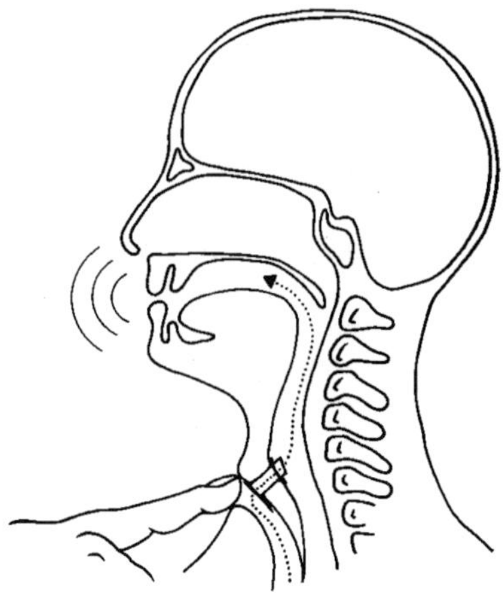

Fig. 1. Schematic drawing of the voice prosthesis in TE-fistula and closure of the tracheostoma with a finger to obtain speech.

basis of surgical and/or technical shortcomings. Optimal results, however, may only be expected if the speech therapist is fully involved and committed, and convinced of the superior early and late voice qualities achievable. Furthermore, good follow-up care is needed to ensure long-term success. In this paper we will briefly summarize the most relevant topics of this intriguing domain of postlaryngectomy rehabilitation, with special attention to the possibilities of voice restoration after more extensive surgical procedures, i.e., total laryngectomy in combination with (near-) total pharyngectomy with or without esophagectomy.

The Provox® indwelling voice prosthesis

In general, two types of voice prostheses can be distinguished, i.e., nonindwelling and indwelling prostheses. The former devices can be removed and replaced by the patient. The latter stay in place until they have to be removed and replaced by the physician at the end of the device life, which is determined by leakage of fluids through the prosthesis or an increased airflow resistance. Indwelling devices have the distinct advantage that the dexterity of the patient plays a less important role in the daily maintenance of the device. This mainly consists of internal cleaning of the prosthesis by the forceful blowing of air through the device or by brushing the lumen of the shaft, while regular replacement of the prosthesis by the patient is unnecessary.

Since 1980, most of the experience with prosthetic voice rehabilitation in our institute concerns indwelling prostheses, in particular during the last 7 years the Provox® voice prosthesis, which, along with a range of special instruments and appliances (Fig. 2), has been developed by us in close collaboration with the manufacturers [9]. Because of our preference for indwelling devices and the fact that the so far available prostheses had a relatively high airflow resistance, we opted to

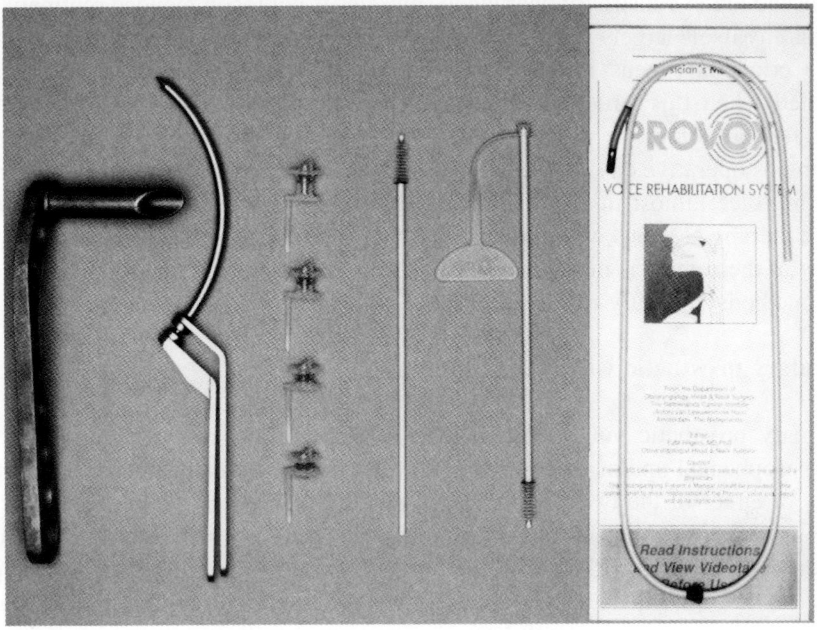

Fig. 2. The Provox® voice rehabilitation system: from left to right the pharynx protector to be used during primary puncture, the trocar and cannula for primary and secondary TE puncture, the voice prosthesis (shaft length 4.5, 6, 8, or 10 mm), the cleaning brush for daily maintenance of the prosthesis, the plug for temporary closure of the prosthesis in case of leakage, and the disposable guide wire for introduction or replacement of the prosthesis, and an extensive manual for the physician (a special patient manual is included in the package as well).

design an indwelling device with improved aerodynamic characteristics [12]. The initial and long-term results with this new device are favorable, as will be briefly summarized below [9,10].

Primary prosthetic voice rehabilitation

We consider primary prosthetic voice rehabilitation the method of choice. As has also been indicated by others, results are superior to secondary prosthetic vocal rehabilitation [8]. However, optimal results of primary voice rehabilitation can only be achieved if the technique of total laryngectomy fulfills certain requirements. Besides keeping in mind the standard oncological principles, care should be taken to create a pharyngoesophageal (PE) segment which is wide and "flexible" enough to enable effortless speech, and to avoid hypertonicity or spasm of the constrictor pharyngeus muscles. Furthermore, the tracheostoma should be wide enough for comfortable breathing and narrow enough to be easily occluded with a finger by the patient when speaking. To avoid hypertonicity or spasm of the PE-segment, a unilateral neurectomy of the pharyngeal plexus is advisable [13]. A myotomy of the middle and lower constrictor pharyngeus muscles is not recommended routinely, since neurectomy itself largely prevents hypertonicity of these muscle groups. A myotomy of the cricopharyngeus muscle (upper esophageal sphincter), however, might be indicated when this structure seems too tight by palpation with the index finger. Voice rehabilitation can start after completion of wound healing, mostly at the 10th to 12th postoperative day. It is our experience that the vast majority of patients regain a useful voice almost instantly and can leave the hospital, mostly after only a few speech therapy sessions, with their communication ability restored satisfactorily. The quality of their voice is more comparable to normal laryngeal voicing than any of the other methods currently available [14].

Secondary prosthetic voice rehabilitation

Secondary prosthetic voice rehabilitation is indicated in case of failure to obtain useful esophageal and/or electrolarynx speech, or in case of dissatisfaction with the results of either of the two. The percentage of successful secondary prosthetic voice rehabilitation procedures seems to be somewhat lower than with primary applications, probably due to the fact that the patient has not been using pulmonary driven speech for some time [8,15]. Nevertheless, with proper training, many secondary patients should be able to acquire a useful prosthetic voice as well. It is our opinion that there are no real medical contraindications for this technique, perhaps with the exception of radiotherapy doses well exceeding 70 Gy in 7 weeks or the equivalent. Severe stenosis of the pharynx or a narrow stoma are relative contraindications since in most patients these problems should be correctable. Also in patients in whom the pharynx and/or esophagus are reconstructed with a gastric pull-up procedure, the colon, or a free revascularized jejunal graft, the method is applicable (see below) [16–18]. If the patient is motivated enough, the method is worth trying.

For preoperative screening, besides regular ENT examination including inspection of the pharynx for the presence of a stenosis or web formation at the base of the tongue, and checking the stomal size, a barium swallow should be performed to check the diameter and mobility of the PE-segment. This is to anticipate possible problems with the introduction of the rigid endoscope and to see whether dilatation of the PE-segment is needed. Whether a preoperative insufflation test should be executed, is controversial [19,20]. The results of this test are not always reliable and a negative result should not be considered as a contraindication against secondary prosthetic voice rehabilitation [19]. A negative insufflation result can be indicative of hypertonicity or spasm of the constrictor pharyngeus muscles, which can be corrected surgically. In general, however, we are not in favor of combining the secondary introduction of a voice prosthesis with a myotomy of the constrictor pharyngeus muscles. We prefer to wait for the results of the speech therapy. Only if hypertonicity of the constrictor pharyngeus muscle becomes apparent, and results do not improve after proper logopedic training, should a myotomy be considered. If a myotomy is needed, the subsequent results of voice rehabilitation can be expected to be considerably improved [21,22]. After secondary puncture, mostly performed under general anesthesia and under broad spectrum antibiotic coverage, speech therapy usually can start the first postoperative day.

Pharyngeal reconstruction and prosthetic voice rehabilitation

Voice rehabilitation after (sub)total laryngopharyngectomy with or without esophagectomy traditionally only has been possible with an electrolarynx. Reconstruction of the pharyngeal defect after subtotal pharyngectomy, with only a small strip of mucosa left, can best be achieved with a pectoralis major myocutaneous (PM) flap. We have experienced that primary insertion of a Provox® voice prosthesis after the application of a PM-flap results in a relatively good voice which is comparable to that after a standard operation. We therefore prefer this reconstruction to the removal of the remaining mucosa strip and reconstructing the pharynx with a free revascularized jejunum flap. The advantages of the PM-flap over the free jejunum flap are obvious: the PM-flap is readily available, is easily harvested, and requires little extra operation time; if constructed properly, there is little chance of stenosis; no abdominal surgery and no special microsurgical expertise are needed. If, however, a total pharyngectomy has to be performed, the free revascularized jejunum reconstruction appears to be very reliable, and combined with a primary insertion of a voice prosthesis results in a fair voice in all patients in whom we have used this type of reconstruction. The voice, however, is sometimes blocked by the autonomous peristalsis of the jejunum segment and sounds "wet" due to the continuous production of secretions. From a prosthetic voice rehabilitation point of view, the jejunum cannot be considered the ideal reconstruction method anymore. Compared to a gastric pull-up operation (if a total esophagectomy is not indicated) the jejunum flap has some advantages: no need for esophagectomy, less abdominal trauma, no intrathoracic trauma, no postoperative dumping syndrome, and primary prosthetic voice rehabilitation is possible.

If the total laryngopharyngectomy has to be combined with total esophagectomy, reconstruction with a gastric pull-up procedure is our method of choice. A relevant observation in this respect is the improved vocalization by using a greater curvature tube instead of the complete stomach. The voice obtained with the tubed stomach clearly has a better intelligibility and loudness. Other advantages of a greater curvature tube over a complete gastric pull-up are: the transposition through the esophageal bed is less difficult, and there is less intrathoracic cardiopulmonary compression, and dumping.

It is our experience that prosthetic vocal rehabilitation after extensive pharyngeal reconstruction is possible in virtually all patients and should be aimed for. Since 1989, positive results with prosthetic voice rehabilitation were obtained after nine pectoralis major flap reconstructions, nine free jejunum transfers, and 11 gastric pull-up procedures. The use of a tubed free radial forearm flap in stead of a jejunum also shows promising results [23].

It can be concluded that in pharyngeal reconstruction, besides oncological and technical arguments, the possibility of applying primary instead of secondary prosthetic voice rehabilitation and the quality of the resulting voice should also play a role in the choice of the reconstruction method.

Long-term results

Between 1988 and 1995 the Provox® voice prosthesis has been used in the Netherlands Cancer Institute in over 200 patients. The study of the long-term clinical results with this device in the first 132 patients and the additional technical developments have provided some interesting data [10]. Our patient population appeared to be comparable to most other reports on prosthetic voice rehabilitation, which show that this technique can be used under virtually all clinical circumstances. The maximum (90 years) and mean (63.3 years) age of our patients seem to be somewhat higher than in most other studies. Many reports indicate that patients over 80 years of age are rarely treated with a voice prosthesis. It seems, however, that there is no real age limit for prosthetic voice rehabilitation. If there is no contraindication for total laryngectomy, primary insertion of a voice prosthesis can be carried out as well. In our series, 10% of the patients were older than 80 years and results of voice rehabilitation are just as good as in the younger age group. In a recent report on defining and predicting "tracheoesophageal success" of the Blom-Singer prosthesis, younger ages appeared to be a significant element, probably because the ability to remove and reinsert the prosthesis appeared to be an important factor [24]. We assume that, especially in older patients, the indwelling nature of the Provox® prosthesis has advantages over nonindwelling devices. The dependence on the dexterity of the patient in the case of the Provox® is low since daily maintenance is easy and mainly consists of brush cleaning the inside of the prosthesis. Although rarely needed, cleaning can be performed easily also by the partner, relative or nurse.

In a recent study, we investigated the patients' subjective ratings of the quality of their speech. The majority of patients reported fair to good intelligibility, both in face-to-face conversation and in speaking on the telephone [25]. Compared with the results of a previous study in our institute, the percentage of patients with a fair or good intelligibility over the telephone increased from 65 to 79%, which is a significant improvement of 14%. Two-thirds of the patients were satisfied with the loudness and slightly more than half with the pitch of their voice. Almost three-quarters of the patients reported satisfaction with the fluency of their speech. Neither radiotherapy before or after surgery, nor age were associated significantly with voice features. Differences between male and female patients were found only for loudness ($p < 0.001$) and pitch, with both being rated lower by the female patients. In general, the fundamental frequency of the voice is too low in female patients. Further analysis showed that patients who were less satisfied with their overall voice quality, reported making fewer telephone calls, being more anxious about speaking with other people ($p < 0.01$), and having fewer friends ($p < 0.001$). A significant negative correlation was also found between the perceived voice quality and feelings of fatigue ($p < 0.01$).

It should be realized that the presence of a voice prosthesis does not prevent the patient from learning esophageal speech and in practice all patients are offered instruction in this form of communication as well. Approximately half of our patients acquire useful esophageal speech in combination with a prosthetic voice [25]. As reported by others, we find that most patients, however, prefer the prosthetic voice because of its better intelligibility, rate, pitch/quality, fluency and availability.

Replacement of the prosthesis

The main reason for replacement of the indwelling Provox® prosthesis during follow-up is leakage through the valve. In general, this replacement can be performed as an outpatient procedure after topical anesthesia. In case of a known or suspected pharyngeal stenosis, dilatation of the pharynx should be performed before replacement of the prosthesis. The special replacement method for this indwelling prosthesis has been described in detail earlier [9,10].

Adverse events and management of complications

In our studies the influence of radiotherapy on the final outcome of the voice rehabilitation seems to be minor, except for the temporary deterioration of the voice during postoperative irradiation [10]. As in other studies [26], we also found no increase in prosthesis-related complications either in the patients who had radiotherapy on the larynx before the laryngectomy, or in the patients receiving postoperative irradiation with the prosthesis already in situ.

As described by others, complications are mostly minor and their treatment is not too difficult [10,11,26]. In applying some form of prosthetic voice rehabilitation one should consider that approximately 25% of the patients occasionally will have problems which need special attention.

A drawback of voice prostheses of a synthetic material is their limited device life, due to *Candida* overgrowth [10,27]. The median device life for the Provox® device is approximately 5 months. Early replacements are almost always needed for leakage caused by *Candida* deposits on the free edge of the hinged valve. It does not seem possible to prevent this completely. The topical application of nystatin on a brush into the voice prosthesis has a positive effect in some patients, increasing the device life sometimes considerably. Other methods are currently under investigation, but definitive solutions have not yet been found. It should be stressed here that the mere presence of *Candida* deposits on a valve, which is still properly functioning, is no reason by itself for replacement of the prosthesis. We have observed that prostheses with extensive *Candida* overgrowth can be left in place for more than 5 years without causing any problem.

Hands-free speech/speech valves

The need to use a finger to close the stoma is an obvious disadvantage of prosthetic speech and for that matter also of other, purely surgical, voice rehabilitation methods. To overcome this problem, speech valves have been developed [28], such as the

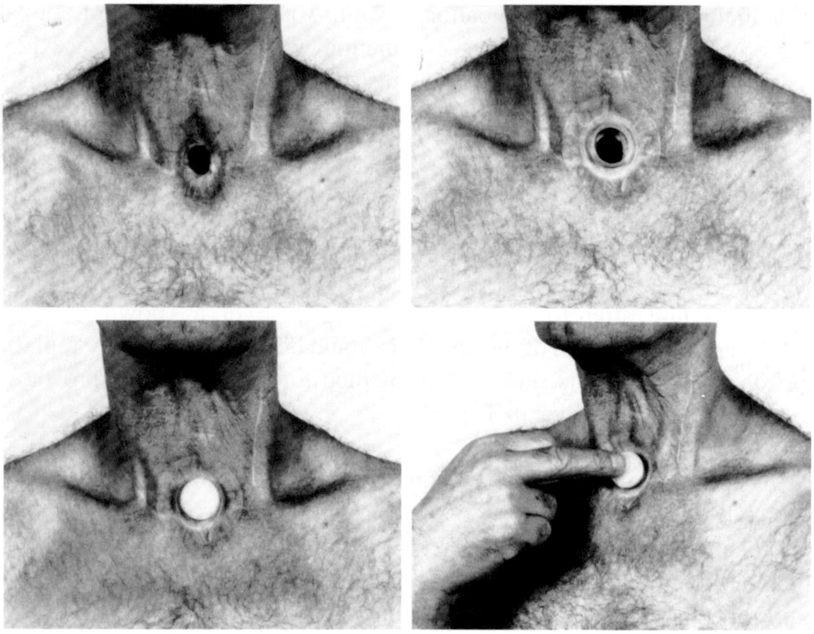

Fig. 3. Provox® Stomafilter: top-left — uncovered stoma; top-right — adhesive housing taped around stoma; bottom-left — heat and moisture exchanging filter with open spring valve in place; bottom-right — stoma occlusion by digital pressure on springed valve.

Bivona valves and the Blom-Singer adjustable tracheostoma valve, which all show promising results. The device is not very user-friendly and requires some dexterity and the application of this device onto the skin around the stoma is somewhat cumbersome. Recently, a new device has been developed (the Provox® stomafilter, Fig. 3) which can be considered to bridge the gap between direct digital occlusion of the stoma and hands-free speech. It contains a heat and moisture exchanger, which clearly has positive effects on the pulmonary problems of laryngectomees [29–31], and a spring valve to be closed with a finger. This device, which is very easy to use in daily practice even for patients of limited dexterity, facilitates stoma closure to a great extent, especially if it is wide, or irregular, or not (yet) healed properly.

Conclusion

Primary prosthetic voice rehabilitation is currently the best option for early and long-lasting successful voice rehabilitation after total laryngectomy, even when combined with total pharyngoesophagectomy. A dedicated multidisciplinary team approach is mandatory for long-term success. The otolaryngologist — head and neck surgeon has to realize that voice rehabilitation has become his prime responsibility again. This means that he/she should be aware of all the surgical and technical aspects of the method. Close collaboration and regular feedback from the speech therapist will ensure the best possible restoration of vocal communication of the laryngectomized patient.

References

1. Gussenbauer C. Ueber die erste durch Th. Billroth am Menschen ausgeführte Kehlkopf-Extirpation und die Anwendung eines Künstlichen Kehlkopfes. Arch Clin Chir 1874;17:343–356.
2. Vuyk HD. Surgical voice rehabilitation after total laryngectomy and Staffieri's procedure. The Hague: Pasmans B.V., 1985. Doctoral Thesis Free University Amsterdam.
3. Singer MI, Blom ED. An endoscopic technique for restoration of voice after laryngectomy. Ann Otol Rhinol Laryngol 1980;89:529–533.
4. Nijdam HF, Annyas AA, Schutte HK, Leever H. A new prosthesis for voice rehabilitation after laryngectomy. Arch Otorhinolaryngol 1982;237:27–33.
5. Panje WR. Prosthetic voice rehabilitation following laryngectomy: the voice button. Ann Otol Rhinol Laryngol 1981;90:116–120.
6. Staffieri M, Staffieri A. A new voice button for posttotal laryngectomy speech rehabilitation. Laryngoscope 1988;98:1027–1029.
7. Manni JJ, van den Broek P, de Groot MAH. Voice rehabilitation after laryngectomy with the Groningen prosthesis. J Otolaryngol 1984;13:333–336.
8. Annyas AA, Nijdam HF, Escajadillo JR, Mahieu HF, Leever H. Groningen prosthesis for voice rehabilitation after laryngectomy. Clin Otolaryngol 1984;9:51–54.
9. Hilgers FJM, Schouwenburg PF. A new low-resistance, self-retaining prosthesis (Provox®) for voice rehabilitation after total laryngectomy. Laryngoscope 1990;100:1202–1207.
10. Hilgers FJM, Balm AJM. Long-term results of vocal rehabilitation after total laryngectomy with the low-resistance, indwelling Provox® voice prosthesis system. Clin Otolaryngol 1993;18:517–523.
11. Schultz-Coulon HJ. Ärtzliche Nachbetreuung von Laryngektomierten mit Stimprothese. HNO 1993;41:597–608.
12. Hilgers FJM, Cornelissen MW, Balm AJM. Aerodynamic characteristics of the Provox low-resistance indwelling voice prosthesis. Eur Arch Otorhinolaryngol 1993;250:375–378.
13. Singer MI, Blom ED, Hamaker RC. Pharyngeal plexus neurectomy for alaryngeal speech rehabilitation. Laryngoscope 1986;96:50–53.
14. Williams SE, Scanio TS, Ritterman SI. Temporal and perceptual characteristics of tracheoesophageal voice. Laryngoscope 1989;99:846–850.
15. Hamaker RC, Singer MI, Blom ED, Daniels HA. Primary voice restoration at laryngectomy. Arch Otolaryngol 1985;111:182–186.
16. Medina JE, Nance A, Burns L, Overton R. Voice restoration after total laryngopharyngectomy and cervical esophagectomy using the duckbill prosthesis. Am J Surg 1987;154:407–410.
17. Izdebski K, Ross JC, Hetzler D, Fontanesi J, Krumpe P. Speech restoration postpharyngolaryngo-esophagectomy using tracheogastric fistula. J Rehabil Res Dev 1988;25:33–40.
18. Maniglia AJ, Leder SB, Goodwin WJ, Sawyer R, Sasaki CT. Tracheogastric puncture for vocal rehabilitation following total pharyngolaryngoesophagectomy. Head Neck 1989;11:524–527.
19. Baugh F, Lewin JS, Baker SR. Vocal rehabilitation of tracheoesophageal speech failures. Head Neck 1990;12:69–73.
20. Blom ED, Singer MI, Hamaker RC. An improved esophageal insufflation test. Arch Otolaryngol 1985;111:211–212.
21. Mahieu HF, Annyas AA, Schutte HK, van der Jagt EJ. Pharyngoesophageal myotomy for vocal rehabilitation of laryngectomees. Laryngoscope 1987;97:451–457.
22. Singer MI, Blom ED. Selective myotomy for voice restoration after total laryngectomy. Arch Otolaryngol 1981;107:670–673.
23. Deschler DG, Doherty ET, Reed CG, Anthony JP, Singer MI. Tracheoesophageal voice following tubed free radial forearm flap reconstruction of the neopharynx. Ann Otol Rhinol Laryngol 1994;103:929–936.

24. Robillard Shultz J, Harrison J. Defining and predicting tracheoesophageal puncture success. Arch Otolaryngol Head Neck Surg 1992;118:811–816.
25. Ackerstaff AH, Hilgers FJM, Aaronson NK, Balm AJM. Communication, functional disorders and lifestyle changes after total laryngectomy. Clin Otolaryngol 1994;19:295–300.
26. Manni JJ, van den Broek P. Surgical and prosthesis-related complications using the Groningen button voice prosthesis. Clin Otolaryngol 1990;15:515–523.
27. Mahieu HF, Saene KF van, Rosingh HJ, Schutte HK. *Candida* vegetations on silicone voice prostheses. Arch Otolaryngol Head Neck Surg 1986;112:321–325.
28. Blom ED, Singer MI, Hamaker RC. Tracheostoma valve for postlaryngectomy voice rehabilitation. Ann Otol Rhinol Laryngol 1982;91:576–578.
29. Ackerstaff AH, Hilgers FJM, Aaronson NK, Balm AJM, van Zandwijk N. Improvements in respiratory and psychosocial functioning following total laryngectomy by the use of a heat and moisture exchanger. Ann Otol Rhinol Laryngol 1993;102:878–883.
30. Hilgers FJM, Aaronson NK, Ackerstaff AH, Schouwenburg PF, van Zandwijk N. The influence of a heat and moisture exchanger (HME) on the respiratory symptoms after total laryngectomy. Clin Otolaryngol 1991;16:152–156.
31. Ackerstaff AH, Hilgers FJM, Aaronson NK et al. Heat and moisture exchangers as a preventative treatment option in the rehabilitation of laryngectomized patients. Clin Otolaryngol 1995;(In press).

Voice therapy

Voice Update.
M. Pais Clemente, editor.

Principles of physiologic voice therapy

Joseph C. Stemple
Institute for Voice Analysis and Rehabilitation, Dayton, Ohio, USA

Abstract. The management of voice disorders by "speech correctionists" began in the 1930s. Since that early beginning a rich and interesting history of voice therapy approaches has evolved, leading to several philosophical orientations of therapy. These orientations include symptomatic, psychogenic, etiologic, physiologic and eclectic voice therapies.

This paper is designed to introduce these management philosophies.

Key words: eclectic, etiologic, physiologic, psychogenic, symptomatic, voice therapy.

Introduction

The management of voice disorders by "speech correctionists" in the USA began in the 1930s. Since that early beginning a rich and interesting history of voice therapy approaches has evolved leading to several philosophical orientations of therapy. These orientations include symptomatic, psychogenic, etiologic, physiologic, and eclectic voice therapies.

Symptomatic voice therapy

The focus of symptomatic voice therapy is on the modification of the deviant vocal symptoms or components which were identified by the voice pathologist during the diagnostic voice evaluation. These symptoms may be breathiness, low pitch, glottal fry phonation, the use of hard glottal attacks, etc. Daniel Boone [1] was the first voice pathologist to organize previous literature and introduce to the profession the symptomatic therapy orientation. Symptomatic voice therapy is based on the premise that most voice disorders are caused by the functional misuse or abuse of the voice components including pitch, loudness, respiration, etc. When identified through the diagnostic process, the misuses are eliminated or reduced through various voice therapy facilitating techniques. Boone [1] stated:

> "In the voice clinician's attempt to aid the patient in finding and using his best voice production, it is necessary to probe continually within the patient's repertoire to find that one voice that sounds "good" and which he is able to produce with relatively little effort. A voice therapy facilitating technique is

Address for correspondence: Dr J Stemple, Institute for Voice Analysis and Rehabilitation, 369 West First Street, #408 Dayton, OH 45402-3065, USA. Fax.: +1-513-496-2610.

> that technique which, when used by a particular patient, enables him to easily produce a good voice. Once discovered, the facilitating technique and resulting phonation become the symptomatic focus of therapy... This use of a facilitating technique to produce a good phonation is the core of what we do in symptomatic voice therapy for the reduction of hyperfunctional voice disorders."

Boone's [1] original facilitating techniques included:

1. altering tongue position,
2. change of loudness,
3. chewing exercises,
4. digital manipulation,
5. ear training,
6. elimination of abuses,
7. elimination of hard glottal attack,
8. establishing new pitch,
9. explanation of the problem,
10. feedback,
11. hierarchy analysis,
12. negative practice,
13. open mouth exercises,
14. pitch inflections,
15. pushing approach,
16. relaxation,
17. respiration training,
18. target voice models,
19. voice rest, and
20. yawn-sigh approach.

From this list, it may be observed that the main focus of symptomatic voice therapy is direct modification of the vocal symptoms. The voice pathologist constantly probes for the "best" voice in the presence of the disorder. When the best voice is found, attempts to stabilize that voice with the various facilitating techniques are made. Symptomatic voice therapy assumes voice improvement through direct symptom modification [2].

Psychogenic voice therapy

Psychogenic voice therapy is based on the assumption of underlying emotional causes for the voice disturbance. The relationship of emotions to voice production has been well documented in the literature starting as early as the middle 1800s [3–5]. West et al. [6] and Van Riper [7] discussed the need for emotional retraining in voice therapy, while Murphy [8] and Brodnitz [9] presented excellent information related to the psychodynamics of voice production.

Aronson [10] first articulated the most complete description of a psychogenic voice disorder when he stated that:

> "A psychogenic voice disorder is broadly synonymous with a functional one but has the advantage of stating positively, based on an explanation of its causes, that the voice disorder is a manifestation of one or more types of psychological disequilibrium – such as anxiety, depression, conversion reaction, or personality disorder – which interfere with normal volitional control over phonation."

Aronson [10], Case [11], and Colton and Casper [12] further discussed the need for determining the emotional dynamics of the voice disturbance from the perspectives of emotions as a cause for voice disorders and voice disorders being the cause of emotional disequilibrium.

Psychogenic voice therapy focuses on identification and modification of the emotional and psychosocial disturbances associated with the onset and maintenance of the voice problem. When the psychogenic causes are resolved, so too will there be a resolution of the voice disorder. Voice pathologists must develop and possess superior interview skills, counseling skills, and the skill to know when the emotional or psychosocial problem is in need of more intensive evaluation and therapy by other professionals [2].

Etiologic voice therapy

Etiologic voice therapy is based on the reasonable assumption that there is always a cause for the presence of the voice disorder. If that cause (or causes) can be identified, then appropriate treatments can be devised for modifying or eliminating those causes. Once modified, the voice production has the opportunity to improve or return to normal [13]. During the diagnostic evaluation, much effort is focused on identifying the direct and indirect causes of the voice disorder. To be successful, the voice pathologist must understand the many etiologic factors that may possibly contribute to the voice disorder. Once the etiologic factors are treated, the vocal symptoms often improve without direct manipulation of the voice components. A common example may be the reduction of the abusive behavior of shouting in children who have vocal nodules. By modifying the shouting behavior, the nodules are given the opportunity to resolve and the voice improves without modification of the voice components which may have resulted from the presence of the nodules (such as lower pitch, breathiness, etc.).

Direct symptom modification (i.e., raising the pitch, reducing breathiness, etc.) is reserved for situations where the inappropriate use of a voice component is found to be the primary etiologic factor. For example, we recently evaluated a patient who attempted to sound more authoritative by using a pitch that was too low with intermittent glottal fry phonation. The use of the inappropriate pitch was found to be the primary cause of the patient's dysphonia and laryngeal fatigue and was therefore modified leading to improved voice production.

Etiologic voice therapy presumes that every voice disorder has a cause. Once identified, the cause can be modified or eliminated leading to improved voice production. If the primary etiologic factor is found to be the inappropriate use of a voice component, then direct symptom modification is used to resolve the problem.

Physiologic voice therapy

Physiologic voice therapy is the term used to describe direct voice therapies which have been devised to alter or modify the physiology of the vocal mechanism. Normal voice production is dependent upon a balance among airflow, supplied by the respiratory system; laryngeal muscular strength, balance, coordination, and stamina; and coordination among these and the supraglottic resonatory structures. In addition, physiologic voice therapy concentrates on developing and maintaining the health of the vocal fold cover. Any disturbance in the physiologic balance of these vocal subsystems may lead to a voice disturbance. As stated by Stemple [2]:

> "These disturbances may be in laryngeal muscle strength, tone, mass, stiffness, flexibility, and approximation. Disturbances may also manifest in respiratory volume, power, pressure, and flow. The overall causes may be mechanical, neurologic or psychological. Whatever the cause, the management approach is direct modification of the inappropriate physiologic activity through direct exercise and manipulation."

Physiologic voice therapy strives to balance the physiology of voice production through direct physical exercise and manipulations of the laryngeal, respiratory, and resonatory systems. In addition special care is taken to account for the health of the vocal fold cover. This care may be related to proper mucosal hydration, attention to voice abuse reduction, or antireflux regimens as examples.

Eclectic voice therapy

Eclectic voice therapy is the combination of any and all of the other orientations of voice therapy. Successful voice therapy is dependent upon the voice pathologist using all of the therapy techniques that seem appropriate for individual patients. Many patients may share the same diagnosis, however, the etiologies and personalities, vocal needs and emotional reactions to their voice problems may be very different. Because of these differences, the same pathologies may require very different management approaches.

Therefore, the voice pathologist is advised not to adhere to any one philosophical orientation of voice therapy, but rather to learn a broad range of management approaches.

The author wishes to thank Singular Publishing Group, Inc. for permission to use this material from Stemple, Glaze, and Gerdeman, (1995) Clinical Voice Pathology: Theory and Management. San Diego: Singular Publishing Group, Inc.

References

1. Boone D. The Voice and Voice Therapy, 1st edn. Englewood Cliffs, NJ: Prentice-Hall, 1971;11.
2. Stemple J. Voice Therapy: Clinical Studies. St. Louis, MO: Mosby Yearbook, 1993;4.
3. Goss F. Hysterical aphonia. J Med Surg Bost 1878;99:215–222.
4. Bach J. Hysterical aphonia. J Med News Phil 1890;57:263–264.
5. Ward W. Hysterical aphonia. J Med Exam Chicago 1877;34:495–505.
6. West R, Kennedy L, Carr A. The Rehabilitation of Speech. New York: Harper and Brothers, 1937.
7. Van Riper C. Speech Correction Principles and Methods. Englewood Cliffs, NJ: Prentice-Hall, 1939.
8. Murphy A. Functional voice disorders. Englewood Cliffs, NJ: Prentice-Hall, 1964.
9. Brodnitz F. Vocal Rehabilitation. 4th edn. Rochester, NY: American Academy of Ophthalmology and Otolaryngology, 1971.
10. Aronson A. Clinical Voice Disorders: An Interdisciplinary Approach. 1st edn. New York: Brian C. Decker, 1980;131.
11. Case J. Clinical Management of Voice Disorders. Rockville, MD: Aspen, 1984.
12. Colton R, Casper L. Understanding Voice Problems: A Physiological Perspective for Diagnosis and Treatment. Baltimore: Williams and Wilkins, 1990.
13. Stemple J. Clinical Voice Pathology: Theory and Management, 1st edn. Columbus, OH: Charles E. Merrill, 1984.

Voice Update.
M. Pais Clemente, editor.

Behavior readjustment voice therapy for the ailing professional voice

M.N. Kotby[1], S.R. El-Sady[1], S.S. Bassiony[1], Y.A. Abu-Ras[2], E.M. Aref[3] and A.A. Orabi[3]

[1]Unit of Phoniatrics, Ain Shaims University, Cairo; [2]Unit of Phoniatrics, Alexandria University, Alexandria; and [3]Unit of Phoniatrics, Assuit University, Assuit, Egypt

Abstract. *Background.* Several techniques of voice therapy have been described and proved successful for the management of the ailing professional voice. Accent method (AM) is one of the holistic approaches for management of voice disorders in general. It may help in establishing a physiological sound base for the aesthetics of the singing voice to be built on.

Methods. In an attempt to evaluate the role of such a treatment modality in helping the ailing professional voice, 10 professional voice users (singers) with variable vocal breakdown were assessed before and after voice therapy. The assessment protocol encompassed elementary diagnostic procedure including interview with patients and auditory perceptual assessment (APA), clinical diagnostic aids (laryngovideostroboscopy and high-fidelity voice recording) and additional instrumental measures including aerodynamic and acoustic measures.

Results. The results indicate a minimal initial pathological profile mainly in the form of phonasthenic manifestations with subtle stroboscopic, aerodynamic and acoustic changes. The vocal breakdown improved posttherapy, both subjectively and objectively.

Conclusion. AM was found capable of reversing and readjusting some of the mechanisms of breakdown of the vocal technique in professional voice users.

Key words: accent method, professional voice, singing voice, voice therapy.

Introduction

Professional voice users include not only singers and actors, but also members of the clergy, Quran recitors, telephone operators and other persons whose ability to earn a living is affected by voice impairment. Being professionals, any trivial changes in their voices may represent a great challenge [1].

There are many manifestations of the breakdown of the singing voice. These include: change of voice quality, reduced pitch range, limited dynamic range, vocal fatigue and prolonged preparatory phase. The expected line of treatment for helping an ailing singing voice is to adjust the aesthetic aspects by the singing teacher. In some instances, however, the breakdown is in the basic physiological control of voice production where management of aesthetics may not be the optimal line of intervention. In such cases reversal of the faulty physiological techniques of voice

Address for correspondence: M. Nasser Kotby, 11 El Ansary Street, Manshiet El Bakry, ET-11341 Cairo, Egypt. Tel.: +20-2–2915434. Fax: +20–2–2915434.

production by behavior readjustment voice therapy may be the logical way to tackle such a problem of the singing voice and to help the professional voice user to resume a career.

The Smith accent method "AM" [2] is one of the holistic approaches for management of a faulty vocal technique. It entails two main tasks:

1. Recommendation of vocal hygiene advice: although vocal hygiene advice is not an integral part of the AM, a few guidelines are given. These are rather limited and simple. Vocal hygiene advice is divided into two categories: 1) "Do/ Don't do" category, including avoidance of alcoholic beverages, smoking, both active and passive, and shouting, both conscious and unconscious. There is, however, no routine recommendation of "complete" voice rest. Such advice is ineffective and difficult to achieve. It is needed only in few acute conditions. 2) "Try to" category, including recommendation of increase of fluid intake, avoidance of frequent throat clearing and sojourn in dry dusty places.
2. Correction of faulty vocal technique [3]. The AM aims at improving voice and speech production. It is a holistic method that restores balance between expiratory phonatory airflow "excitor" and vocal fold muscle adjustment "vibrator". Through the restoration of the physiological balance and timing between the airflow, P_{sub}, and laryngeal muscle contractions, the optimal habitual and comfortable pitch usually emerges. The dynamic range of voice intensity is enhanced by the loudness variations during the accent exercises. Further, AM establishes a better coordination between voice produced at the glottis and the resonatory articulatory activities. Thus, it improves such final aspects of speech production as projection, sonority and prosody through indirect work on coordination.

   AM entails a dynamic integration of:
   a) abdominodiaphragmatic breathing,
   b) accentuated rhythmic vowel play, phonation, and later articulation, and
   c) body and arm movements.

It is important to point out that AM does not give special attention to relaxation exercises. Breathing exercises coordinated with the rhythmic dynamic body movement inherent to the AM are the main tools used for achieving general relaxation.

The AM has a place in the management of professional voice problems. It helps the professional voice by correcting a faulty vocal production technique, thus providing an optimal physiological base for the aesthetics of voice to be built on.

The aim of this work is to evaluate the role of AM as a treatment modality in helping the ailing professional voice.

Material and Methods

The subjects of this study comprised 10 professional voice users, one Quran recitor (a cappella singer), four Arabic ballad singers, two pop and three operatic singers. There were seven males and three females aged between 22 and 59 years (mean = 40). The main presenting symptom was a variable degree of failure of the singing and/or the speaking voice.

The protocol of voice assessment encompassed the following items:

I. Elementary diagnostic procedures including:
   1. Patient interview, comprising among other things:
      a) The patient's own grading of severity of voice dysfunction on a 5-point scale (1 very good and 5 very bad) [4].
      b) Search for possible predisposing factors.
   2. Auditory perceptual assessment (APA) as assessed by a group of expert judges following a modified GRBAS scale [5,6] with four grades from 0 (normal) to 3 (severe dysphonia). The following voice quality characteristics are included in this evaluation (GSLBI): overall grade "G", strained "S", leaky "L", breathy "B" and irregular "I".

II. Clinical diagnostic aids including:
   1. Laryngovideostroboscopy using either the microscope, nasofibroscope and/or rigid telescope [7].
   2. High fidelity voice recording.

III. Additional instrumental measures including:
   1. Aerodynamic measures including vital capacity (VC), maximum phonation time (MPT), phonatory quotient (PQ), habitual frequency (Fo), habitual sound pressure level (SPL), Fo range, SPL range, mean flow rate (MFR), subglottic pressure (P_{sub}), glottal efficiency (GE) and glottal resistance (GR) [8].
   2. Acoustic analysis included measurements of frequency and amplitude perturbation (jitter and shimmer, respectively) and harmonic to noise (H/N) ratio [7].

All of the subjects were given a voice-therapy program utilizing the AM. The program was administered in individual sessions of 20 min each, three times per week. The subjects were evaluated initially and on two follow-up occasions.

Results

The initial diagnostic profile of the subjects showed the following characteristics: the symptomatology was in the form of a change of speaking and singing voice in the form of voice fatigue in four of the subjects. The other six subjects complained of change of singing voice only; three had voice fatigue, two were unable to reach higher tones, and one was unable to reach the lower tones. The APA showed little departure from normality (Table 1).

The instrumental tools of assessment, aerodynamic and acoustic measures, did not show significant change from the normative data. Frequency perturbation, however, showed a highly significant departure from normality (Table 2).

The subjects were diagnostically categorized as: seven dysodia, one phonasthenia with dysodia, two hyperfunctional dysphonia with dysodia, one vocal fold polyp and one with vocal nodules.

The changes in the diagnostic data that occurred in response to voice therapy were calculated as a difference between the initial recording and the last follow-up findings using the paired Student's t test.

The improvement in the patient's symptoms showed a positive grade shift in all

Table 1. Auditory perceptual assessment (APA) (n = 10).

	G	S	L	B	I
0	4	5	4	10	9
I	1	1	1	–	–
II	3	2	2	–	1
III	2	2	3	–	–
IV	–	–	–	–	–

Table 2. Comparison between acoustic measures before therapy and the control group.

	Control	Before	p	Sig.
Jitter (%)	0.100	0.3965	<0.01	HS
Shimmer (dB)	1.005	1.5309	>0.05	NS
H/N ratio	15.020	12.8340	>0.05	NS

Table 3. Changes in stroposcopic parameters.

Parameter	Findings	Before (%)	After (%)
Amplitude	Normal	0	50
	Unilat. decreased	33.3	0
	Bilat. decreased	66.6	50
Mucosal wave	Normal	0	50
	Unilat. decreased	33.3	0
	Bilat. decreased	66.6	50
Symmetry	Symm.	16.6	66.8
	Asymm. (amplit.)	33.3	16.6
	Asymm. (phase)	16.8	16.6
	Asymm. (both)	33.3	0
Phase closure	Normal	16.6	83.4
	Pred. open	50	0
	Pred. inconsist.	33.3	16.6
Glottic closure pattern	Normal	0	50
	Longitud. gap	16.6	16.6
	Fusiform gap	16.6	0
	Hour-glass gap	33.3	16.6
	Ant. waste	16.6	0
	Post. waste	16.6	16.6

10 patients (100%) ($p < 0.001$). The number of grade shifts varied from two (n = 1) to one (n = 9). The APA, as judged by the authors, showed a highly significant improvement in (G) ($p < 0.01$). The voice quality parameters of strained (S) and leaky (L) voice showed highly significant improvement ($p < 0.01$), while irregular (I) quality showed nonsignificant improvement ($p < 0.05$).

Changes in the laryngovideostroboscopic picture showed an asymmetrical, relatively small glottal wave, with variable phonatory gap (Table 3). The changes in

Table 4. Aerodynamic results using paired t test.

	Before	After	p	Sig
Vital capacity (ml)	3004	3252.5	<0.05	S
MPT (s)	19.57	25.44	<0.05	S
PQ (ml/s)	183.14	163.099	>0.05	NS
Hab Fo (Hz)	150.3	156.3	>0.05	NS
Hab SPL (dB)	73.2	69.4	>0.05	NS
MFR (ml/s)	156.8	129.6	<0.01	HS
Fo Range (Hz)	335.7	394.1	>0.05	NS
SPL Range (dB)	19.6	26.4	<0.01	HS
Psub (cm H_2O)				
GE (XE^{-05})	8.76	11.05	>0.05	NS
GR (cm H_2O/	61	143	>0.05	NS
ml/s)	75	59	>0.05	NS

Table 5. Acoustic results using paired t test.

	Before	After	p	Sig.
Jitter (%)	0.3965	0.388	>0.05	NS
Shimmer (dB)	1.5309	0.981	<0.05	S
H/N Ratio (dB)	12.834	12.56	>0.05	NS
Av. pitch (Hz)	142.257	146.97	>0.05	NS

the aerodynamic parameters varied in the degree of significance (Table 2). The VC and MPT were significantly improved, MFR and SPL range showed a highly significant change, while habitual Fo, habitual SPL, Fo range, P_{sub}, GE, GR and PQ did not show a significant change (Table 4). The acoustic analysis of voice showed significant improvement in shimmer, while the jitter and H/N did not show a significant change (Table 5).

Discussion

The initial pathological profile of the subjects indicated that only a small sector had clear auditory perceivable changes of voice. When present, these involve the extreme aspects of the vocal function rather than major change in the quality of voice. The vocal complaint was mainly in the form of subjective feelings of vocal fatigue (phonasthenia). This means that the vocal problem might not be perceived by the clinician while it still undermines the professional performance. The stroboscopic changes observed in this patient's material (mainly a glottal gap) were found to improve with better breath control, and well-synchronized timing between the onset of phonatory exhalation and phonatory coaptation at the glottis. The aerodynamic measures were mainly nonsignificant since the normative range of data is rather wide. This tool is still useful, however, in comparing data of the follow-up studies within the same subject. The only change in acoustic measures was the increased frequency perturbation. This supports the APA observation of only a little change in voice quality, and may reflect an explanation for the nature of the vocal breakdown.

There are several mechanisms through which a breakdown of the singing voice may occur: 1) excessive vocal, physical and emotional effort of the performance, 2) poor acoustical conditions of the hall, and microphones, 3) inadequate professional skill of the performer [9]. Sataloff [10] reported that the most common technical singing errors involve excessive muscle tension in the neck and laryngeal muscles, inadequate abdominal support, and efforts to use the voice beyond the singer's limits. White, being a singer, experienced the status of "acceptable sounds, accompanied by an unacceptable vocal fatigue" [11]. He found that controlled tension in the "breathing" muscles could minimize the tension in the laryngeal muscles.

The beneficial effects of the AM in correcting the vocal pathology may be achieved through:

- Reduction of hyperfunction through better air support and better timing. This may lead to reduction of the phonatory gap evidenced by stroboscopic observation and MFR measurement in the posttherapy readings. The same mechanism may also help in resuming the symmetry and increasing the amplitude of the glottal wave, as evidenced in the posttherapy observations.
- Reduction of muscle tension through the rhythmic abdominodiaphragmatic breathing, dynamic rhythmic body and arm movements coupled with activated articulatory movements (with secondary better projection), may allow the subject freedom to expand the pitch and the dynamic ranges.

Behavior readjustment voice therapy may not be, however, the only line of treatment for the ailing professional voice. Phonosurgery and pharmacotherapy may be attempted when strictly indicated.

In this study, two of the singers had minor morphological lesions. A polyp was treated conservatively since it was of recent onset, small and reddish in color. The nodules, in a female singer, were small and soft, accordingly a conservative line was also adopted. Hasty phonosurgical intervention could impair or end a musical career (Ford, 1994).

Two of the female singers reported in this study were approaching menopause. In one of them, estrogen replacement therapy was attempted. The results await final evaluation. Sataloff reported [10] that estrogen may "forestall the appearance of disturbing changes in postmenopausal singers by many years."

References

1. Sataloff RT, Spiegel JR, Hawkshaw MJ, Heuer RJ. Professional voice users: obtaining the history. In: Benninger MS, Jacobson BH, Johnson AF (eds) Vocal Arts Medicine: The Care and Prevention of Professional Voice Disorders. New York: Thieme Medical Publishers Inc., 1994:72–78.
2. Smith S, Thyme K. Accent Metoden. Herning: Special Paedagogisk Forlag, 1978.
3. Kotby MN. The Accent Method of Voice Therapy. California: Singular Publishing Group, Inc., 1995.
4. Kotby MN, El-Sady SR, Bassiony SS, Abu-Ras YA, Hegazi MA. Efficacy of the accent method of voice therapy. J Voice 1991;5,4:316–320.
5. Hirano M. Clinical Examination of Voice. New York: Springer-Verlag, 1981.
6. Kotby MN. Voice disorders: Recent diagnostic advances. Egypt J Otolaryngology 1986;3(1):69.

7. Kotby MN, El-Sady SR, Abd El-Rahman AG, Abd El-Nasser H, Dawood AA, Helal EH. Pediatric vocal fold nodules: diagnostic profile and alternative lines of management. In: Jacob Sade (ed) Infections in Childhood Ear, Nose and Throat Aspects. Amsterdam: Elsevier Science B.V. 1994:354–361.
8. Kotby MN, Barakah MA, Abou El-Ella MY, Khidr AA, Hegazi MA. Aerodynamic analysis of voice disorders. In: Sacristan T, Alvarez-Vicent J, Bartual J, Antoli-Candela F, Rubio (eds) Otorhinolaryngology, Head and Neck Surgery. Proceedings of XIV World Congress of Otorhinolaryngology, Head and Neck Surgery, vol 2. Amsterdam: Kugler and Ghedini Publication, 1990:20–41.
9. Novak A, Dlouha O, Capkova B, Vohradnik M. Voice fatigue after theatre performance in actors. J Folia Phoniatr 1991;43:74–78.
10. Sataloff RT. Common diagnosis and treatment in professional singers. J Ear Nose Throat 1987;66:278–288.
11. White RC. On the teaching of breathing for the singing voice. J Voice 1988;2,1:26–29.
12. Ford CN. Phonosurgery. In: Benninger MS, Jacobson BH, Johnson AF (eds) Vocal Arts Medicine: The Care and Prevention of Professional Voice Disorders. New York: Thieme Medical Publishers Inc., 1994:344–355.

Voice Update.
M. Pais Clemente, editor.

Principles and outcome of voice therapy in pediatric and younger populations

Anita McAllister and Elisabeth Sederholm
Department of Speech Pathology, Danderyd Hospital, Danderyd, Sweden

Introduction

Dysphonia and hoarseness in children's voices have been the focus of a number of studies since the beginning of this century. The importance of the symptom and thus the relevance of treatment has, however, been questioned. Many researchers and clinicians have felt that the problem clears up by itself during puberty without any treatment [1]. The other opinion – that it could be important to recognize and treat children with voice disorders – has been advocated by Sédlacková [2], among others. She claimed that chronic child hoarseness could occasionally cause organic voice disorders.

In spite of considerable research efforts, investigations of the prevalence of child hoarseness have arrived at widely diverging results (Table 1). The number of children included in these studies varied greatly, ranging from 80 to 32,500. The large difference in sample size suggests that varied research methods have been used.

The morphology of children's vocal cords is quite different from that of an adult. The differentiation of the layers in lamina propria continues through puberty and is not considered fully established until around the age of 15–16 [3]. This might imply an increased sensitivity to vocal abuse. If the child has repeated infections or allergies the edematous mucosa needs higher pressure to accomplish vibratory onset. This increased vocal effort can produce organic lesions like vocal nodules.

A close link between voice problems and psychological conditions such as stress and anxiety has been pointed out by Toohill [4], and several other researchers.

In a previous investigation on hoarseness in children we studied 58 10-year-old children in the Stockholm area [5]. The voices were evaluated by a listener panel of seven speech and language pathologists, all experts on voice disorders. They rated the voices along 16 voice parameters represented by visual analogue (continuous) scales on a test form. Rank-ordered rating means revealed a discontinuity in the distribution for most parameters (for an example see Fig. 1). This discontinuity was used as an operational definition between hoarse and normal voices.

Chronic hoarseness was established in 14% of the children by recording and

Address for correspondence: Anita McAllister, Department of Speech Pathology, Danderyd Hospital, S-182 88 Danderyd, Sweden. Tel.: +46-8-622-5857. Fax: +46-8-622-5857.

Table 1. Prevalence studies on child hoarseness (adapted from [3]).

Name	Year	Ages	N	Prevalence (%)	Terms used
Flatau & Gutzman	1908	7-15	575	42	Chronic hoarseness
Weinberg	1914	7-14	800	26	Hoarse vs. husky vs. clear
Fröschels	1920	4-14	380	0.5	Organic hoarseness
Curry	1949	10	40	55	Hoarse-husky
Curry	1949	14	40	80	Hoarse-husky
Pont	1965	5-14	639	9	Hoarseness
Baynes	1966	6-12	1012	7	Hoarseness
James & Cooper	1966	8	718	6	Voice disorders
Senturia & Wilson	1968	5-18	32500	5	Voice deviation
Gillespie & Cooper	1973	2-18	5054	1	Voice problem
Silverman & Zimmer	1974	5-13	162	23	Hoarseness
Yairi et al.	1974	6-12	1549	5	Unpleasant, husky
Pannbacker	1975	6	93	9	Chronic hoarseness
Sonninen, Sonninen	1976	8	90	65	Unclear voice
Warr-Leeper et al.	1978	11-13	999	8	Vocal deviation
Leeper et al.	1980	6-11	1481	7	Percept. dev. fr. normal
Casper et al.	1981	6-16	96	4;12	Hoarseness
Krahulec et al.	1985	5-6	81	75	Voice dysfunction
Michailova	1987	1-15	3000	6	Dysphonia
Powell et al.	1989	6-10	847	17	Phonatory disorders
Sederholm et al.	1993	10	58	24	Acute hoarseness
McAllister et al.	1994	10	58	14	Chronic hoarseness

evaluating the voices on two separate occasions with a 2-month interval [6]. All children were examined by a phoniatrician, the late Patricia Gramming, using videolaryngostroboscopy. Fifty percent of the chronically hoarse children had longitudinally extended edematous vocal nodules. No other organic laryngeal pathologies were found.

The hoarse group of children were different from the normal group with regard to: sex — they were all boys; and personality — they were regarded as boisterous, talkative, unstable and sensitive to changes in their daily environment. They also spent more time in large groups/day than the children with normal voices. Fifty percent of the hoarse group were bilingual whereas only 20% in the nonhoarse group were of immigrant descent.

Internationally, Wilson [7], Andrews [8], Ørsted [9] and several others have proposed different programs for the treatment of voice disorders in children. Most programs advocate a step by step evaluation and therapy. The aim of the therapy is to modify or change breathing patterns, habitual pitch, loudness, resonance, tension and to increase vocal awareness. These goals are met using different age-related strategies like progress charts, yelling charts, listening exercises, tension — over tension — relaxation exercises, positive vocal images and role play.

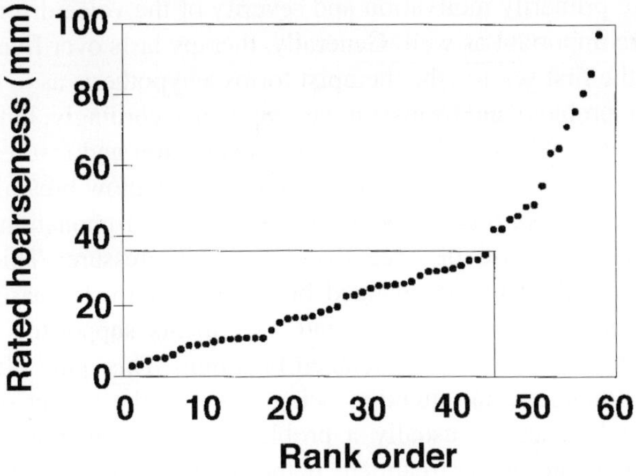

Fig. 1. Rated mean hoarseness values for the 58 voices plotted in rank order. Note the marked discontinuity at the hoarseness value of approximately 35 mm.

Voice therapy for children in Sweden

In general few children receive professional voice therapy in a clinical setting before voice change in puberty. However, most children with voice deviations who turn to the hospital clinics receive regular examinations by an ENT doctor or a phoniatrician at least once a year to check vocal fold status. The traditional outlook has been that voice use is closely linked to personality and thus voice therapy has to be very sensitive to the specific child in question. Furthermore, the children are often unaware of the problem and not motivated to start voice therapy. According to the saying that our children behave as we do, not the way we tell them to, indirect therapy with the parent as a model has been a favored method.

Those children who do get therapy usually are either the more severe cases or those highly motivated, maybe with a special interest in music and singing. They might want to apply to schools with special programs in music and singing. In order to be accepted they want voice therapy in order to normalize their vocal behavior. However, most dysphonic children probably never turn up in the special clinics since they are taken care of by special teachers within the school setting.

Working with children requires other strategies than traditional voice therapy for adults. Adults that begin therapy are very aware of their voice problems. In the case of a child it may be the parents or a teacher that has initiated the contact and pointed out the problem. This makes it necessary for the clinician to work in close collaboration with the parent.

At our clinic at Danderyd hospital we have had a special interest in children's voices due to the research project conducted in cooperation with Johan Sundberg at the Royal Institute of Technology in Stockholm. Quite a few children have received therapy, more recently also in groups, with an age range from 3–13 years. Criteria for treatment are primarily motivation and severity of the voice disorder but age and social factors are important as well. Generally, therapy lasts over five to 10 half-hour sessions. After the first session the therapist forms a hypothesis as to the main factors behind the voice problem and forms a treatment plan accordingly, but anytime during therapy something may occur that causes a re-evaluation and results in a change of treatment strategies. The focus often lies on reducing shallow breathing patterns and then obtaining good coordination between breathing and phonation. Another main focus is to reduce the use of excessive subglottal pressure. This is sometimes achieved as a side-effect of the changed breathing pattern. Increased awareness of natural, well grounded body postures and movements supporting a low point of gravity is closely related to a deep, relaxed breathing. This quite often produces an optimal pitch without special attention being given to the notion of habitual pitch itself. Excessive loudness is usually a problem initially but not an area of main interest until fairly late in the treatment if the problem still persists. Children who have persistent use of excessive loudness should of course be referred to an audiologist for a hearing test. The problem with excessive loudness is quite often closely related to a high-pitched and strained voice. If measured, the voice usually is within normal limits for speaking but is perceived as loud due to the strained quality. With a good vocal technique the child can be loud without harming the vocal cords but it may of course still be disturbing. Quite often these children also have hard/sharp glottal attacks on vowels in initial position. This problem is dealt with in exercises with breathy attacks or /h/-like beginnings. It also continues in the exercises dealing with the sonority of the voice that mainly focus on a relaxed low larynx achieved with prolonged-b-exercises and increased awareness of tension-relaxation. It is quite important to create positive vocal images for these children. Awareness of vocal behavior is achieved via listening exercises and role play where doing right and doing wrong can help the children feel the difference.

Extirpation of vocal nodules in children is very rare and not recommended.

Discussion

Better education of class and preschool teachers with regard to voice use could surely serve as preventive programs as pointed out by several researchers [10–12]. By being positive models of communication the teacher sets the trend in the group. How do you take turns? What do you do when you listen? What are the pragmatics of communication? Other areas of importance can be the selection of songs for the choir. Is this well adapted to the age group and their pitch capabilities? Increasing the class- and singing-teacher's ability to identify children with hoarseness and other voice disorders would enhance the possibilities of an early intervention. Problems detected at an early stage are generally supposed to clear up faster, since the child has not had a chance to firmly establish his or her vocal behavior.

Wilson [7] has stated that improvement should be noted within 3 months. However, in most Swedish clinics this perspective is too long due to demands today of cost effectiveness.

References

1. Håkansson BÅ, Kitzing P. Do hoarse children get voice problems in adulthood? J Acta Otolaryngol (Suppl) 1984;412:43–45.
2. Sédlacková E. Les dysphonies hypercinétiques des enfants, causées par surmenage vocal. J Folia Phoniatr 1960;12:48–60.
3. Hirano M, Kurita S, Nakashima T. Growth, development, and aging of human vocal folds. In: Bless DM, Abbs JH (eds) Vocal Fold Physiology. San Diego, CA: College-Hill, 1983;22–43.
4. Toohill RJ. The psychosomatic aspects of children with vocal nodules. J Acta Otolaryngol 1975;101:591–595.
5. Sederholm E, McAllister A, Sundberg J, Dalkvist J. Perceptual analysis of child hoarseness using continuous scales. Scand J Log Phon 1993;18:73–82.
6. McAllister A, Sederholm E, Sundberg J, Gramming P. Relations between voice range profiles and physiological and perceptual voice characteristics in ten-year-old children. J Voice 1994;8(3):230–239.
7. Wilson DK. Voice Problems of Children, 2nd edn. Baltimore: Williams & Wilkins, 1979.
8. Andrews ML. Voice Therapy for Children. Singular Publishing Group Inc., San Diego, 1991.
9. Ørsted Å. Det logopædiske arbejde med børnestemmer. In: Kølle I, Severinsen KM, Tommerup D, Kjær B (eds) Børnestemmer II. København: Audiologopædisk Forening, 1993;47–60.
10. Deal RE, McClain B, Sudderth JF. Identification, evaluation therapy and follow-up for children with vocal nodules in a public school setting. J JSHD 1976;41:390–397.
11. Cook JV, Palaski DJ, Hanson WR. A vocal hygiene program for school age children. J Lang Speech Hear Serv School 1979;10:21–26.
12. Nilson H, Schneiderman CR. Classroom program for the prevention of vocal abuse and hoarseness in elementary school children. J Lang Speech Hear Serv School 1983;14:2,121–127.

Voice Update.
M. Pais Clemente, editor.

Voice treatment for patients with Parkinson's disease

Lorraine Olson Ramig

Department of Communication Disorders and Speech Science, The University of Colorado-Boulder, Boulder, Colorado; and William James Gould Voice Research Center, The Denver Center For The Performing Arts, Denver, Colorado, USA

Abstract. At least 75% of patients with Parkinson's disease have disordered speech and voice. Previous approaches to speech treatment have been unsuccessful and approximately 4% of patients with Parkinson's disease currently receive speech therapy. This paper summarizes a speech treatment program with established short and long-term efficacy for improving vocal intensity and speech intelligibility in patients with Parkinson's disease. The rationale for this program called the Lee Silverman voice treatment (LSVT) is provided. The essential concepts of the LSVT include: focus on phonation, high effort, intensive treatment, with calibration and quantification. These concepts are described and treatment techniques are suggested. Prognostic factors, follow-up recommendations and early intervention issues are addressed.

Key words: aging voice, neurological voice disorders, treatment efficacy.

Introduction

At least 75% of patients with Parkinson's disease have disordered speech and voice, with every patient developing speech and voice disorders as the disease progresses [1,2]. Reduced vocal loudness may be one of the first signs of Parkinson's disease [3] and is a classic speech symptom together with monotone, imprecise articulation, hoarse and breathy voice, vocal tremor and short rushes of speech [3,4]. It has been suggested that these characteristics are associated with rigidity, hypokinesia and tremor in the muscles of the speech mechanism. For example, reduced loudness has been related to rigidity in laryngeal musculature and bowed vocal folds [5]. Decreased range of tongue, lip and jaw movement attributed to rigidity has been associated with imprecise articulation [6].

While previous approaches to speech treatment for patients with Parkinson's disease have had limited effectiveness [7–9], this paper will present a new method of intensive voice treatment with well-documented short and long-term efficacy [10–13]. The rationale, experimental documentation of efficacy, key treatment elements and considerations for implementation of this approach will be discussed.

Traditional approaches to speech therapy for patients with Parkinson's disease

The typical patient with Parkinson's disease who seeks or is referred for speech

Address for correspondence: Lorraine Olson Ramig PhD, CCC-SP, Department of Communication Disorders and Speech Science, Campus Box 409, University of Colorado, Boulder, CO 80309, USA.

therapy has a moderate to severe speech disorder and complains of reduced speech intelligibility. He and his family express frustration at not being able to communicate effectively and frequently report that the patient withdraws from conversations and many social situations because people cannot understand him.

The traditional speech treatment approach for patients with Parkinson's disease has involved therapy which is delivered once or twice a week in an outpatient clinic. Typically the focus of treatment has been on improvement of articulatory precision, reduction of rate, and enhancement of intonation [14,15]. Patients, their families and speech clinicians will report some degree of speech improvement during the course of therapy, but carry-over or maintenance of the treatment-related changes once therapy is discontinued is generally disappointing. Consequently the ability to communicate deteriorates in many patients with Parkinson's disease as their disease progresses [16,17]. This communication impairment may limit full participation in society of patients with Parkinson's disease.

Intensive voice treatment for Parkinson's disease

In 1987, Ramig and Mead developed a treatment program for patients with Parkinson's disease which focused on voice therapy rather than speech therapy. Their approach was shaped by a number of factors: the high incidence of disordered voice in Parkinson's disease (e.g., Logemann [17] reported 89% of 200 patients with Parkinson's disease had disordered voice), the apparent role of reduced loudness in limiting communication intelligibility, and reports that intensive speech therapy focusing on phonation has been of value to patients with Parkinson's disease [18,19]. Ramig and Mead designed a treatment program to improve perceptual characteristics of voice and functional communication by targeting the underlying laryngeal physical pathology associated with the voice disorder [12,20]. This approach is summarized in Table 1. For example, the breathy, weak voices of patients with Parkinson's disease have been associated with glottal incompetence (e.g., bowed vocal folds [5], anterior vocal fold gaps). A primary therapy goal is to increase loudness and decrease breathiness by increasing vocal fold adduction. The monotonous voices of patients have been associated with rigidity in the cricothyroid muscles. A second goal of therapy is to improve intonation by increasing cricothyroid muscle activity. The hoarse voices of patients have been associated with vocal fold vibratory instability. A third goal of therapy is to improve voice quality by increasing stability of vocal fold vibration.

The specific tasks used in treatment were designed to address these goals through enhanced phonatory effort with immediate carry over into functional communication. This treatment program has come to be known as the Lee Silverman voice treatment for Parkinson's disease (LSVT), named for an early patient.

Documentation of voice treatment efficacy

Given the limited efficacy of previous methods of speech therapy for patients with

Table 1. Logic for development and rationale for therapy goals and tasks for the LSVT. Treatment philosophy is high phonatory effort with immediate carry-over into functional communication.

Perceptual characteristics of speech	Hypothesized laryngeal and/or respiratory physical pathology	Therapy goals and tasks
Reduced loudness	Reduced vocal fold adduction (e.g., bowed vocal folds)	– Increase vocal fold adduction via isometric effort (pushing, lifting) during phonation
Breathy, weak voice	Reduced respiratory support	– Increase maximum duration vowel phonation at greater vocal intensity – "Think loud/shout"
Hoarseness	Rigidity, hypokinesia, in laryngeal and/or respiratory muscles	– Improve vocal quality during sustained phonation and speaking
Monotone	Rigid cricothyroid muscle	– Increase maximum fundamental frequency range – High/low pitch glides – Sustained phonation at highest and lowest pitches

Parkinson's disease, an essential component in the development of the LSVT was to objectively quantify pre- to posttreatment improvement as well as long-term maintenance of treatment-related changes. Statistically significant increases on the variables of maximum duration of phonation, maximum phonation range, and fundamental frequency in reading have been documented following this intensive voice treatment [10,12]. The magnitudes of these pre- to posttreatment differences were significantly greater than those measured in an untreated control group [21]. Three to 6-month follow-up data support maintenance of these posttreatment increases [12]. Corresponding improvements in perceptual aspects of speech production, e.g., intelligibility and loudness, have been reported pre-, posttreatment and at follow-up as well [11].

Ongoing efficacy studies have addressed the underlying physiologic bases for improved communication in patients following voice treatment [22]. Measurements have been made of vocal fold closure [23], intensity [13], subglottal air pressure and glottal airflow [24] as well as speech intelligibility before and after intensive voice treatment. Findings to date support statistically significant posttreatment increases in vocal fold adduction (quantified from videolaryngostroboscopy) [23] and sound pressure level (quantified from the acoustic signal) [13] and suggest that increased vocal fold adduction is a key element in treatment success.

Key elements of voice treatment for Parkinson's disease

The LSVT for Parkinson's disease differs from previous approaches to speech therapy in a number of ways. The treatment focuses on voice production, is intensive (four times a week for 1 month), it requires that patients be habituated to a high effort level during speech production and teaches the patient to be comfortable – calibrated to the new vocal effort level.

Increasing vocal effort

The singular focus of treatment is on increasing vocal effort in order to enhance vocal fold closure and loudness. While patients with Parkinson's disease do have disordered articulation and rate, the consistent focus for all 16 sessions of treatment is vocal effort. It has been observed that even in a mild patient, a consistent vocal effort focus during all 16 sessions is necessary to reach the habitual use of the louder voice. When the focus remains on increased phonatory effort, vocal loudness is increased and this effort generalizes to enhanced articulation as well [24]. Both vocal and articulatory contributions to enhanced speech intelligibility have been documented following treatment which focuses on vocal effort alone [11].

The singular focus on increased vocal effort makes an immediate impact on vocal loudness and speech intelligibility with a relatively simple carry-over task – "speak loud" or "shout". After the first session of treatment, patients are often able to use a louder voice in simple greetings such as, "Hi Honey!" In many cases, this provides the initial positive feedback patients and families need to enhance their motivation and confidence to focus intently on treatment.

The primary goal of treatment is to elicit a louder voice with good quality. This is accomplished through adduction exercises which may include "pushing" exercises [25] and loud phonation. Once the louder voice is established, respiratory and laryngeal coordination at increased loudness levels is trained. Exercises such as maximum duration vowel phonation targeting duration, constant loudness and steadiness are practiced 10–15 times per session with the patient being constantly urged to "go longer, louder and steadier". Fundamental frequency range is another maximum phonatory effort task that is practiced six to 10 times per session. Both of these maximum effort tasks are carried out during each of the 16 sessions and on-line duration and frequency range data are collected on each patient's performance. These daily clinical data are useful for both patient and clinician reinforcement as well as for documentation of treatment efficacy for insurance reimbursement. Patients are encouraged to use the same vocal effort level they use during sustained phonation when they speak. This focus on increased phonatory effort offers a simple target for speech production tasks with the focus being "speak loud" or "shout". Beginning with the first day of treatment, patients identify 10 functional phrases frequently used in their daily environment and immediately practice daily use of their louder voice in these phrases.

Patients with Parkinson's disease have a well-established difficulty in simultaneously executing two different movements [26,27] and many experience impaired cognitive function [28,29]; this may be one explanation why previous speech therapy approaches for patients which focused on multiple levels of speech production (articulation, rate, intonation) have not been consistently successful. In the LSVT treatment approach the simple focus of increased loudness in speech production is targeted hierarchically from words, phrases, sentences and conversation on a week-by-week basis. The goal for dismissal from treatment is adequate loudness during 90% of spontaneous utterances or targeted task during treatment sessions and reports of 80% carry-over outside of treatment. In most cases, this goal can be reached by the 4th week of treatment.

High effort intensive treatment

Additional keys to treatment success include: high effort, intensive treatment and calibration. The treatment style is highly energetic and intensive both on the part of the patient as well as the clinician. The clinician serves as an energetic motivator, constantly urging the patient to sustain phonation "longer, louder, higher and lower". The use of high effort, intensive treatment is based upon neurology and physical therapy practices [30–32] that suggest when pushed to higher effort levels, patients with Parkinson's disease can compensate for bradykinesia and improve task performance. The daily training of high effort to increase magnitude of speech motor output is based upon the similar problems in scaling the magnitude of output (e.g., stride length in walking, letter stroke in writing) observed in patients with Parkinson's disease [33–35]. We speculate that intensive high effort voice treatment teaches patients to rescale the magnitude of speech motor output [12,13] and that daily treatment with intensive practice [36,37] and feedback (knowledge of results) [38,39] facilitates this training. It is therefore essential that patients use this high effort level throughout the majority of each treatment session. Thus, individual, daily treatment is necessary for at least the first 16 sessions of treatment. This enables the clinician to monitor closely the level of effort of each patient and continuously motivate the patient to increase and maintain effort levels. If the patient does not achieve these effort levels during treatment, he will surely not achieve them on his own outside of treatment. In order to habituate this high effort level outside of the treatment room, homework is assigned from the first day of treatment.

Calibration

Habituation and calibration of the patient to the new phonatory effort level is another key component to treatment success. Initially, when using the louder voice, patients complain that they feel like they are "shouting or talking too loud". The clinician should view this as a positive sign because it indicates that the patient is using a higher effort level. The next critical phase is to teach the patient that this effort level is desirable and is not "too loud". This calibration phase is essential for successful treatment. If the patient is not comfortable with his louder voice he will not use it habitually. Activities that are helpful in this calibration phase include feedback with a tape recorder, activities in self-monitoring and group therapy (after the initial 16 sessions). We have found it useful to provide patients with objective feedback through instruments such as the Voice Light [40,41].

Critical considerations

Because the majority of patients with Parkinson's disease have disorders of articulation and rate, a speech clinician not trained in the LSVT will be tempted to spend therapy time treating these disorders. This will diffuse the focus from increased phonatory effort and reduce the magnitude of the treatment effect. In order to achieve habituation of the louder voice, it essential to keep the focus on phonation throughout all 16 sessions of treatment. It has been documented that increased phonatory effort generalizes to improved articulatory precision [24] and reduced rate [13] without diffusing treatment focus to articulation or rate.

Urging the patient with Parkinson's disease to a higher phonatory effort level may be challenging for the clinician. The style of the treatment is positive, energetic and consistently high effort. The clinician has the role of "infusing the patient with enthusiasm." Given the reduced affect and low-energy style of many patients, clinicians may find this to be a challenge. However, it has been reported that even on days when patients report medication problems or fatigue, if the clinician takes a directive, energetic approach, the results are positive. Patients learn that even when they do not feel their best, they can still produce intelligible speech. In order to keep the patient at a high-effort level throughout the therapy session, the clinician must closely monitor the patient's output and continuously encourage this increased effort. If the patient is not continuously urged to high phonatory effort levels during 90% of each therapy session, the resulting improvement in speech and voice will not be maximal.

The clinician may be concerned that increased phonatory effort may be abusive to voice production. Recent data document significantly improved glottal competence posttreatment with no significant supraglottal hyperadduction [23]. All patients must receive an otolaryngological examination before initiating this treatment to rule out any contraindications and posttreatment laryngeal examinations are useful to document treatment-related improvements in glottal competence.

The clinician cannot underestimate the significance of calibration and habituation of the patient to this new phonatory effort level. The patient may use the louder voice in the treatment room, but if he is not completely comfortable with it, he will not use it in functional communication. Calibration and habituation begin with the first treatment session and continue daily throughout all sessions.

Follow-up recommendations

Once the patient has demonstrated the ability to speak with increased loudness 90% of the time in spontaneous conversational speech or during tasks in the treatment room, and reports 80% carry-over outside of the treatment room, therapy can be terminated. This goal requires no less than sixteen sessions of individual treatment. We recommend to the patient and his family that he continue to practice his voice exercises for 10–15 min at least three times a week. Many patients have found a video tape of home exercises useful [40,41].

Long-term maintenance and follow-up treatment

Research data has documented a clear maintenance of treatment effects up to 6–12 months without additional treatment [42]. After 6 months, the maintenance varies depending upon the patient. We recommend that all patients be re-evaluated 6 months' posttreatment. Given the progressive nature of Parkinson's disease, treatment targets may need to be modified. If the voice has deteriorated 6–12 months after treatment, the most common observation is that the patient has "fallen out of calibration". Frequently, two or three voice treatment sessions with encouragement to do homework (at least three maximum "ahs" at the beginning of the day to get calibrated for the day) will get the patient back on track.

Early voice treatment

Early in the course of Parkinson's disease, patients may have a monotonous, hoarse voice which is reduced in volume. If voice treatment is initiated before speech intelligibility is reduced, patients may be able to develop vocal habits which will allow them to maintain communication. Improved and maintained speech intelligibility may enhance and sustain employability for patients with Parkinson's disease in the workforce.

Prognostic factors

A number of factors which increase the likelihood that patients will improve with the LSVT have been identified. This does not eliminate the possibility of improvement for patients who do not have these characteristics. It may mean that in those cases therapy may be more challenging.

Patients with idiopathic Parkinson's disease and the classic voice that is reduced in loudness or is hoarse respond well to treatment. This may be accompanied by glottal incompetence (e.g., bowed vocal folds or anterior gap). The efficacy of intensive voice treatment on nonidiopathic forms of Parkinsonism has been investigated [43,44]. Motivated patients who feel speech is important are good candidates for the LSVT. However, many patients who were not motivated at the beginning of treatment become motivated when they learn that they can improve their voices. Patients who are active communicators are good candidates; however, patients who had withdrawn from communication prior to treatment report that after therapy they talk more because they feel more confident. Patients who are stimulable to generate a louder voice are also very good candidates. While patients with adequate cognition respond well to treatment, positive posttreatment results have been observed in patients who were mildly or moderately demented [45].

Patients with atypical Parkinson's disease

Patients with atypical Parkinson's disease have been treated with the LSVT and improvements have been documented on a case-by-case basis. Pre- to posttreatment results from a patient having had a bilateral thalamotomy [44] and patients having the Parkinson's plus syndromes of Shy-Drager, progressive supranuclear palsy, and multisystem atrophy [43] documented improvements in phonation but of a lesser magnitude and reduced long-term maintenance than observed in patients with idiopathic Parkinson's disease. Patients with laryngeal hyperadduction resulting from either physical pathology or secondary compensatory behavior, have responded well to treatment when the focus is directed toward increased respiratory effort.

Voice treatment: drug treatment interaction

While neuropharmacological interventions have proven effective in the management of many motor symptoms of Parkinson's disease, the speech and voice problems of these patients are not consistently or significantly alleviated by these interventions [5,46,47]. In fact, in some cases, drug-related dyskinesias effect respiratory, laryngeal and oral motor musculature and are severely detrimental to speech production. Since it cannot be assumed that neuropharmological interventions will enhance speech production, it is important that patients receive speech therapy in order to maximize their communication intelligibility.

Swallowing

Swallowing disorders (dysphagia) have been identified in all phases of the swallow (oral preparatory, oral, pharyngeal and esophageal) in patients with Parkinson's disease [48]. While there is a tendency for swallowing disorders to increase as the disease progresses, a one-to-one correlation has not been established. Additionally, it has been documented that patients with Parkinson's disease frequently aspirate but are unaware of their swallowing difficulties or aspiration [49]. Therefore, early diagnosis through videofluoroscopy is necessary to document the presence of a swallowing disorder. This evaluation, usually done in collaboration with a speech pathologist and radiologist, provides objective data on the status of the swallowing mechanism. If a disorder exists, the speech pathologist can teach the patient compensatory techniques in order to prevent aspiration or other swallowing difficulties and monitor the patient changes. Maximum phonatory effort tasks used to increase vocal fold adduction and improve voice production may be useful in reducing aspiration. Clinical reports suggest improved swallowing and less choking following the LSVT.

Conclusion

The majority of patients with Parkinson's disease can benefit from speech therapy designed to maintain and increase their vocal loudness. The LSVT for Parkinson's disease has documented short- and long-term effectiveness. The ability to communicate plays an important role in the self-concept and well-being of an individual.

Therefore speech treatment can play a key role in enhancing the quality of life of a patient with Parkinson's disease. A detailed guide to the LSVT may be useful in administration of this treatment program [50].

Acknowledgements

This work was supported in part by grant from NIH R01 DC01150, The National Center for Voice and Speech P60 DC00976, The Hearst Foundation and The Family of Lee Silverman.

References

1. Oxtoby M. Parkinson's disease patients and their social needs. London: Parkinson's Disease Society, 1982.
2. Streifler M, Hofman S. Disorders of verbal expression in Parkinsonism. J Adv Neural 1984;40:385–393.
3. Aronson AE. Clinical voice disorders. New York: Thieme Stratton, 1985.
4. Darley FL, Aronson A, Brown J. Differential diagnostic patterns of dysarthria. J Speech Hear Res 1969;12:246–269.
5. Hansen DG, Gerratt BR, Ward PH. Cinegraphic observations of laryngeal function in Parkinson's disease. J Laryngoscope 1984;94:348–353.
6. Weismer G. Articulatory characteristics of Parkinsonian dysarthria: Segmental and phrase-level timing, spirantization and glottal-supraglottal coordination. In: McNeil M, Rosenbek J, Aronson A (eds) The Dysarthrias: Physiology, Acoustics, Perception, Management. San Diego: College Hill Press, 1984;101–130.
7. Sarno MT. Speech impairment in Parkinson's disease. J Arch Phys Med Rehab 1968;49:269–275.
8. Allan CM. Treatment of nonfluent speech resulting from neurological disease: treatment of dysarthria. Br J Dis Commun 1970;5:3–5.
9. Weiner WJ, Singer C. Parkinson's disease and nonpharmacologic treatment programs. J Am Geriatr Soc 1989;37:359–363.
10. Ramig L, Horii Y, Bonitati C. The efficacy of voice therapy for patients with Parkinson's disease. National Center for Voice and Speech: Status and Progress Report, vol 1. 1992:61–86.
11. Ramig L. The role of phonation in speech intelligibility: preliminary data from patients with Parkinson's disease. In: Kent R (ed) Intelligibility in Speech Disorders: Theory, Measurement and Management. Amsterdam: John Benjamin, 1992;119–155.
12. Ramig L, Bonitati C, Lemke J, Horii Y. Voice treatment for patients with Parkinson's disease: Development of an approach and preliminary efficacy data. J Med Speech Lang Pathol 1994;2(3): 191–209.
13. Ramig L, Countryman S, Thompson L, Horii Y. A comparison of two forms of speech treatment for Parkinson's Disease. J Speech Hear Res (In press).
14. Hoberman SG. Speech techniques in aphasia and Parkinsonism. J Michigan St Med Soc 1958;57:1720–1723.
15. LeDorze G, Dionne L, Ryalls J, Julien M, Ouellet L. The effects of speech and language therapy for a case of dysarthria associated with Parkinson's disease. Eur J Dis Comm 1992;27:213–324.
16. Morley DE. The rehabilitation of adults with dysarthric speech. J Speech Hear Dis 1955;20:58–64.
17. Logemann JA, Fisher HB, Boshes B, Blonsky ER. Frequency and concurrence of vocal tract dysfunctions in the speech of a large sample of Parkinson patients. J Speech Hear Dis 1978;42:47–57.
18. Scott S, Caird FL. Speech therapy for Parkinson's disease. J Neurol Neurosurg Psych 1968;46:140–144.

19. Robertson S, Thompson F. Speech therapy in Parkinson's disease: a study of the efficacy and long-term effect of intensive treatment. Br J Disord Commun 1984;19:213–224.
20. Ramig L, Scherer R. Speech therapy for neurological disorders of the larynx. In: Blitzer A, Sasaki C, Fahn S, Brin M, Harris K (eds) Neurological Disorders of the Larynx. New York: Thieme, 1992;248–278.
21. King J, Ramig L, Lemke J, Horii Y. Parkinson's disease: longitudinal changes in acoustic parameters of phonation. J Med Speech Lang Pathol 1994;2(1):29–42.
22. Ramig L. Voice therapy for Parkinson's disease: it's worth the effort. A video tape produced by The National Center for Neurogenic Communication Disorders. University of Arizona-Tucson, 1993.
23. Smith M, Ramig L, Dromey C, Darby K, Samandari R. Vocal dysfunction in Parkinson's disease: videolaryngostroboscopic findings pre- and postvoice treatment. J Voice (In press).
24. Dromey C, Ramig L, Johnson A. Phonatory and articulatory changes associated with increased vocal intensity in Parkinson's disease: a case study. J Speech Hear Res (In press).
25. Froeschels E, Kastein S, Weiss DA. A method of therapy for paralytic conditions of the mechanism of phonation, respiration and glutination. J Speech Hear Dis 1955;20:365–370.
26. Benecke R, Rothwell JC, Dick JRR, Day BL, Marsden CD. Performance of simultaneous movements in patients with Parkinson's disease. Brain 1986;109:739–757.
27. Yanagisawa N, Fujimato S, Tamaru F. Bradykinesia in Parkinson's disease: disorders of onset and execution of fast movement. J Eur Neurol 1989;29(Suppl):19–28.
28. Loranger AW, Goodell H, Leo JE. Levodopa treatment of Parkinson's syndrome. J Arch Gen Psych 1972;26:163–168.
29. Pollock M, Hornsbrook RN. The prevalence, natural history and dementia of Parkinson's disease. J Brain 1966;89:429–448.
30. England AC, Schwab RS. The management of Parkinson's disease. JAMA Arch Int Med 1959;104:439–468.
31. Hallett M, Khosbin S. A psychological mechanism of bradykinesia. J Brain 1980;103(2):301–314.
32. McDowell FH, Lee JE, Sweet RD. Extrapyramidal disease. In: Baker AB, Joynt RJ (eds) Clinical Neurology. Philadelphia: Harper & Row, 1986:24–26.
33. Brooks VB. The neurological basis of motor control. New York: Oxford University Press, 1986.
34. Muller F, Stelmach GE. Scaling problems in Parkinson's disease. In: Requin J, Stemach GE (eds) Tutorials in Motor Neurosciences. Dordrecht: Kluwer Academic Publishers, 1991:161–174.
35. Stemach GE. Basal ganglia impairment and force control. In: Requin J, Stemach GE (eds) Tutorials in Motor Neurosciences. Dordrecht: Kluwer Academic Publishers, 1991:137–148.
36. Schmidt RA. A schema theory of discrete motor skill learning. J Psychol Rev 1975;82:225–260.
37. Schmidt RA. Motor control and learning. Champaign, IL: Human Kinetic Publishers.
38. Adams JA. Use of the models knowledge of the results to increase observer's performance. J Hum Move Stud 1986;12:89–98.
39. Adams JA. A closed-loop theory of motor learning. J Motor Behav 1971;3:111–150.
40. Ramig L, Bonitati C, Winholtz W. The Lee Silverman voice treatment. A video tape produced by Wintronix, PO Box 514, Blue Springs, MO 64014.
41. Wintronix, PO Box 514, Blue Springs, MO 64014.
42. Ramig L, Countryman S, O'Brien C, Smith M. Efficacy of voice treatment for Parkinson's disease. J Neurology 1995.
43. Countryman S, Ramig L, Pawlas A. Speech and voice deficits in Parkinsonian plus syndromes: can they be treated? J Med Speech Lang Pathol 1994;2(3):211–225.
44. Countryman S, Ramig L. Effects of intensive voice therapy on voice deficits associated with bilateral thalamotomy in Parkinson's disease: a case study. J Med Speech Lang Pathol I993;1(4):233–250.
45. Mead C, Ramig L, Beck J. Parkinson's disease with severe dementia: effectiveness of intensive voice therapy. J ASHA 31:10–118.
46. Leanderson R, Meyerson BA, Persson A. Lip muscle function in Parkinsonian dysarthria. J Acta Otolaryngol 1972;34:271–278.
47. Larson K, Ramig L, Scherer R. Acoustic and glottographic voice analysis during drug-related

fluctuations in Parkinson's disease. J Med Speech Lang Pathol 1994;2(3):227–239.

48. Logemann J. Dysphagia in movement disorders. J Adv Neurol 1988;49:307–316.
49. Robbins J, Logemann J, Kirshner HS. Swallowing and speech production in Parkinson's disease. J Adv Neurol 1986;19:283–287.
50. Ramig L, Pawlas A, Countryman S. The Lee Silverman Voice Treatment (LSVT): a Practical Guide to Treating the Voice and Speech Disorders in Parkinson's disease. National Center for Voice and Speech; University of Iowa; Iowa City, Iowa (In press).

Voice Update.
M. Pais Clemente, editor.

Preoperative voice therapy: indications, basis, strategies

Rebecca Leonard and Krzysztof Izdebski
Department of Otolaryngology, Head and Neck Surgery, University of California, Davis Medical School, Sacramento, California, USA

Abstract. Laryngeal imaging has significantly enhanced the potential for conservative management of dysphonic patients with benign glottal pathology secondary to vocal hyperfunction. The inclusion of imaging in the voice clinician's evaluative protocol has improved differentiation between those patients likely to benefit from conservative treatment, i.e., voice therapy, and those likely to benefit from surgery. This paper describes pertinent observations derived from the visualization of laryngeal function which facilitate treatment decisions. Information obtained from these observations is considered, firstly, as a basis for prognostication in the choice between conservative vs. surgical treatment and, secondly, as a critical underpinning of conservative treatment.

Key words: benign pathology, preoperative, voice therapy.

Treatment of the dysphonic patient with benign laryngeal pathology related to vocal hyperfunction presents a unique challenge to the otolaryngologist and voice clinician. Both are likely to agree that the patient is an immediate candidate for counseling regarding the causes and consequences of vocal hyperfunction, and that any management plan which fails to consider prevention of future pathology is negligent. But indications for conservative treatment vs. immediate surgical resolution may not be straightforward. Questions regarding the potential response of the pathology to conservative measures, the amount of time allowed for these measures before considering other treatment alternatives, and the specific content of a trial voice therapy program, must all be balanced against the potential risks of surgery for voice recovery.

Recently, a number of treatment decisions have been significantly aided by the inclusion of laryngeal imaging (phonoscopy) [1–3] in the voice clinician's evaluative protocol. The intent of this paper is to discuss the contribution of imaging observations in choosing between conservative and surgical treatments, and in planning effective strategies for those patients selected for a trial of voice therapy.

Comprehensive assessment of the preoperative patient includes a battery of phonatory function studies, including perceptual, acoustic, aerodynamic and perhaps other measures. However, clinical experience suggests that rigid and flexible endoscopic observation of the larynx, and its pathology, at rest and during a variety

Address for correspondence: Rebecca Leonard, Department of Otolaryngology, Head and Neck Surgery, University of California, Davis Medical Center, 2521 Stockton Blvd., Sacramento, CA 95817, USA.

of vegetative and phonatory tasks – we refer to this as a "phonoscopic" evaluation – may provide the best input to prognostic decision making regarding the potential value of preoperative voice therapy. The objectives of this assessment are to:

1. Describe the characteristics of the pathology, particularly as these relate to phonatory physiology.
2. Identify specific vocal practices which may be producing or exacerbating the pathology.
3. Explore new vocal practices which facilitate resolution of the pathology.
4. Prognosticate and implement the most efficacious treatment plan.

Let us consider the first goal: describing the pathology. Most lesions which affect the vocal folds will occasion at least some of the tissue changes noted here – the addition of mass to the vibratory source, increases in viscosity and friction of, in particular, the vocal fold "cover", possible increases in tension in nonmuscular and perhaps even muscular components of laryngeal structures, as well as alterations in blood flow, glandular products and sensation.

On phonoscopic examination, a number of these tissue changes are apparent, and provide clues regarding a lesion's amenability to voice therapy. In general, greater compressibility, evidence of acuteness and lack of organization, greater integrity of the mucosal wave and lack of other pathology can be considered positive prognostic indicators for preoperative therapy. Our experience suggests, further, differential responses to preoperative treatment depending on type of pathology, with outcomes for nodules/mucosal swellings, excellent; granulomas, fair; and polyps, poor.

Another factor which must be considered, often related to the size or extent of pathology, is the patient's degree of disability. That is, if a patient's phonatory or communication skills are seriously compromised by the pathology, earlier surgical intervention might be indicated even if other factors point toward a positive outcome from preoperative voice therapy.

A critical aspect of this stage of assessment is observation of the pathology during phonation at different frequencies and intensities. Consider, for example, the characteristic of compressibility. As presented in Fig. 1A, a lesion on the left fold gives the impression of being soft and polypoid. But as observed in Fig. 1B, during the patient's production of loud voice at comfortable pitch, the lesion appears incompressible and, in fact, seems to deform the softer tissue of the right fold. In another example shown in Fig. 2A–C, bilateral lesions (Fig. 2A) appear somewhat compressible on maximum adduction at comfortable phonation (Fig. 2B); but with a small increase in intensity and a slight decrease in pitch (Fig. C), are completely compressed.

The vibratory edges of the vocal folds should also be examined (stroboscopically) across a range of frequencies and intensities for evidence of thickness or stiffness. It can be noted in Fig. 3, for example, that closure between the true folds appears, at a comfortable pitch, complete and with no evidence of pathology (Fig. 3A). When the folds are observed at a very high frequency (Fig. 3B), however, a stiff, immobile area in the midmembranous portion of both folds is apparent. Stiffness or mucosal thickening which is variably apparent according to phonatory task is indicative of

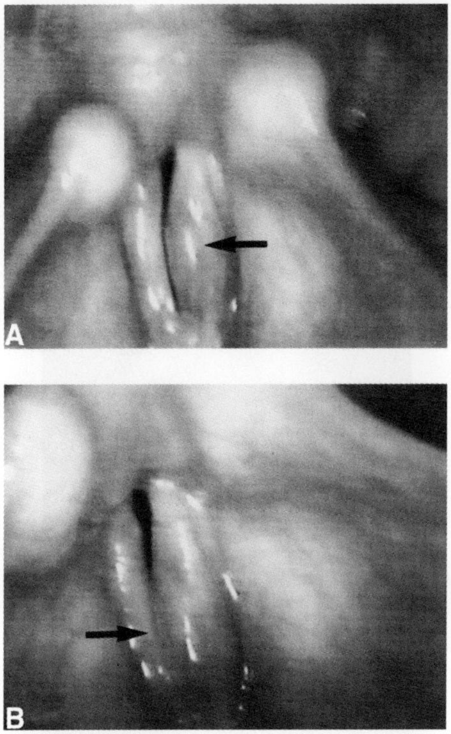

Fig. 1. **A**: Lesion on left fold appears compressible just prior to contact with right fold. **B**: Adduction of folds reveals lesion on left to be incompressible.

pathology which may be amenable to conservative treatment, as opposed to a lesion which demonstrates constant stiffness across all or most tasks.

Observation of the folds during opening and closing phases of vibration provides additional prognostic information. For example, the vocal folds shown in Fig. 4A represent a point just prior to initiation of the closed phase of a vibratory cycle and, in Fig. 4B a point within the closed phase of the cycle. The impression is that the mucosa of the left vocal fold is somewhat irritated, but without lesion. However, in Fig. 4C, the same vocal folds have just begun to separate, and a small lesion becomes apparent on the left. The inconsistent presence of the lesion suggests that it is confined to a small area of the fold, perhaps just below the most superior edge of the cover, and is also compressible, and hence, likely to be amenable to voice therapy.

A second focus of the phonoscopic examination is the identification of specific vocal practices which are producing or exacerbating pathology. Hyperfunctional behaviors which produced the pathology are likely to still be present. In addition, the presence of the pathology itself, however, may occasion other practices which are abusive.

For example, a lesion mass may differentially "load" the vocal folds, requiring increased effort to initiate or maintain voicing, and producing asymmetries in

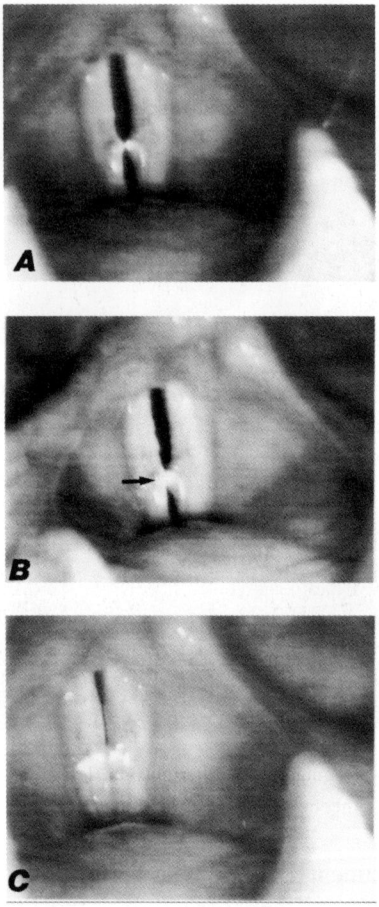

Fig. 2. **A**: Bilateral lesions, larger on left than right, are apparent. **B**: Lesions appear compressible at maximum adduction, comfortable pitch. **C**: With increase in intensity and decrease in pitch, lesions appear completely compressed.

vibratory behavior and a loss of periodicity in glottal pulsing. Pathology may also reduce the efficiency of opening and closing phases of vibration; and, depending on its size and extent, produce early or excessive loss of air through the glottis. Any of these conditions might represent a mechanical overload for the laryngeal machine [4,5].

One example of a hyperfunctional vocal practice is presented in Fig. 5. In the illustration at the top in this figure, the patient is talking, and the true vocal folds appear normally adducted. In the middle frame the patient is still speaking on the same exhalation but with compromised pulmonary support. It will be noted that the arytenoids approximate the epiglottis. By the point represented in the illustration at the bottom of Fig. 5, still on the same exhalation, supraglottic constriction is so great

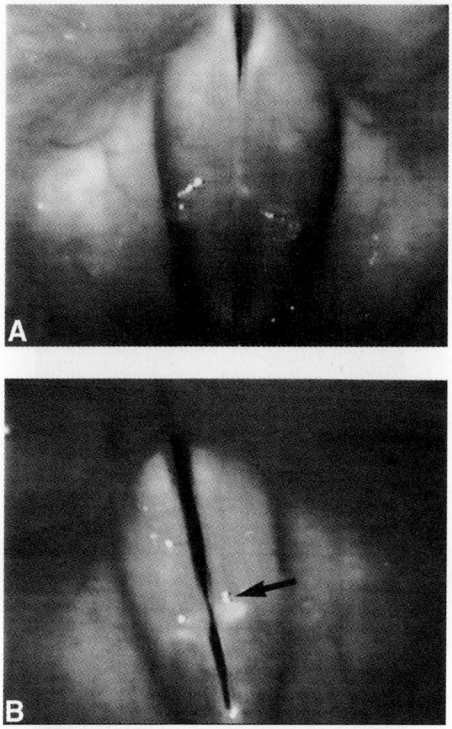

Fig. 3. **A**: At comfortable pitch, contact between right and left folds appears complete. **B**: At high frequency, stiff, immobile areas along both folds are apparent.

that the true folds are difficult to see — and the patient is still talking. This hyperfunctional activity needs to be eliminated, and can be by determining how many syllables per exhalation can be produced before the arytenoid constriction is elicited. Fiberoptic examination on a variety of speaking tasks will allow this determination, and will also allow the patient to associate other sensory experiences — such as contraction of the abdominal muscles or a deterioration of voice quality — with the onset of the aberrant behavior.

In another patient with pathology (presented in Fig. 6) it is apparent that the onset of voicing following an inspiration is associated with false fold constriction (Fig. 6A). This behavior is associated, acoustically, with a "hard glottal attack". Once voicing is initiated (as illustrated in Fig. 6B) the false folds relax. On phonoscopy, reducing the effort associated with voicing onset, perhaps with slight breathiness or passive exhalation, can be explored and, if successful, related to other perceptions which the patient can use to avoid the abusive behavior.

During this portion of the examination, laryngeal behaviors on vegetative tasks, such as coughing or straining, and on tasks which may be typical of a patient's daily nonspeech voice use, such as vocalization associated with exercise, hard physical labor or sport, should also be scrutinized for hyperfunction.

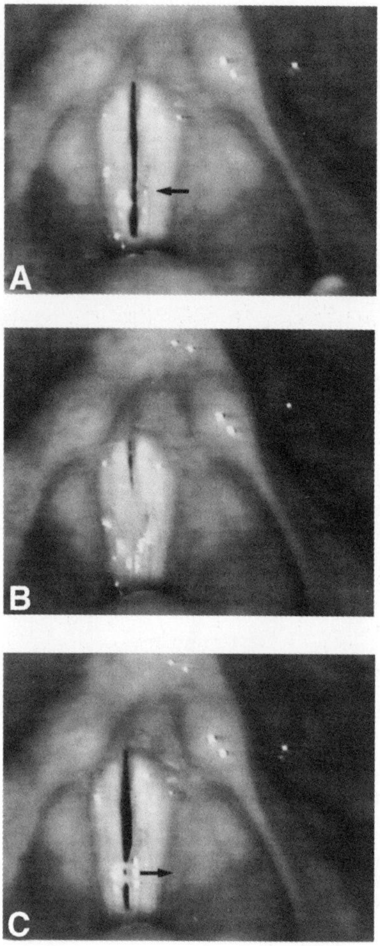

Fig. 4. **A**: During "closing" phase of vibratory cycle, left vocal fold reveals some mucosal changes. **B**: Closure between folds appears complete. **C**: As folds begin to separate for opening phase of vibratory cycle, a small area of thickened mucosa is apparent on the left.

The clinician's third task on phonoscopic exam is to explore new vocal practices which may be conservational, that is, which prevent exacerbation of pathology by minimizing phonatory stress. If identified, these vocal practices will become objectives of preoperative therapy. One example of such a practice is the alteration of adduction patterns in ways that minimize collision forces at the site of pathology.

Presented in Fig. 7A are vocal folds demonstrating broad-based mucosal swelling. The patient is phonating at comfortable pitch and intensity levels. It will be noted that the vocal folds, maximally adducted, contact only at the site of the lesion. With a slight increase in pitch (as illustrated in Fig. 7B) contact between the folds is more extensive, and at a site shifted slightly anterior to that previously shown.

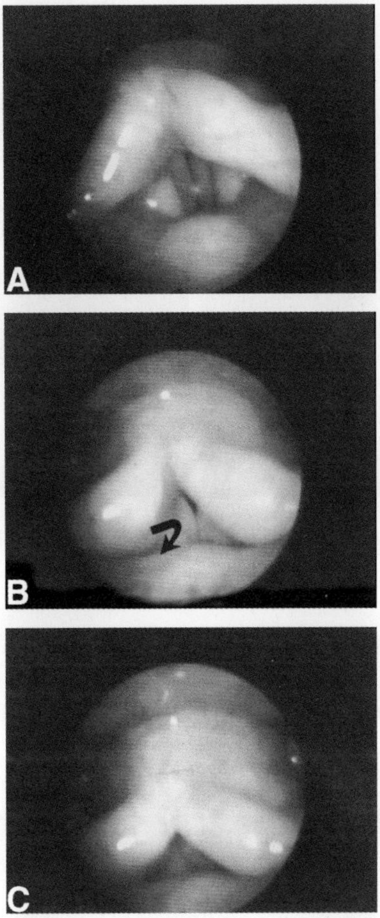

Fig. 5. **A**: Normal vocal fold behavior early in a breath group (all syllables on one exhalation). **B**: Constriction of false folds as speaker continues talking on same exhalation. **C**: Severe constriction of supraglottic structures as speaker's pulmonary support is exhausted.

In another example shown in Fig. 8, a granuloma (indicated by the arrow in Fig. 8A) on the left fold is a constant collision site when the patient is instructed to vocalize at comfortable pitch. A small increase in pitch (demonstrated in Fig. 8B) allows the collision or compression site to be displaced anteriorly, and away from the pathology. Decreasing amplitude of the voice, or a slight increase in breathiness, of course, might be combined with the new pattern of contact to further decrease collision forces between the folds.

An additional conservation strategy involves reducing phonatory stress by dispersing the lesion load. That is, if the mass-loading effects of the lesion can be more evenly distributed across the vibratory mechanism, the collision impact at the site of pathology should be reduced. Consider the example of a patient with mucosal

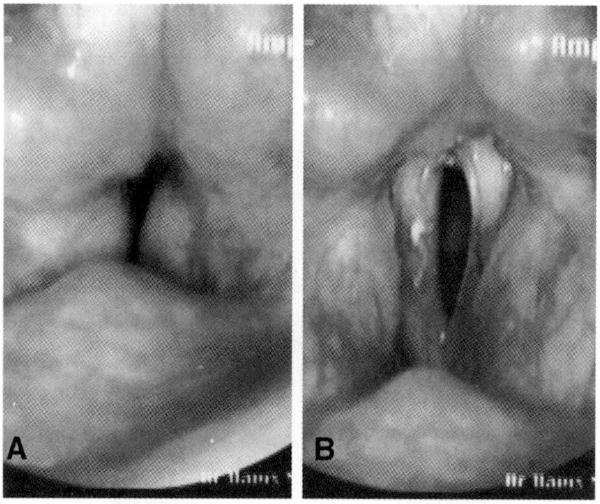

Fig. 6. **A**: Onset of voicing is associated with false fold constriction. **B**: Following onset, false folds relax, and true vocal folds are visible.

changes of the vocal folds presented in Fig. 9A. The pattern of contact shown in Fig. 9B represents maximum adduction of the folds at comfortable pitch and loudness levels. Compare this with the patient's contact pattern presented in Fig. 9C, also at

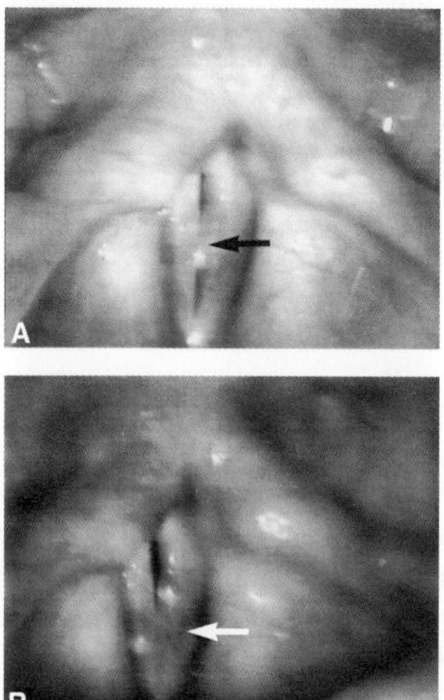

Fig. 7. **A**: Broad-based mucosal swellings are apparent on both true vocal folds. Contact occurs only at site of lesion when patient is phonating at comfortable pitch and intensity levels. **B**: Contact between folds is more extensive, anterior to previous contact point. Pitch has been slightly elevated.

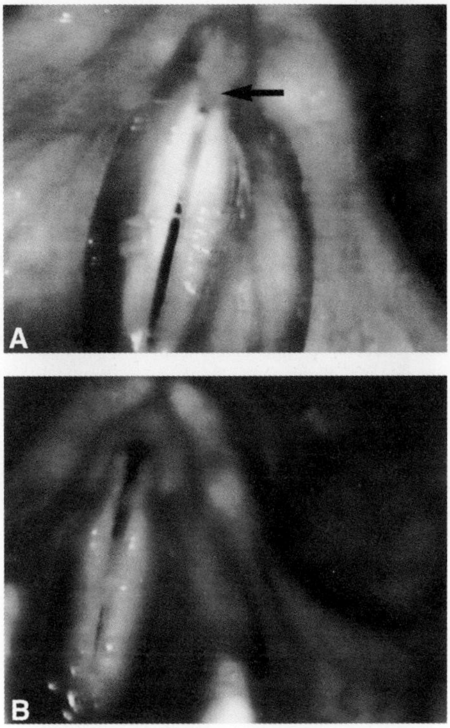

Fig. 8. **A**: Granuloma on left fold (at arrow) is at collision site between folds during phonation at comfortable pitch. **B**: With small increase in pitch, collision site is shifted anteriorly, away from lesion.

maximum adduction, but at a slightly lower pitch and reduced amplitude. The more extensive contact between the folds in the latter illustration reflects a more even distribution of pathology, and perhaps, less forceful collision at the previous point of contact. A similar situation would seem to obtain in another patient presented in Fig. 10. Small changes in the phonatory parameters which produced the pattern in Fig. 10A resulted, as shown in Fig. 10B, in greater dispersal of the lesion across the contact area of the vocal folds. In both of these patients, greater symmetry in vibratory phenomena was also noted with the altered patterns of adduction.

Following the phonoscopic evaluation and the integration of imaging data with other phonatory function data, case history and clinical findings, the clinician's final task – prognostication and implementation of the most efficacious treatment plan – can be reasonably considered. Assuming a trial period of therapy is recommended, the clinician must design a therapeusis which reflects an appropriate balance between restricted voice use, i.e., voice rest and (modified) conservational voice use.

In our experience it has been helpful to consider conservative vocal practices as they relate, separately, to the "body" and other muscular components of the vibratory source, and to the "cover" or nonmuscular components of the mechanism. This distinction seems reasonable because of the different roles of these structures in

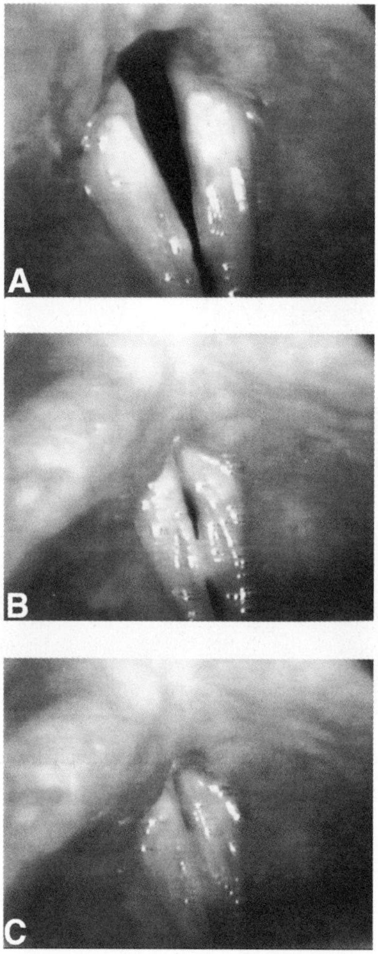

Fig. 9. **A**: Lesions noted on both right and left vocal folds. **B**: Maximum closure between folds at comfortable pitch and loudness levels. **C**: Maximum closure between folds at slightly lower pitch and reduced loudness.

phonation, and also because they are typically affected differentially by pathology (i.e., in pathology of the larynx caused by vocal hyperfunction it is very often the case that the lesion affects the cover, or mucosa, directly, but neither invades nor arises from muscle tissue, so that effects on body and other muscular components are indirect).

With respect to the body, phonatory stress may be lowered by reducing overall tension, and by maintaining uniform tension levels within and across breath groups, i.e., all the syllables or words produced on one exhalation during speech. Vocal practices which should facilitate these goals include:

1. Decreasing the speed and extent of pitch and intensity changes during speech. For

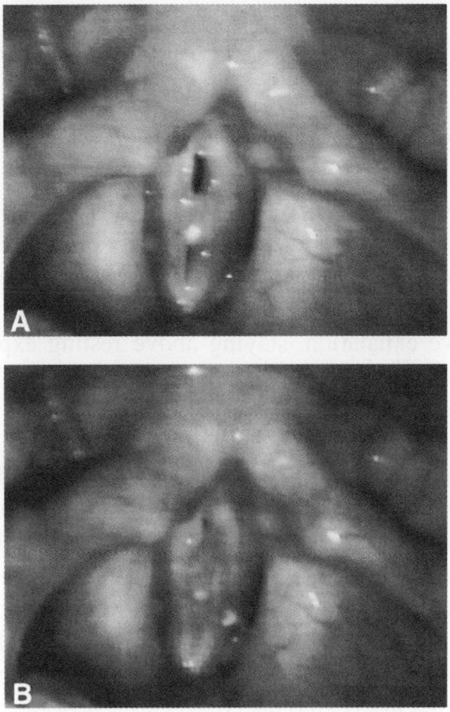

Fig. 10. **A**: Maximum closure between vocal folds at comfortable pitch and loudness levels. **B**: Maximum closure between folds is more extensive with small changes in pitch, loudness and effort.

example, note the "melody plots" of pitch and intensity presented in Fig. 11. On the left are typical, pretreatment plots in a patient with vocal nodules. Compare

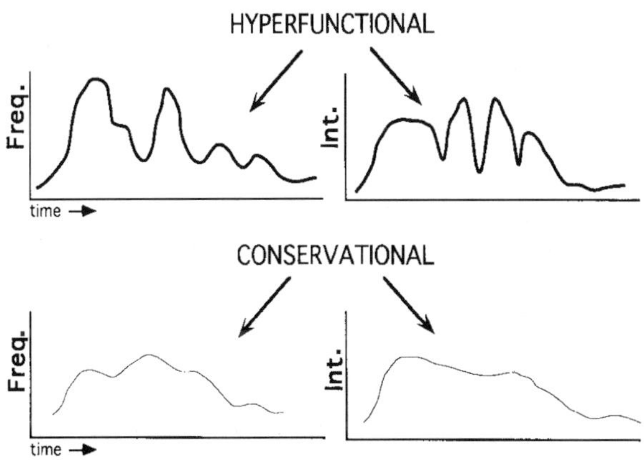

Fig. 11. Melody plots revealing, at top, hyperfunctional patterns of pitch and intensity change over one breath group. Plots at bottom are conservational, reflecting reduced phonatory stress as compared to patterns at top.

this to the plots on the right, produced by the same patient repeating the utterance. The "conservational" patterns on the right reflect reduced "phonatory stress", that is, slower and less extreme changes in F_0 and I_0 and, it follows, a decreased workload on the body.

2. Reduced vocal loudness is another conservational practice to consider. Decreasing vibratory phenomena in the "cover" which are transmitted into the body should facilitate the body's maintenance of a particular length-tension posture, and perhaps also decrease the workload of the respiratory system.
3. Conservation of both laryngeal and respiratory muscular components can also be facilitated by restricting the number of syllables produced on an exhalation. Speaking on passive exhalation, staying above resting expiratory level (or 30% VC) and avoiding abdominal compression, are strategies which may be taught to a patient to achieve this goal.

With respect to conservation of the cover, a number of the same objectives described previously should be considered. Previous experience with the patient during phonoscopic evaluation is critical, since it will have revealed which, or which combinations, of these strategies are most useful to the task. In our experience, periodic therapy sessions in which both patient and clinician observe the larynx while the patient attempts various therapeutic maneuvers can also be extremely valuable.

The outcome of preoperative treatment, which may be clear even within 2–4 weeks, is especially successful if the need for surgery no longer exists, or if the extent of surgery required has been reduced. Regardless of the outcome, however, the patient's experience with preoperative treatment is likely to ensure a better and more expedient postoperative result.

In summary, we would suggest that the role of preoperative voice therapy is one that goes well beyond simply telling a patient to "rest your voice" for 1 or 2 weeks and, if the pathology does not resolve, surgery will take care of it. A well-designed and well-executed preoperative treatment program is a powerful tool, and, in our opinion, should always represent the first treatment option for this patient population. It is, of course, incumbent on the physician to recognize the possibilities of conservative therapy, and to recommend them when they are appropriate. Beyond this, it is equally incumbent on the voice clinician to plan and execute a therapeusis tailored accurately and appropriately both to the patient, and to the pathology.

References

1. Scherer R. Physiology of phonation: a review of basic mechanics. In: Ford C, Bless D (eds) Phonosurgery: Assessment and Surgical Management of Voice Disorders. New York: Raven Press, 1991;77–93.
2. Izdebski K, Ross JC, Klein JC. Rigid transoral larngovideostroboscopy (phonoscopy). In: McFarlane S (ed) Seminars in Speech and Hearing. New York: Thieme-Stratton, Inc., 1990;11(1).
3. Scherer R, Titze I. Vocal fold contact stress during phonation. J Acoust Soc Am 1982;71:S55.
4. Cooper D, Pinczower M, Rice D. Throarytenoid intramuscular pressures. J Ann Otol Rhinol Laryngol 1993;102:167–175.
5. Cooper D, Partridge LD, Fariborz AH. Muscle energetics, vocal efficiency, and laryngeal biomechanics. In: Titze I (ed) Vocal Fold Physiology, Frontiers in Basic Science. San Diego: Singular Publishing Group, Inc., 1993;37–92.

Voice Update.
M. Pais Clemente, editor.

Adjunctive voice therapy in the management of dysphonias in premalignant conditions

Vicki L. Hammen[1], Patricia Waugh[2], Carol Grigg[2] and Allen D. Hillel[2]

[1]*Purdue University, West Lafayette, Indiana; and* [2]*University of Washington, Seattle, Washington, USA*

Abstract. The management of dysphonia in premalignant conditions presents a challenge to an otolaryngologist and a voice therapist alike. While medical/surgical management of the condition is of prime importance, the accompanying dysphonia that typically occurs also should be addressed. The multiple surgeries often required to treat these conditions can significantly change the vibratory and perceptual characteristics of the voice, and hence, affect the dysphonia. However, the extent of phonatory changes occurring postsurgically can be compounded by presurgical vocal use habits. Through a series of case studies, phonatory behaviors that may impact the postoperative voice are identified. An adjunctive voice therapy program will be described that can facilitate the preservation of optimal voice while patients undergo surgical treatment for these premalignant conditions.

Key words: intervention papillomatosis, leukoplakia, voice disorders.

In this paper, the role of adjunctive voice therapy in the management of two cases with potentially premalignant conditions will be discussed. The first case presented with papillomatosis, a viral condition resulting in rough, warty growths in the larynx and surrounding areas. The second case presented with leukoplakia, patchy areas of hyperplasia. While some voice pathology textbooks [1,2] suggest these conditions could benefit from voice therapy, many practitioners manage them with an exclusively medical or surgical approach. A speech or voice pathologist may be consulted only after the completion of medical or surgical treatment, if the resulting voice was not satisfactory. The purpose of this paper is to illustrate that adjunctive voice therapy can have a beneficial impact on both the medical care of these individuals as well as the voice. It is important to state at the outset that it is critical that behavioral intervention be conducted as part of a close partnership with otolaryngology.

Case #1

The first case is KO, a 38-year-old male, a singer and a keyboardist. He had been hoarse for 2 years at the time of his first evaluation. He had been diagnosed with recurrent papillomatosis and a different otolaryngologist performed the first surgical

---

Address for correspondence: Vicki L. Hammen PhD, Department of Audiology and Speech Sciences, Heavilon Hall, Purdue University, West Lafayette, IN 47907-1353, USA. Fax: +1-317-494-0771.

removal of the papilloma. Our voice evaluation, using laryngovideostroboscopy and perceptual judgments, indicated that this individual had extensive bilateral papilloma resulting in a severe dysphonia. The dysphonia was characterized by harshness, strain and breathiness. CO_2 laser surgery was performed to resect the papilloma, but the otolaryngologist indicated that location of true vocal folds was difficult as the patient also had edema.

A 1- and 2-month follow-up examination with laryngovideostroboscopy showed severe vocal hyperfunction. The signs of hyperfunction during the examination were anterior-posterior compression, false fold approximation, and possible ventricular phonation. Voice therapy was recommended at this time. KO was scheduled for therapy on a twice weekly basis for approximately 3 months, however, he attended only about 50% of the sessions. At 4 months postsurgery he was seen again in the clinic. Videostroboscopy showed slight improvement in voice use, however, he also had increased papilloma present. It was felt that the patient may have been responding to the the papilloma by attempting to increase the force of vocal fold adduction to achieve closure. Therefore, further progress in voice therapy was judged to be unlikely until the additional papilloma was removed. Subsequently, a second surgery was performed to resect the additional papilloma.

Patient KO was again seen for a 1-month postsurgical follow-up evaluation. Vocal quality continued to be severely hoarse and strained. Unfortunately, he had dropped out of voice therapy by this time and returned to working as a keyboardist for a musical group that appeared in local bars and clubs. He was unable to resume his work as a singer, but did acknowledge that he talked quite a bit during the shows. He also expressed a great deal of anger and frustration with this condition. Although he had found additional employment as a gardener, he wanted to continue his career as a singer.

During the videostroboscopic examination vocal hyperfunction was again observed. When light, easy phonation was requested, severe anterior-posterior compression occurred. Mucosal wave was absent and the vocal folds appeared enlarged. It was difficult to determine what proportion of the abnormal phonatory function we observed was due to increased papilloma or edema. The otolaryngologist informed KO that further surgical management of the papillomatosis would be quite difficult until he reduced or eliminated his poor vocal-use habits. He then started voice therapy again, this time with a contract that specified both what he and the clinician would contribute to the therapeutic process.

Since this patient presented with frequent throat clearing, a strained vocal quality, and hard glottal attack, the adjunctive voice therapy program focused on these issues. He received education regarding gastroesophageal reflux and was started on an antireflux regimen. A vocal hygiene program was developed that included scheduling of his voice use. That is, he was to limit voice use during the day to preserve his voice for when he needed to communicate during performances at night. Two approaches were used to address his throat clearing. KO needed to increase his hydration, so whenever he felt the need to clear his throat he was instructed to take sips of water instead. Secondly, we hypothesized that some of the sensations triggering the throat clearing may have been related to the increased mass of the vocal folds from the edema and/or papilloma. Therefore, if the desire to clear was not alleviated by drinking water, he was instructed to use an air cough. That is, a cough that is produced by rapidly forcing air through a slightly approximated, not closed glottis. Finally, easy onsets of phonation and a slightly breathy mode of phonation was taught to eliminate the hard glottal attacks. The main goal of intervention was to optimize phonatory function (and, hopefully, vocal quality) between episodes of papilloma recurrence.

While actively participating in voice therapy, he subsequently had two more surgeries to remove additional papilloma. A videostroboscopic examination following 1.5 years of surgical management with adjunctive voice therapy showed a reduction in anterior-posterior compression and ventricular fold approximation, however, these behaviors were not eliminated. Perceptually KO would be characterized as having a mild-moderate dysphonia with a low pitch and breathiness. Perhaps most important is that the patient now feels he has his best voice in 3 years.

Case #2

The second case is WS, a 69-year-old retired male. The patient indicated that he had be intermittently hoarse for 25 years. He also reported a long history of alcohol use. He sought medical attention at another facility because he had had two recent upper respiratory infections with hoarseness that did not resolve. Another otolaryngologist in the area performed a complete resection of severe dysplasia bilaterally. Following surgery an antigastroesophageal reflux regimen was initiated and radiation therapy was recommended. At this time WS sought a second opinion and was evaluated by the authors. A laryngoscopic examination showed bilateral erythema, thickened true vocal folds, and spotty areas of leukoplakia. During videostroboscopy, severe anterior-posterior compression, false fold approximation and ventricular phonation was observed. Vibratory function of the true vocal folds during phonation was not able to be assessed since the hyperfunctional behaviors prevented adequate visualization. Perceptually, WS was moderately hoarse with a low, rough vocal quality. It was also noted that he initiated phonation from low lung volumes. Therapy probes showed a reduction in vocal hyperfunction and improved visualization of his vocal folds during a slightly high-pitched hum.

The otolaryngologist's decision was to monitor his condition for 1 month. However, since it was difficult to view the vocal folds the otolaryngologist was concerned that monitoring the effects of medical or surgical intervention on phonation would be difficult. The patient's apparent lack of compliance with the antireflux regimen also was of concern. Therefore, voice therapy was recommended and the patient agreed to participate. This adjunctive voice therapy program addressed gastroesophageal reflux, respiratory patterning, and tone focus. The antireflux regimen and vocal hygiene program included recommendations and encouragement to discontinue his alcohol use. Other antireflux approaches such as small frequent meals, elevation of the head of the bed, elimination of irritants (such as spicy and fatty foods) were presented during therapy. He was taught to take in an adequate prephonatory inspiration and to recognize the need to replenish his air supply. Tone focus was shifted from the larynx/pharynx to the oral cavity which also resulted in slightly elevating his fundamental frequency. WS participated in three voice therapy sessions over the course of the 1-month interval prior to re-evaluation of the leukoplakia by the otolaryngologist. That evaluation showed no change in the leukoplakia, however, the full length of the true vocal folds were able to be seen as a reduction in the hyperfunctional vocal behaviors had occurred. The otolaryngologist recommended WS initiate radiation therapy, which he did at a location close to his home, therefore additional follow-up examinations were not completed.

What would be some indications that an adjunctive voice therapy program should be pursued? Individuals in vocally demanding professions are prime candidates for adjunctive voice therapy since they need to use their voices and will do so at all costs. Therefore, they are more likely to develop maladaptive compensatory behaviors, such as anterior-posterior compression, and ventricular fold approximation. Certainly these maladaptive behaviors may arise in part from the individual's response to these pathologic conditions. These premalignant conditions will cause alterations in the mass characteristics and, hence, phonatory characteristics of the vocal folds. The individual may be responding to these changes in such a way that a strained, harsh vocal quality is developed. Voice pathologists need to instruct the patient in methods to eliminate these maladaptive compensatory behaviors so the already taxed phonatory mechanism can function as optimally as possible under adverse conditions. Finally, poor vocal use habits, or traditional vocally abusive behaviors would likely predispose individuals to additional dysphonia with premalignant conditions.

In conclusion, it is important to restate what was pointed out at the start of this paper. That is, adjunctive voice therapy with premalignant conditions requires close cooperation between the otolaryngologist and voice pathologist. It is critical that the voice pathologist always keeps in mind that the cause of the dysphonia in these cases is a medical condition that is potentially malignant. So, close communication and interaction between the otolaryngologist and voice pathologist is essential to determine if continued voice therapy is in the best interest of the patient's overall health. However, well-timed adjunctive voice therapy can be beneficial in maximizing phonatory function and providing an optimal base for the repeated surgical procedures often needed to manage these conditions.

References

1. Greene M, Mathieson L. The Voice and its Disorders, 5th edn. London: Whurr Publishers, 1989.
2. Stemple JC, Glaze LE, Gerdeman BK. Clinical Voice Pathology: Theory and Management. San Diego: Singular Publishing Group, 1995.

Integrated treatment of dysphonias

Voice Update.
M. Pais Clemente, editor.

Integrated approach to the treatment of benign dysphonias: pharmacology, voice therapy and manipulation. Problems with suitable trial design in a multidisciplinary clinical setting

Tom Harris, Jacob Lieberman, Sara Harris and Dinah Harris
Lewisham Hospital and Queen Mary's Hospital, Sidcup, UK

Key words: drugs, granuloma, hyperfunction, multidisciplinary, reflux.

Why, when most problems of a medical nature are brought to one doctor, do we think that managing dysphonia requires several specialists from different disciplines to listen to the history and examine the patient at an initial interview. What makes dysphonia so special?

Most diseases have multiple symptoms, while dysphonia, a symptom, may have multiple causes. Moreover, not all patients with a given dysphonic symptom will be suffering from the same predisposing factors.

A patient may have a husky voice which is related to their work/overuse/gastro-oesophageal reflux/a cyst or poor technique which may be either habitual or learned. Listening to the voice quality may suggest a possible aetiology but it usually requires a combination of examining skills to identify all the factors which may be involved.

The dysphonia may be due to local, distant, or generalized disease or diseases. Organic lesions may be a product of somatization.

This is something that doctors are trained to identify. Most laryngologists are on less certain ground when it comes to psychological factors. An example of this is an arytenoid granuloma, which is a well characterized lesion which responds very poorly to surgery, only moderately well to speech therapy but often surprisingly well to some medications and manipulation. There are several suggested factors in the etiology: trauma, due either to iatrogenic or patient dysfunction causes, gastro-oesophageal acid reflux with or without laryngeal overspill [1,2] and there is almost certainly a psychological input, which renders the patients vocal behavior such that the lesion tends to recur unless all the contributory factors are addressed [3,4].

Management

Let us briefly discuss management decisions. Clearly the most important factor is to

Address for correspondence: Tom Harris MA, FRCS, Consultant Otolaryngologist, 59 Southbrook Road, Lee, London, SE12 8LJ, UK. Fax: +44-181-852-9629.

exclude life-threatening disease, and any possibility that the airway might be compromised. In either of these cases surgery is inevitable. Where lesions are benign with no threat to the airway, management decisions are made on the basis of clinical judgement and the responses of the patient to "probe" therapy techniques (both manipulative and vocal) that are carried out at the initial assessment.

It is very clear that most acute insults to the laryngeal mucosa do not result in chronic granulating lesions [5], e.g., "Intubation Granuloma". Why, then do some patients progress to a chronic condition while others do not?

Careful endoscopic and palpatory examination of vocal function shows evidence of continuing muscle misuse resulting in physical trauma to the mucoperichondrium of the interarytenoid area which needs to be resolved if progress is to be made.

Let us consider the management options open to us in the treatment of arytenoid granuloma.

Surgery

Most of the patients with arytenoid granuloma seen in the voice clinic at Queen Mary's Hospital, Sidcup, are secondary referrals. In general, the patients have already undergone attempts at surgical removal either by knife or laser between two and nine times, despite the general experience of all ENT surgeons that conservative surgery alone is ineffective.

There are other extremely important factors in the etiology and maintenance of these lesions, and without addressing these "other factors", the lesion will regrow in around 3 weeks in the postoperative period.

Speech therapy

Speech therapy may be helpful especially if the therapist is mindful of the multifactorial genesis of the lesion. Voice therapy will be aimed at reducing the sharp arytenoid closure at the onset of phonation and the subsequent tight vocal gesture of the posterior supraglottic configuration which squeezes the arytenoids together during phonation. Usually, however, patients have difficulty in altering these habitual voicing patterns and the lesion may regress only slowly if this is the single treatment modality used. While the strength of speech therapy techniques lies in introducing new and more efficient vocal behavior it is less effective for rapid eradication of pre-existing abusive patterns where active disease exists.

Osteopathic manipulative techniques

In our clinic we have been looking at the ways in which manipulative treatment can reduce existing vocal hyperfunction and hence fatigue and discomfort [6]. We find that in the case of arytenoid granuloma, manipulation reduces the considerable vocal hyperactivity. We believe that this helps to break up the cycle of recurrent damage allowing the lesion to resolve.

Voice coaching

While it is rare for singers or actors to produce arytenoid granulomas, where they exist, the voice coach will need to attend to the transfer of the new voicing patterns into performance work.

Counselling

In the authors' voice clinic, the resident osteopath is also a trained psychotherapist well able to recognize contributing psychological patterns and with the skill to help the patient gain insight into these areas. While it is not appropriate in a clinic dedicated to the management of a particular set of symptoms to enter into long-term counselling/psychotherapeutic work patients can be referred on for counselling from other sources.

A recent well-conducted trial from Germany confirms our clinical experience that there is a strong psychological element in the formation and maintenance of arytenoid granuloma [3]. While counselling may not resolve the lesion alone, it does appear that where patients do not address the psychological factors, such as anger or depression or fail to gain insight into these areas, the lesions not only fail to regress, but tend to recur, often on the contralateral side to the original site.

Medication

In the voice clinic we use very few drugs. However, we keep coming back to gastro-oesophageal reflux as a precipitating and maintaining factor in all sorts of vocal hyperfunction. Certainly there seems to be a strong relationship between GOR and generation and maintenance of an arytenoid granuloma.

As far as oesophageal acid reflux and dysphonia are concerned, mechanical reflux suppressants, agents for reduction or suppression of acid production, prokinetic agents and cytoprotectants all have their place [7].

All these classes of drugs are useful, but we find the proton pump inhibitors such as omeprazole over a period of 3 months are the most successful in reducing granulomata.

Misoprostol

Our preferred medication in the management of arytenoid granulomata, however, is misoprostol, a semisynthetic E1 prostaglandin which is normally associated with the healing of NSAID-induced stomach ulcers. The actions of misoprostol are to reduce the amount of resting and stimulated gastric acid secretion, to promote earlier emptying of the stomach and locally at the site of the lesion to produce a paracrine effect increasing blood flow and promoting healing. This too will slowly reduce and heal arytenoid granulomas.

Problems that will be encountered in the design of trials to demonstrate the effectiveness of multimodality management of dysphonias

It is clear from our clinical experience that multimodality treatment is most effective in treating these lesions. However, we feel it is important to provide scientific evidence that is reliable and valid in order that this approach may become acceptable and effective and worthy of adoption in any voice clinic. Herein lies a difficulty: The normal scientific methodology for research into these treatment modalities may not be appropriate or possible.

Normally scientific research in medicine requires multitailed double-blind crossover prospective trials. However, applying these techniques to the multidisciplinary treatment of dysphonia creates many problems. These could be:

1) It is extremely difficult to find reliably matched groups of patients who share not only the same physical condition and socioeconomic background but also show matched personality traits.
2) The number of patient groups needed to deal with the multifactorial nature of dysphonia would take many years to assemble especially from the throughput of a single clinic.
3) The difficulty with multicentre studies is that there is at present, no way to standardize the skills of the practitioners involved nor to quantify like a drug, the therapeutic output. It is hard even to define the goal or goals of therapy. Medical oncologists are able to arrange multicentre trials because all participants are able to follow exactly the same protocols, goals are clear and the trial techniques are therefore appropriate.

Arytenoid granuloma has been chosen as an example of the effectiveness of multidisciplinary work because it lends itself nicely to the application of different treatment modalities and the aim of treatment is clear, i.e., resolution of the lesion on endoscopic inspection. Therefore the effects of treatment are easily discerned by whether the lesion regresses or not. If the patient has a long history of surgical intervention with the lesion recurring within weeks to its original size, and manipulation alone resolves it in three to four sessions it is reasonable to suggest that manipulation has been effective. What is more difficult to discover is the nature of the effectiveness. As yet, no generally accepted criteria exist for identifying or quantifying changes produced by laryngeal manipulation, let alone counselling.

For the future what is then needed is a new generally acceptable research paradigm that can encompass the multifactorial etiology of most dysphonias, and the development of improved, reliable and practical methods to measure changes brought about by treatment modalities such as manipulation and counselling.

References

1. Jones NS, Lannigan FA, McCullagh M, Angiannsah A, Owen W, Harris TM. Acid reflux and hoarseness. J Voice 1990;4(4):355–358.
2. Lumpkin SMM, Bishop SG, Katz PO. Chronic dysphonia secondary to gastroesophageal reflux disease (GERD): diagnosis using simultaneous dual-probe prolonged pH monitoring. J Voice

1989;3(4):351–355.
3. Kiese-Himmel C, Kruse E. Das Laryngeale Kontactgranulom – ein psychosomatisches Storungsbild? (Gottingen). Folia Phoniatr Longop 1994;46(6):288–297.
4. Mans EJ. Psychotherapeutische behandlinng von patienten mit funktionellen stimmstorungen. (Dusseldorf). Folia Phoniatr Longop 1994;46(1):1–8.
5. Harris TM, Johnston DF, Collins SRC, Heath ML. A new general anaesthetic technique for use in singers: the brain laryngeal mask airway vs. endotracheal intubation. J Voice 1990;4(1):81–85.
6. Harris TM, Lieberman J. The cricothyroid mechanism and its relation to vocal fatigue and vocal dysfunction. J Voice – J Br Voice Assoc 1993;2(2):89–96.
7. Harris TM. The pharmacological treatment of voice disorders. Main report for IALP XXII World Congress. Folia Phoniatr Logop 1992;3–4(Suppl 44):143–154.

Voice Update.
M. Pais Clemente, editor.

Treatment of dysphonias in the geriatric population

Thomas Murry and Gayle E. Woodson
Department of Otolaryngology – Head and Neck Surgery, University of Tennessee, Memphis, Tennessee, USA

Abstract. The clinical spectrum of voice disorders in the older adult requires an understanding of both vocal function and the aging process. This presentation explores the concepts of disease vs. disorder and normal lifespan changes vs. abnormal vocal function in the older adult. Medical, surgical, pharmacological and traditional voice therapy approaches will be discussed. Data are presented to illustrate aspects of aging normal and abnormal voices. Problems relating to vocal variability and need for multiple baseline assessment are discussed. Etiologies, pathophysiologies and treatment rationales are examined in relation to the needs of the older person with a voice disorder.

Key words: aging voice, aging, dysphonia, geriatrics.

Treatment of dysphonias in the geriatric population

Voice production in the geriatric population combines a number of physical functions with perceptual, experiential and environmental factors. Like most motor functions of the body, phonation is affected by anatomical, physiological, neurological and behavioral synthesis. When one or more of these systems functions less efficiently, decays or becomes diseased, phonation will change. Study of the elderly voice requires discriminating normal phonatory variation from disease onset, and short-term changes related to other physical systems from long-term changes which may continue to degrade the phonatory system. The clinician as well as the scientist is faced with the dilemma of sorting out the old voice from new pathology.

The voice of the elderly has been the subject of considerable investigation by neurologists, physiologists and gerontologists. Thus, substantial information exists on the normal voices of elderly [1–3] as well as on the physiological parameters associated with vocal aging [4]. By contrast, less information exists on the parameters associated with elderly voice disorders. Moreover, although we may be tempted to attribute hoarseness in an elderly patient to presbyphonia, retrospective studies have shown that careful examination will separate diseases, both focal to the larynx and systemic, from the normal aging process [5,6]. The aging process in the larynx and its associated structures is similar to aging in other systems. Muscle activity is reduced, restricted, and often weakened, despite the lack of a disease or disorder. Aging may alter function in both normal and disordered voices in the elderly. A

Address for correspondence: Thomas Murry PhD, Department of Otolaryngology – Head & Neck Surgery, University of Tennessee, 956 Court Ave., B-220, Memphis, TN 38127, USA.

management model of the aging voice may be viewed in stages that progress from normal phonation to impaired phonation and finally to a voice disorder. Management of the disorder is primarily by the speech pathologist and otolaryngologist with support from the neurologist, gerontologist and psychologist. This paper describes the effects of aging on phonation.

Vocal fold anatomy and physiology

The vocal folds undergo structural changes as one goes from infancy, through adulthood to old age. Anatomic [7,8] and histologic studies [9,10] have shown that differences in structure and function do exist in the larynx as a result of aging. However, the significance of those differences on the strength and quality of the voice has not yet been adequately determined. Structural changes occur with aging in the cover and body of vocal folds, which are comprised of epithelium, lamina propria and vocalis muscle. Mucosal drying may occur from medications, poor mucosal hygiene, or decreased salivary function. Within the lamina propria, changes in each of the three layers has been identified. The superficial layer becomes thick and edematous. The intermediate layer thins out and may become atrophic. The deep layer develops a fibrotic characteristic so that this layer thickens, more in men than in women. The vocalis muscle tends to atrophy in the aging process, as one might expect. Again this may be seen earlier and to a greater degree in males than females. The normal aging process by itself will account for changes in vocal output. These may be summarized in the data provided by Hollien et al. [1,2] and by Murry and Doherty [11] who suggest that speaking fundamental frequency, frequency variability and speaking rate will vary from childhood to elderly in relation to anatomical and physiological changes of the vocal folds as well as to changes in the respiratory mechanism.

Geriatric voice disorders

Voice disorders in the elderly may be related to laryngeal as well as nonlaryngeal factors. The clinician must determine the presence of disease vs. normal aging processes. Once determined, the level of care must be related to the disease process, if present, and the needs for communication. Laryngeal changes leading to vocal dysfunction include joint stiffness, vocal fold paralysis, laryngeal sicca, benign lesions, bowing and atrophy. Although malignant lesions occur more often in the elderly than in a young population, benign lesions and other voice disorders still far exceed the number of vocal fold malignancies in old age.

Disorders of the voice may be present, alone or in some combination. For example, long-term vocal fold paralysis is often accompanied by atrophy on the nonparalyzed side [12]. This results in less ability to compensate for the paralytic condition. Bowing may also be a part of the paralytic condition. However, it may not be clear if the bowing results from the paralysis alone or if it represents a functional repositioning of the vocal fold to compensate for the lack of closure. In such cases, medialization surgery as well as behavioral voice therapy may be required to achieve satisfactory glottic closure and correct the compensatory behavior.

Nonlaryngeal factors must also be considered when assessing the voice of the elderly. Most prominent are neurological diseases and disorders and pulmonary dysfunctions. Both have significant effects on voice. Logemann et al. [13] reported as many as 79% of Parkinson's patients experience voice disorders. Pulmonary diseases and dysfunctions account primarily for reduced volume but may result in other voice changes as well. Hearing loss, CNS disorders and drug regimens contribute to changes in the voice. Each must be addressed when deciding which treatment modality is best.

Voice assessment

Assessment of the geriatric voice should include perceptual, acoustic, endoscopic and physiologic evaluation. Objective measures of phonatory function may be the most efficacious for determining treatment effectiveness. Also important, however, is subjective assessment of loudness, endurance and fatigue which may be more related to the patient's desired outcomes. In the elderly voice, perceptual parameters that are typically encountered include weakness, reduced volume, pitch changes, unsteady voice, breathy voice quality and fatigue-induced changes. The related acoustic events can be seen in increased jitter and shimmer, a reduction in harmonic to noise ratio, a decrease in amplitude over time and increases in SD Fo. Table 1 summarizes the primary features obtained from voice analysis in 25 consecutive elderly patients (ages 63–79) seen over a 3-month period. The features were included if they were outside the normal range of values seen in our voice center. In general, these findings support the results of Shipp et al. who identified acoustic and temporal changes in the elderly through controlled perceptual listening experiments [14,15]. When assessing the elderly patient with a voice disorder, such factors such as noise, amplitude variability, intensity range, control of frequency, intensity and the presence of a compensated

Table 1. List of features obtained from voice analysis in 25 consecutive patients, ages 63–79 (mean = 69.6) seen over a 3-month period. Patients may have more than one feature.

Feature	n
Increased airflow rate	23
Phonational range less than two octaves	20
Decreased harmonic/noise ratio	19
Amplitude decrease after 30 s of oral reading	17
Increased shimmer	17
Reduced rate of speaking (<150 wpm)	15
Increased SD Fo	15
Voice breaks	12
Increased jitter	12
Abnormal range of speaking fundamental frequency	8
Phoneme distortion	4

falsetto voice quality should be addressed.

It is also necessary to look at the physiological changes that accompany the perceptual and acoustic parameters. These include air escape, laryngeal tension, voice tremor, imprecise consonants, rate of speaking, fundamental frequency, other tremors and generalized fatigue over time. While not all of these factors are strictly laryngeal, they do affect vocal function and therefore can play a role in geriatric voice disorders. Neurological disorders and pulmonary changes can significantly impair the voice, even in the absence of laryngeal pathology [16,17].

Examination of the larynx and related structures is usually done via office endoscopy. Stroboscopic examination is reserved for looking at mucosal wave motion, symmetry of vibration and microscopic vibratory characteristics. The laryngeal examination should evaluate laryngeal edema, glottal gap, adequate vocal fold mass, bowing, false vocal fold involvement, and the mucosal wave. In the aging voice, it may be expected that these parameters will change in relation to other neuromuscular changes. As yet no objective measures have documented the prevalence of these changes in the normal geriatric population.

Treatment of the elderly voice

Examination of the larynx and related structures is important to obtain diagnostic information and determine the need for, and type of, treatment. Equally important is the need to understand the patient's communicative problems. Table 2 summarizes the self reports of 25 patients seen in our clinic over a 3-month period (these are the same patients as reported in Table 1). Each patient was asked to identify his or her primary vocal concern. It is clear that the overwhelming consideration is the need for adequate volume. The importance of voice quality is secondary. Thus, it is important to address the issue of vocal volume in the treatment program whether it be through voice therapy or surgical procedures to approximate the vocal fold.

Changes in the aging voice do not always represent a true voice disorder. There is considerable variability in the voice as it becomes older and this variability is enhanced when the older person has another illness and infirmity. Fundamental frequency of phonation, intensity of phonation and the variability associated with these two parameters have long been the outcome measures for the study of normal phonation. However, there are numerous sources of variation which must be taken into account when using these measures to study the aging voice beyond simply age

Table 2. Patient self reports of treatment needs.

Loss of volume/loudness	24
Fatigue while talking	22
Difficulty breathing while talking	18
Raspy or hoarse voice	14
Swallowing difficulty	9

This survey is from 25 patients, ages 63–79 (x = 69.9).

and gender. In two recent studies, we have shown that constancy varies from young to old, from males to females and from normal to pathological older patients [18,19]. Variation is significantly related to the type of voice sample used. In older females, the fundamental frequency for reading is generally lower than that for extemporaneous speech. Vowels tend to have the highest mean Fo of the three types of samples. The results for males are somewhat different. Young males consistently produce vowels with the lowest mean Fo, unlike the older males or the females. It should be pointed out that vowels are consistently the most variable sample from day-to-day and within any 1 day for young and older males and females. Table 3 summarizes the results from the younger and older groups.

Patients with vocal fold paralysis vary greatly in the severity of symptoms. Recent evidence indicates that in most cases of laryngeal paralysis, the muscles are not totally denervated. Severity seems related to the amount of residual innervation and configuration this imparts to the glottis. Woodson and Murry [12] looked at subjects with defined vocal fold paralysis using endoscopic, aerodynamic, acoustic and electromyographic criteria. In paralytic dysphonia, the paralyzed vocal fold was generally found to be shortened and patients used compression of the glottis in the sagittal plane to shorten the normal vocal fold to achieve improved closure. While this maneuver generally approximates the vocal fold processes, it is done with increased effort which often leads to bowing of the normal fold. Furthermore, elderly patients frequently have a reduced capacity for compensation, because of general muscle weakness. Through rotation of the vocal process using the arytenoid adduction technique originally proposed by Isshiki [20], both the length of the membranous vocal fold and the angle between the membranous and cartilaginous segments of the vocal fold were increased following surgery. Woodson and Murry [12] found that mean airflow rate obtained from the speech segment was significantly related to the angle and length measures, both prior to and following arytenoid adduction surgery.

Table 3. Results of fundamental frequency variation produced by young and older males and females for three types of speech samples, sustained phonation, reading and 30 s of extemporaneous speech.

Group	Sample type						
	/a/			Reading		Extemporaneous speech	
	n	mean	SD	mean	SD	mean	SD
Young males (25–35 years)	9	123	1.8	137	0.9	136	1.2
Young females (25–35 years)	10	209	1.4	195	1.2	189	1.8
Older males (65–75 years)	6	142	1.5	139	6.9	134	1.1
Older females (65–75 years)	7	189	1.8	170	2.3	175	2.2

Mean values are in Hz; SD in semitones (ST).

The acoustic measures obtained from the sustained vowel samples were not significantly related to the angle or length measures. It is also noteworthy to point out that in the severe voices, acoustic measures also did not relate well to the subjects' perception of their voice changes.

Summary

The geriatric voice is best studied as a manifestation of aging. By understanding the aging process from infancy to old age, we gain an understanding of the changes that occur in vocal fold function and the pathophysiology requiring treatment. The components necessary for phonation must be considered as a unit. That is, assessment of normal phonation as well as voice disorders in the geriatric population must account for physiologic and acoustic measures which validate the output as well as the patient's subjective impressions of use and function. In searching for outcome measures, it is necessary to consider the interrelationship of objective measures as they relate to functional voice use. There is a need to improve objective measures with regard to this population, as well as a need to study outcomes of treatment through controlled clinical trials.

References

1. Hollien H. In: Huntley RA, Helfer KS (eds) The Normal Aging Voice. Successful Aging in Communication. Baltimore: Andover Medical Pubs, 1993;(In press).
2. Hollien H. "Old Voices": What do we really know about them? J Voice 1987;1(1):2–17.
3. Ptacek P, Sander E. Age recognition from voice. J Speech Hear Res 1966;9:273–277.
4. Ringel RL, Chodzko-Zajko WJ. Vocal indices of biological age. J Voice 1987;1:31–37.
5. Woo P, Casper J, Colton R, Brewer D. Dysphonia in the aging: physiology vs. disease. J Laryngoscope 1992;102:139–144.
6. Morrison MD, Gore-Hickman P. Voice disorders in the elderly. J Otolaryngol 1986;15:231–234.
7. Hirano M, Kurita S, Yukizane K et al. Asymmetry of the laryngeal framework: a morphonologic study of cadaver larynges. J Ann Otol Rhinol Laryngol 1989;98:135–140.
8. Kahane JC. Connective tissue changes in the larynx and their effects on voice. J Voice 1987;1:27–30.
9. Luchsinger R, Arnold GE. Voice-Speech-Language: Clinical Communicology: its Physiology and Pathology. Belmont, CA: Wadsworth Publishing Co., 1965;69–81.
10. Rosenberg S, Malmgren LT, Woo P. Age related changes in the internal branch of the rat superior laryngeal nerve. J Arch Otolaryngol Head Neck Surg 1989;115:78–86.
11. Murry T, Doherty ET. Selected acoustic characteristics of pathologic and normal speakers. J Speech Hear Dis 1980;23:361–67.
12. Woodson GE, Murry TM. Glottic configuration after arytenoid adduction. J Laryngoscope 1994;104(8):965–969.
13. Logemann JA, Fisher HB, Boshes B, Blonsky R. Frequency and co-occurance of vocal tract dysfunctions in the speech of a large sample of Parkinson patients. J Speech Hear Dis 43(1):59–75.
14. Shipp T, Hollien H. Perception of the aging male voice. J Speech Hear Res 1969;12:704–710.
15. Shipp T, Qi Y, Huntley R, Hollien H. Acoustic and temporal correlates of perceived age. J Voice 1992;6(3):211–216.
16. Close LG, Woodson GE. Common upper airway disorders in the elderly. J Geriatr 1989;44:67–72.
17. Ward PH, Colton R, McConnel F, Malmgren L, Kashima H, Woodson GE. Aging of the voice and swallowing. J Otolaryngol Head Neck Surg 1989;100:283–286.
18. Morris RJ, Brown WS. Age-related voice measures among adult women. J Voice 1987;1:38–43.

19. Murry T, Brown WS, Morris R. Patterns of fundamental frequency for three types of voice samples. J Voice 1995;(In press).
20. Isshiki M, Tanabe M, Masaki S. Arytenoid adduction for unilateral vocal fold paralysis. J Arch Otolaryngol Head Neck Surg 1978;14:555–558.

1996 Elsevier Science B.V.
Voice Update.
M. Pais Clemente, editor.

Differential diagnosis and treatment of psychogenic dysphonia

Janina K. Casper
Department of Otolaryngology and Communication Sciences, State University of New York Health Science Center, Syracuse, New York, USA

Abstract. The presenting perceptual symptomatology of psychogenic dysphonia is diverse and shared with various other disorders of voice. Laryngoscopic and stroboscopic findings may not differentiate the psychogenic problem from other categories of voice disorders, particularly musculoskeletal dysphonia and neurogenic problems. Acoustic and physiological analyses may help us to understand the "differences" in the voice signal, but may not be particularly helpful in identifying the psychogeneity of the problem. Thus, the differential diagnosis of psychogenic problems presents a particular challenge for the otolaryngologist and the speech-language pathologist. The suspicion of a psychogenic disorder usually arises when the vocal symptoms, the history and the examination findings do not "match". This suspicion demands careful exploration. The characteristics of the symptoms of psychogenic dysphonia are contrasted with those of spasmodic dysphonia and musculoskeletal tension dysphonia, problems which also share many characteristics. There is some general agreement on the basic treatment approach to psychogenic dysphonia although the specific techniques may vary from clinician to clinician. This discussion will center on the philosophy of our approach to these patients. Attention is also paid to the often overlooked malingering patient whose motivations differ significantly from those of the psychogenic patient and whose treatment course may thus be different as well.

Key words: conversion dysphonia, dysphonia, hysterical aphonia, psychogenic dysphonia, psychogenic voice disorder.

Introduction

The diagnosis of a voice disorder is made after careful history taking and examination of the patient and it is the diagnosis that then determines the treatment protocol. The diversity of the symptoms and signs of psychogenic dysphonia defies simple categorization. Thus, when the diagnostic steps lead to the suspicion of a possible psychological or psychogenic etiology, it is essential that full consideration be given to other diagnoses which may share some of the same or very similar symptoms and signs. The perceptual signs, for example, can be similar to those heard in musculoskeletal tension dysphonia or spasmodic dysphonia. Laryngoscopic and stroboscopic findings do not readily differentiate the psychogenic voice problem from other dysphonias. Acoustic analysis may help us to understand the "differences" in the voice signal, but are not particularly helpful in identifying the psychogeneity of the problem or in differentiating among the possible diagnoses. The otolaryngologist and

Address for correspondence: Janina K. Casper PhD, Department of Otolaryngology and Communication Sciences, SUNY Health Science Center, 750 East Adams Street, Syracuse, NY 13210, USA.

the voice clinician share the challenge of making the diagnosis and may, on occasion, need to include other professionals in the process.

What is a psychogenic voice disorder?

Our use of the term psychogenic dysphonia is reserved for a specific group of patients who differ from the many patients whose voice problems may be stress related and expressed through excessive musculoskeletal tensions. Excluded also are those patients who experience stress as a result of a dysphonic voice. We believe that the nature of those stresses is different from the underlying emotional conflict of the psychogenically dysphonic patient whose dysphonia can be expressed in such a variety of vocal forms – from total aphonia to excessively tense and explosive voicing.

Psychogenic dysphonia is thought to be a sign, a vocal manifestation of psychological disequilibrium, or a somatization of an emotional conflict. A conversion disorder, a term sometimes used synonymously with psychogenic disorder, is defined [1] as an alteration or loss of physical functioning that suggests physical disorder, but that is apparently an expression of a psychological conflict or need. The symptom, in this case a dysphonia or aphonia, is intentionally produced with the primary gain being to keep internal conflict out of awareness, and secondary gain being realized from avoidance of a noxious activity while yet getting support from the environment that otherwise might not be there. Psychogenic or conversion disorders must be differentiated from the classical conversion hysteria which refers to a personality type or behavior pattern that is evidenced repetitively in the individual's life.

Malingering is another type of conversion that mimics psychogenic dysphonia in presentation. However, malingering has a very specific underlying motivation and is a totally conscious act. It is a conscious faking of a disability for a goal that is usually obvious when the environmental circumstances are known. In the USA, the most obvious goal is to obtain a legal judgment against someone identified as being to blame for the loss of voice and the suffering attendant upon it and, of course, to receive a monetary settlement or judgment. Malingering or faking a voice disorder may also be used to avoid expected behaviors, such as going to work, while gaining sympathy, not unlike the child who fakes a stomach ache in order to avoid going to school.

Differential diagnosis

There is no specific relationship between the type of underlying psychogenic problem a person is experiencing and the type of laryngeal symptomatology that is exhibited. Furthermore, the severity of the symptoms is not necessarily equivalent to the severity of the underlying psychological problems, nor is severity differentially diagnostic. Patients with very mild symptoms may be equally as resistant or more resistant to abandoning those symptoms than some with extremely disabling dysphonia, who sometimes may surrender the symptoms with startling ease.

Although psychogenic dysphonia may share certain characteristics with spasmodic dysphonia and musculoskeletal tension dysphonia, differences do exist. It is necessary to consider those differences in order to arrive at a proper diagnosis.

The patient with spasmodic dysphonia will have symptoms that are both consistent and constant. The nature of the symptoms does not vary although patients report some increase or decrease in their presence related to situation, stress level, emotional state or fatigue. They rarely experience total absence of symptoms for any period of time. The patient with musculoskeletal tension also exhibits consistent symptoms, reports constancy in their presence, again with some variability of severity often related to amount of use, and the symptoms are consistent with the hyperfunctional movement. In contrast, the patient with psychogenic dysphonia may report much variability in symptoms and the clinician may be aware of much variability of symptoms during the course of the evaluation or in response to various diagnostic probes. It is not unusual for the patient with a psychogenic disorder to report an "on and off" pattern. The symptoms may come and go during a day or may be absent for weeks at a time, often with return of normal voice during those periods. Such reporting is not heard from either the patient with spasmodic dysphonia or with musculoskeletal tension dysphonia.

The symptoms of the spasmodic patient are consistent with the particular movement that is affected. Thus, the voice stoppages heard in the patient with adductor spasmodic dysphonia typically occur on initiation of vowels but not during sustained vowel production. The spasm, or the hyperadduction of the vocal folds is the movement that is affected and usually exhibited at the initiation of voicing and production of vowels, but that abates as the voicing is sustained, as in a prolonged vowel production. The abductor spasmodic patient displays symptoms on voiceless consonants. Ludlow (1995) [2] describes this behavior as "prolonged voice offset during voiceless consonants". Perceptually there is a delay in initiating voicing after the production of the voiceless consonants; the vocal folds are unable to close quickly and smoothly and a breathy quality is perceived. This consistency of symptom with underlying movement disorder is not present in patients with psychogenic dysphonia. There is no specific pattern that is seen to relate to any movement disorder. For example, a patient with normal vocal folds structurally and normal movement on nonspeech tasks may present as aphonic with incomplete glottal closure during attempts at voice production. There is neither a movement or a structural deviation present to explain the aphonic voice production.

Vocal symptoms of the malingerer compared to the patient with psychogenic dysphonia are not differentially diagnostic. The diagnosis of malingering must be made with extreme care and caution as it may well impact on legal issues. The patient who is faking a voice problem in the hope of some direct gain must attempt to tie the onset of the problem to a very specific event. For example, "They were using a strong chemical outside of my window and I suddenly lost my voice", might be a typical history given by a malingerer (obviously it is necessary to make sure that the person has not had an allergic reaction). Patients who are malingering often have limited knowledge of voice production and do not present a cohesive history. Often malingerers have difficulty maintaining their symptom and much variability may be observed. They may give themselves away by inconsistency of vocal behavior. For example, they may produce normal voicing on a cough or throat clearing while presenting as aphonic, or they may be heard to speak normally to a spouse when not aware of being overheard by others.

Videolaryngostroboscopic examinations of patients with adductor spasmodic dysphonia reveal hyperadduction or over adduction during phonation especially at the onset of voicing and vowel production. This movement is consistent with and reflective of the audible interruption of voicing. Similarly, a slowing of adduction or an extension of adduction following production of voiceless consonants is the visible movement that corresponds to the perception of intermittent breathiness in the patient with abductor spasmodic dysphonia.

A variety of interesting observations can be made during videolaryngostroboscopic examination of the patient with psychogenic dysphonia. In some instances, the technique of the examination itself, either anchoring the tongue forward during rigid endoscopy, or inserting the nasendoscope, is sufficiently distracting or disrupting to the patient that control of the dysphonic voice cannot be maintained. Even when the symptoms are not totally eliminated during the testing, the symptoms may be variable and inconsistent. Some patients make a valiant effort to maintain the symptom and, in so doing, actually produce voice that is much worse during the examination than in conversation. Still other patients are so fearful of not being able to control their symptom that they simply refuse to follow instructions about change of pitch or loudness that might disturb that control.

There are additional subtle – sometimes not so subtle – distinctions among these dysphonias that are elicited by history. We have already mentioned the aspects of consistency vs. variability of symptoms. This is an area worthy of very specific exploration, beyond a single answer to a single question because a pattern may emerge providing insight into the motivation for the dysphonia. Reporting of onset of the problem can also be revealing. The linking of an emotional or disturbing event that occurred at about the same time or immediately prior to the onset of the dysphonia is common to many dysphonias and thus is not diagnostically differentiating. Nevertheless, it must be considered and particularly so when the patient provides excessively precise information about the very moment that the voice "went" or the symptoms "turned on". Patients with musculoskeletal tension dysphonia and those with spasmodic dysphonia usually describe more gradual onset and/or worsening of symptoms over time.

Examination procedures and protocol

It is important that the examination procedures and protocols include tasks that will sample a variety of phonatory behaviors. Flexible endoscopic examination is the procedure of choice to examine laryngeal movement during speech. Much information will be lost if examination is limited to the use of the rigid endoscope with prolongation of the vowel /i/ as the only task. The speech stimuli must include sentences containing vowel-initiating words and no devoicing (e.g., Every morning a man and a woman eat out), as well as some loaded with voiceless consonants (e.g., He saw half a shape), in order to observe adductory and abductory movements associated with spasmodic dysphonia. A variety of tasks that require adjustments in phonatory behavior, such as changes of pitch, pitch glides, siren sounds, changes in intensity and an extended speech task are useful in detecting inconsistency of symptomatology typical of the psychogenic patient and the malingerer. Observation of nonphonatory tasks should be included in the test protocol. These can include acts that elicit vocal fold abduction (e.g., deep inhalation, sniffing in), vocal fold adduction (e.g., effort closure, swallow, cough, throat clear), and alternating ab/ad duction as in whistling. Examination of these behaviors will give information about the control of movement in the absence of phonation and in the health of the vocal fold mucosa. Patients with psychogenic problems are often "disturbed" by being asked to engage in these behaviors because they are so afraid of losing control over their symptoms and do not understand the nature of these tasks. And finally, the examination procedure should involve the use of some diagnostic probes with the nasendoscope in place to determine whether the phonatory physiology is accessible to change through a behavioral approach.

Important information can be obtained from sensitive observation and interaction with the patient. The patient's affect, interactive style (e.g., guarded, open), and response to inquiries and to testing should be noted carefully. Patients' responses to positive changes in the voice can also be instructive in differentiating among the diagnoses. Patients with musculoskeletal tension dysphonia are anxious to change behavior and pleased with any decrease of the hyperfunctional symptoms. Patients with spasmodic dysphonia are willing and eager to try anything to improve vocal function but rarely get relief from behavioral changes. Although some patients with psychogenic dysphonia become excited and relieved by the emergence of the "normal voice", others give no sign of awareness of a change and minimize it if questioned, often reverting into the dysphonic voice. They resist making the phonatory adjustments requested of them and may appear justified when a technique does not work.

An interesting additional element to the diagnostic process is the use of a sodium amytal interview, as reported by Ludlow [2]. Sodium amytal is a drug that reduces volitional cortical control. Preliminary results of patient interviews using this drug reveal that there is either no change or a worsening of symptoms in patients with spasmodic dysphonia who are correctly aware of the changes; that there is a remission of symptoms in patients with vocal tremor which the patients accurately recognize; and that there is improvement of the voice in the psychogenic patients, but with lack of awareness of the improvement by the patient. We have observed a similar reaction in patients who produce normal voice during some examination tasks but fail to recognize the difference and, indeed, may deny it.

Treatment philosophy

Restoring normal voice in the patient with psychogenic dysphonia can be accomplished in a variety of ways. According to Aronson [3] and others, patients may give up their symptoms spontaneously as they are carefully interviewed and allowed to unburden themselves of what has been troubling them. There are, however, many patients who do not behave in this manner. It is essential that patients be prepared to relinquish or surrender their dysphonia in order for the symptom-based therapy combined with the support and empathy provided by the voice clinician to be effective. Normal phonation may be elicited through a variety of techniques, such as laughing, coughing, throat clearing, etc. Once elicited, the sound can then be shaped into phonation for speech production. The clinician must have considerable clinical skill and sensitivity in order to guide the patient through this process so as to provide him or her with a "face-saving" means of abandoning the symptom. This occurs when the patient's problem is legitimized by being taken seriously and when various vocal "exercises" or techniques are used. Probing into the possible motivations for the dysphonia must be interwoven with the direct attention to the voice so that the patient gains insight and understanding of the underlying problems.

The types of "exercises" used may be extremely variable. Some clinicians use hands-on manipulation of the larynx while others use phonation-based activities. Some clinicians are comfortable and skilled in dealing with psychological problems and rely on those techniques to a great extent. This therapy is usually short term and effective.

There are patients who need to maintain their symptoms because of the purpose they serve and the psychological gains they provide. They are not prepared to surrender their symptoms and will resist doing so. This type of therapy will be ineffective for those patients, or if effective the problem may recur. If, after three sessions, the patient has failed to make the anticipated progress, it is necessary to question the diagnosis, to re-examine the therapy and to make recommendations for further examination and/or treatment. This may include referral for psychiatric consultation. Psychological counselling may also benefit those patients who regain their voices but continue to have unmet needs.

Treatment of the patient who is suspected of malingering also requires great skill. It is not wise, nor is it necessary, to confront these patients with knowledge of their malingering. It is important to carefully document and tape record all instances of normal voicing. It is possible to make it clear to the patient and others that the examination fails to reveal any abnormality, and that you believe that the phonatory mechanism is capable of normal voice and requires no further treatment. Providing ongoing treatment in such cases suggests that there is a legitimate problem that requires this treatment and does not recognize the fakery involved.

For those patients whose diagnosis remains somewhat in question despite skilled examination, a short trial period of voice therapy can be extremely helpful. Such therapy can be exceedingly useful in determining the contribution of psychogenic elements to the problem.

References

1. Diagnostic and Statistical Manual of Mental Disorders: DSM IV, 4th edn. Washington, DC:

American Psychiatric Association, 1994.
2. Ludlow C. Differential Diagnosis of Neurogenic and Psychogenic Voice Disorders, presented at Annual Academy of Neurology, May 6–13, 1995, Seattle, WA.
3. Aronson AE. Clinical Voice Disorders: an Interdisciplinary Approach. New York: Brian C. Decker, 1985.

Voice Update.
M. Pais Clemente, editor.

Treatment of dysphonias secondary to stress and psychogenic factors

Mara Behlau
Department of Otolaryngology and Human Communication Disorders, Universidade Federal de São Paulo, Escola Paulista de Medicina, Unifesp-EPM; and Centro de Estudos da Voz-CEV, São Paulo, Brazil

Abstract. Stress and psychogenic factors can trigger a voice alteration and/or a laryngeal disorder. 277 adult patients were analysed and classified into four different groups: I – psychogenic dysphonias (79 patients); II – functional cases (39 patients); III – organic functional dysphonias (45 patients); and IV – minor structural changes dysphonias (40 patients). Females were more likely to develop the classic psychogenic dysphonias (98% of cases), usually in one isolated episode with no related psychiatric disorder; good results with symptomatic vocal rehabilitation can usually be obtained. Both sexes can develop a secondary organic lesion or a minor structural change dysphonia. There are different personality and vocal behavioural patterns that lead to a certain kind of lesion; moreover, there are certain anatomic configurations that seem to select the type of mucosal alteration (glottic proportion, glottic chink, and vocal fold opening angle). These lesions require eclectically oriented therapy with a multiprofessional team approach, since some degree of recurrence and failure of treatment may occur. Finally, minor structural changes may have been silent for a long time and have had their vocal component triggered by psychogenic and/or stress factors. In some cases it was difficult to distinguish the etiological aspect of the lesion, however, the treatment happened to be an important tool for diagnosis.

Key words: emotions, personality, vocal rehabilitation, voice.

"It is due to stress that we reach even higher degrees of physical and mental progress". *Selye, 1974.*

sometimes the price is a dysphonia...

The relationship between voice and personality is common knowledge and ancient understanding, even before the basic anatomic data on voice production, has been described. We use our voices in the same way we function psychologically. One of the most frequent causes of voice change is related to stress and psychoemotional issues. These factors can trigger a voice alteration and/or a laryngeal disorder. Stress originally meant mechanical tension. This concept was enlarged by the health science area by Selye [1]. Recently, Vasconcelos [2] offered the following concept of stress: "a physiological alteration in the organism that occurs in a situation which requires a stronger reaction than the usual organic activity". The stress process can be viewed as having three phases: alarm, resistance and exhaustion [2–4]. The alarm phase is

Address for correspondence: Mara Behlau PhD, Director Centro de Estudos da Voz, Rua Diogo de Faria 231, São Paulo 04037-000, Brazil. Fax: +55-11-575-9649.

a total mobilization of the organism, which can include the following related symptoms: tachycardia, perspiration, paleness, high blood pressure, fatigue and insomnia. Those symptoms represent a healthy reaction of the organism and belong to the so-called "eustress" phase, a "good stress". The second step is the resistance phase which means a specific mobilization where the physical symptoms disappear, being replaced by psychological correlates, such as irritation, social isolation and feelings of impotence. The third and last phase is the exhaustion which indicates an energetic collapse of a specific vulnerable organ that usually develops an organic pathology. Phases 2 and 3 are parts of "distress", a "bad stress". In a previous study [5], 81 patients with functional and organic functional dysphonias and a control group of 40 normal voice individuals were submitted to five inventories (life events units (LEU), body resonance tendency (RESCORP), list of stress symptoms (LSS), state-trait anxiety inventory (STAI) and behavior patterns type A (BEPATYA)). Some very interesting conclusions could be derived from such analysis. The number of life events was similar in the two studied groups but the value of the past negative events was still higher nowadays for the dysphonic group, which means that coping is less efficient for the voice-disordered patient. The dysphonic group showed a stronger tendency towards somatization; moreover, they also showed a stronger tendency to a "type A" pattern, i.e., extroversion, competitiveness, impatience, intolerance, high overload and aggressiveness. On the other hand, they were shown to have an equivalent number of stress symptoms. Anxiety, as a personality trait, was equivalent for both groups. It is interesting to observe that the dysphonia itself was pointed out as a meaningful stressor, which reinforces the importance of an approach that can quickly offer the patient a better voice.

The objective of this study was to perform a retrospective analysis of 277 Brazilian adult patients, ranging from 22 to 49 years old, belonging to the middle and upper-middle classes (Table 1). The basic criterion for selecting individuals for the group was the assumption that the voice disorder was due to mainly psychogenic or stress factors. The individuals were divided into four groups (Table 1).

Group I: psychogenic conversion

This group included all patients with typical psychogenic voice alterations. A sudden

Table 1. Patient distribution according to etiological category and sex.

Etiological category	Female		Male	
	n	%	n	%
Psychogenic conversion	79	28.5	3	1.1
Functional cases	39	14.1	11	4.0
Organic functional disorders	45	16.2	40	14.4
Minor structural changes dysphonia	40	14.4	20	7.2
Total	203	73.2	74	26.7

dysphonia onset is the main characteristic for this group. The patients usually present recent complaints, from days to weeks. Female patients comprise 98% of cases, the psychogenic voice conversion being a typical female manifestation. It is interesting to point out that 70% of patients do not relate the dysphonia to a psychological event in the first consultation. The vocal emission can be very bizarre, ranging from total collapse of the sound source, to a whispered phonation, an intermittent voice phonation ("on-off" laryngeal effect – not to be confused with adductory spasmodic dysphonia), hysterical falsetto and a divergence of registers (frequently between modal and high register, but also between modal and fry). The laryngeal evaluation can show a hypotonic image but more often we can see a hypertonic constriction with false fold dislocation towards the midline or also a typical posterior whispering triangle. In 10% of patients it can be seen that laryngeal organic signs or lesions whose presence does not exclude the diagnosis of psychogenic conversion. The best choice of treatment is vocal rehabilitation. As a rule these cases show good evolution in a short period of therapy (1.5–3 h treatment) under a symptomatic orientation approach.

Our experience [6] and literature [4] do not show a displacement of the symptoms to another organ due to the specificity of the related symbolism with a communication problem, but there can be some recurrence of the dysphonia. In our population 5% presented with more than one episode. Frequently, after the symptom removal and the return to the habitual voice quality, the disclosure of the real history of the case takes place.

Group II: functional cases

This group included all patients with vocal alterations where the most important data consisted of faulty vocal behaviour and/or a laryngeal asymmetry (laryngeal phonatory inadaptation). The patients in this group present a diffuse and gradual onset of the vocal alteration, with periods of normal voice and a short duration of complaints, usually a few months. A high incidence of patients (85% of cases) related the beginning of the symptoms to an increase in voice use, problems at work/home, career promotion and more responsibility and too much tension. The voice is not always so altered and the patients usually complain of loss of potency, reduced vocal resistance and an effort to speak. The main goals in a vocal rehabilitation program are to achieve an effortless phonation, reduce the vocal fatigue and prevent secondary lesions since these patients are "candidates" for mass lesion development. A gradual return to a normal stable voice is usually seen within a short period of treatment (4–6 h). Some degree of progression to secondary lesions can be noticed which reinforces the importance of an early prevention approach.

Group III: organic functional disorders

This group included all patients with secondary mass lesions from behavioural origin. These cases exhibit a long period of voice and related symptom complaints, from months to years, with fluctuating vocal quality. The voice alteration range is very wide. The goal of the rehabilitation is the reabsorption of the lesion and the basic criterion is a team effort attitude. The most frequent observed lesions are nodules, polyps, Reinke's edema and contact ulcers. Different personality traits, vocal behaviour patterns and anatomic configuration practically select the mucosal alteration. For example, vocal fold nodules are bilateral lesions, typically female, age ranging from 25 to 35 years old, and not always showing an evident disturbed vocal output. The patient with vocal fold nodules has long-term disturbed vocal behaviour, with an anatomic predisposition such as lower glottic proportion (short phonatory dimensions when compared to the respiratory dimensions of the glottis), and a large vocal fold opening angle. As main personality characteristics these individuals are responsible, overloaded and perfectionists. For secondary lesion treatment the best approach is an eclectic program with a strong etiological orientation and a complete voice training program. The evolution is usually moderate to good but there is some degree of recurrence since certain patients identify themselves with the altered voice (idiosyncratic dysphonias).

Group IV: minor structural changes dysphonia

This group consisted of all patients whose larynx showed organic structural congenital lesions, such as sulcus vocalis and cysts. The goal in this group is obviously to reduce the vocal impact of the congenital lesion and to enhance the voice resistance. These patients indicate that they have had a typical voice for a long time, and 40% of them refer to having a "different" voice since childhood. The current episode was usually triggered after a period of time below 1 year, after a higher tension period, increase of voice usage and/or a upper tract infection. The best vocal rehabilitation orientation is a symptomatic approach, using specific voice techniques, a modified vocal rest program and hydration as a coadjuvant. The evolution is moderate to good, but there is an inherent degree of confusion between these lesions and secondary laryngeal lesions, mainly between cysts and nodules. In several cases, a surgical exploratory approach was the diagnostic tool to differentiate the category of lesion.

As a general conclusion we can state that stress and psychological factors can trigger a voice alteration with or without an associated laryngeal lesion. The vocal correlates of the psychogenic conversion cases are usually typical. Mass lesions from mechanical phonotrauma can be the result of a stressful life, a faulty vocal pattern plus an anatomical laryngeal predisposition. On the other hand, congenital minor structural changes of vocal fold cover can have their vocal component triggered after stress events or psychological factors. It seems to us that the best choice of treatment is still vocal rehabilitation with psychotherapy if needed (particularly with recurrence). Some patients have their larynx as a stress target – laryngoreactors – and they will always be "dysphonic", even if their voices sound normal. Stress is the "habitual pattern" of today's life. Besides the development of a stress reduction program, we need to have a better understanding of the laryngeal and personality factors that can trigger a voice disorder.

References

1. Selye H. A syndrome produced by diverse nocuous agents. Nature 1935;July 4.
2. Vasconcelos EG. O modelo psiconeuroimunológico de stress. In: Seger L (ed) Psicologia e odontologia, 2nd edn. São Paulo: Santos, 1992.
3. Selye H. Stress in Health and Disease. Boston: Butternworth, 1976.
4. Spiegel H. Is symptom removal dangerous? Am J Psychiat 1967;123:1279–1282.
5. Behlau M, Coelho MA, Vasconcelos E. Considerations on the relationship between stress and dysphonia. Paper presented at The 22nd Annual Symposium: Care of the Professional Voice, 1993, Philadelphia, USA.
6. Behlau M, Pontes P. Disfonias psicogênicas. In: Ferreira LP (ed) Um pouco de nós sobre voz. Barueri: Pró-Fono, 1992.

Professional voice

Voice Update.
M. Pais Clemente, editor.

Healthy voice training for all age groups and all singing styles

Hermann LeRoux
Voice Chair, San Francisco Conservatory of Music, San Francisco, California, USA

Abstract. Twenty-four years of education, habituation and follow-up observations as to the efficacy of appropriate warm-up and other related techniques covering the full sequence of voice training and voice maintenance, has shown excellent results in singers with major operatic careers, musical theatre careers, careers as cantors in Synagogues and Cathedrals, recitalists, impersonators, rock singers, professional choral singers, jazz singers and gospel singers. These techniques have also successfully been used to restore problem voices in collaboration with scientists and medical experts.

The goals of this presentation are to demonstrate various techniques and stress the importance of proper stretches, warm-up exercises and other related techniques as an integral part of voice training, voice building and voice maintenance.

With a background of the physiological and psychological phenomena of various life stages, these techniques can be used in voice training from childhood through puberty and adulthood to more advanced ages.

Introduction

The human voice is an instrument consisting of a power supply, the lungs, an oscillator, the vocal folds and resonators, the larynx, the pharynx and the mouth.

The singing gesture originates in the brain. From there the thought impulse is conveyed to the central nervous system. Nerve fibres, originating in the central nervous system are inserted into the muscular system. To allow a singer to perform with effective and specialized skills, only the essential nerve fibres must fire in precise sequence and in split-second precision timing. Sensory feedback for the singer is limited and we cannot see the mechanism at work[1].

To allow for the smooth transmission from the brain to the sound production, appropriate exercises covering the full sequence of voice training, voice building and voice maintenance must be designed and habituated.

Address for correspondence: Prof Hermann LeRoux BM, MM, TLD, PDM, Voice Chair, San Fransisco Conservatory of Music, 1201 Ortega Street, San Fransisco, CA 94122, USA.

[1]Feedback and visual confirmation of the mechanism in action are available using several instruments and computer programs and will hopefully become standard studio equipment during the next few decades.

The sequence of voice training[2], voice building and voice maintenance

1. Relaxing and focusing of the mind.
2. Good posture.
   a) Large postural muscles (skeletal alignment)
   b) Inner postural muscles (open throat – palate, larynx, tongue, pharynx)
3. Good breathing – inhalation and efficient exhalation (breath flow and support).
4. Phonation – efficient flow phonation and the noninterference in the activation, phonation and connection of the tone to the airflow coupled with diction, enunciation and articulation.
5. Registration – the balance and coordination of the various vocal registers.
6. The development of sound qualities[3] such as speech, falsetto, twang, sob, operatic ring, belting, vocal intensities and articulations through the entire range and consistent with each individual singer's endowed capacities.
7. The development of a subtext and related techniques to explore, transfer and project a singer's innermost feelings to a given text.
8. The use of the spoken voice to establish a clear link between the speaking voice and the singing voice.
9. To build and maintain self-confidence.

Rules for using the exercises

1. Vocal warm-up and other related exercises must be tailor-made to suit the needs of each individual singer.
2. The exercises must be executed correctly – only a teacher's outstanding ear and eye can help here in analyzing and identifying problems, designing exercises, implementing and habituating the correct use of the exercises.
3. The total time spent on warm-up and building exercises should be 10–15 min, 5 min minimum, with 15–20 min spent on more vigorous exercises and voice building (where appropriate); 30–60 min can then be spent working and developing the repertoire to performance standard. All these elements depend on the individual student's capacity, age, needs and experience.
4. As the human being consists of physical, emotional and intellectual components and as the body is interconnected and interdependent on all these elements, it is important for the singer to become aware of the interdependence. Singers must

---

[2]Interrelated areas of study that must be part of the voice training sequence (as a prerequisite or concurrent study) are: thorough knowledge and application of the International Phonetic Alphabet, study of frequently used foreign languages, word by word translations (when appropriate), research (time period, composer, character analysis, musical style) and musical excellence in musicianship skills (rhythm, ear training, sight-singing, solfege, keyboard facility, analytical skills, harmony) and skills in presentation, stage craft and acting.

[3]Jo Estill.

become aware of appropriate voice use (including the FACH system), vocal hygiene, voice care and a good balance between the physical, emotional and intellectual components of their makeup.

Stress some general rules for voice hygiene, appropriate voice use and voice maintenance. These rules include:

1. If it feels bad, don't do it.
2. Keep it simple – less is more.
3. Avoid screaming, loud laughter, heavy throat clearing or singing too heavily or too loudly for too long. Learn to "mark" correctly.
4. Hold down coughing and sneezing; do it silently and gently.
5. Do not talk in noise, cars, planes, buses or noisy restaurants.
6. Limit your voice use before a performance.
7. Avoid singing in a tessitura that is continually near the extremes of your range and vocal capacity.
8. Be acutely aware of register extremes. Do not push one register into the next, i.e., chest into the upper register.
9. Learn to use your voice with as little effort as possible.
10. Do not sing with a sore throat. Consult your ENT as to what is appropriate.
11. Maintain good health, exercise regularly – this is an excellent way to reduce stress. Eat a balanced diet with vitamin supplements in moderation. Sleep at least 7–8 h every night. Establish regular hours for your restful sleep. Maintain good body hydration, eight glasses of water every day (the best is to Pee Pale). Try to keep a 40–50% humidity level. Maintain hydration when you breathe in dry air in air-conditioned rooms, cars, planes, heated rooms. Do not smoke anything. Do not breathe in polluted air. Avoid the use of over-the-counter preparations for colds, flu, etc. Do not use aspirin or aspirin products when you sing. Consult your physician about the use of birth control pills and singing before or during menstruation or when you have a viral or bacterial infection. Reduce stress levels – resolve conflicts quickly, exercise regularly! Think positively!!

Remember, singers are different. As singers, we are vocal athletes. No athlete will ever do strenuous exercises or exert effort without proper stretches and warm-up exercises. Appropriate warm-up and related exercises can:

1. elicit better vocal qualities;
2. reduce the possibility of vocal misuse;
3. elicit a wider spectrum of vocal intensities in a healthy manner;
4. improve pitch accuracy;
5. stimulate deep breathing;
6. supply the brain with oxygen, which in turn increases alertness;
7. give us energy; and
8. make us feel good.

Always begin with less strenuous exercises and proceed to more taxing exercises.

Exercises covering the voice training sequence

1. Exercise to relax and focus the brain through deep breathing and visualization.

2. Body stretches for vocal athletes.
3. Alignment exercises.
4. Exercises for good breathing.
5. Exercises for flow phonation.
6. Exercises for register blending and coordination.
7. Exercises for vocal qualities.
8. Exercises for developing subtexts.
9. Exercises for building self-esteem.

Examples of exercises

To relax and focus the mind through deep breathing and relaxation

Lie flat on your back with your arms next to your body, the palms of your hands touching the floor. Follow your breath. Allow any thought to enter the mind. Do not hold on to any thoughts.

Begin to direct your breath flow to all the body parts, starting with the feet. Breathe into the body part, "shake them out", relax them. Continue with the ankles, calves, knees, thighs, pelvic area, pubic bone, buttocks, lower abdominal muscles, lower ribs, epigastrium, rib cage, breastbone, clavus bones, shoulders, neck, jaw, tongue, palate, larynx, cheeks, eyes, forehead, skull, upper arm, lower arm, hands and fingers. Once you are relaxed, visualize a place where you want to be, i.e., the beach.

a) Visualize yourself singing on the beach.
b) Visualize yourself singing in the lesson.
c) Visualize yourself singing in Carnegie Hall, etc. Observe your feelings and be aware of your breath. Discuss your feelings and tensions afterwards.

Body stretches for vocal athletes

All these exercises should be repeated two or three times and should begin with establishing good breathing.

1. Place the feet apart, about shoulders' width. Breathe in. Stretch up on the toes with arms stretched past the ears, fingertips reaching for the sky on the exhalation.
2. Interlock the fingers of both hands in front of you. Turn the palms out. Breathe in. Stretch out on exhalation.
3. Bend over to the front with the knees slightly bent. Place the hands over the lower back and rib cage. Inhale. Feel the expansion in the back. Exhale. Feel the lower abdominal muscle involvement. Keep the space open as you exhale.
4. Bend over again. Begin to breathe into the back, swinging the arms from left to right and eventually describing a circle to the left and to the right on expiration.
5. Stand up straight. Feel as if you are dangling from the ceiling on a string, like a puppet. Keeping the spine aligned, the knees and lower abdominal muscles relaxed, breathe in. Describe a circle with your head. If you feel any tension in

the neck, stay with it. Breathe into the tension. Lower your head slowly.

6. Align the body. Inhale while raising the palate, lowering the larynx and pushing the tongue out. Exhale through the same position. Relax this posture so that the tongue is not pushing the larynx down or suppressing it.
7. Take your tongue in your hand with a piece of cloth. Pull it out gently while raising the palate and lowering the larynx.
8. Let the head and neck hang over in a forward bend. Shake the head from side to side with the tongue hanging out. Stand up straight. Inhale with palate raised and larynx down and tongue flat with the tip touching the lower front teeth.
9. Stand in front of a mirror. Align the body. Stand in a performance posture. Check the alignment checklist:
   a) Feel your feet. Where are they? Are you balanced? Can you move into another position with ease?
   b) Are your knees unlocked?
   c) Is your spine aligned? Are you "off the hips?"
   d) Is your rib cage expanded, your breastbone high and your tailbone tilted?
   e) Are your lower abdominal muscles relaxed?
   f) Is your neck loose, free and the cervical crane stretched?
   g) Is your jaw unhinged and not jutting out?
   h) Are your lips relaxed and free?
   i) Are your shoulders back and down?
   j) When you inhale, do you feel the cheeks pulled towards the ears, palate raised, larynx down, the tongue relaxed with the tip of the tongue touching the lower front teeth?
   k) Are your hands relaxed and behind the seams in your pants?

To confirm this checklist, stand against a wall with one heel flat against the wall, the other heel pulled up, resting on the ball of that foot. Stretch out your arms with the palms flat against the wall. Push yourself away from the wall so that nothing touches the wall except your palms through the elbows. Stretch the cervical crane. Relax in this posture and breathe deeply, leaving the lower muscles open when you exhale. Drop the arms, thumbs touching behind the seams of your pants or skirt. Look and feel full of energy and enthusiasm.

Breathing exercises

1. Inhale as if you are sucking through a straw, drinking a thick milkshake. Feel the low breath and support. Exhale on a silent lip trill.
2. Stand aligned and relaxed. Get rid of all the air in the body. Allow the body to "open up" for air. Feel how low the breath goes. Exhale on a "sss" sound, 20–40 counts.
3. Repeat the previous exercise, panting on "f-f-f" until all the air is out and the body opens up for the next inhalation.
4. Repeat any of the inhalation exercises. Exhale while pumping the epigastrium. Be aware of support and "gripping."

Phonation

1. Repeat the inhalation exercise and exhale on "S".
   a) Lip trills on "phrr" and "bhrr".
   b) Yawn-sighs, from high to low
   c) Five note exercises, 5-4-3-2-1, starting in the middle range, then moving lower, then back to the middle range, then higher, as:
      - lip trills
      - hum and chew
      - hum and chew and clean the teeth with the tongue, upper and lower, from left to right.
      - all nasal sounds with "O" vowels, "NO, MO, NGO", on 5-4-3-2-1.
      - all vowels with diphthongs, "ia, io, ii, ie, iu".
      - using a hum on 1 5-4-3-2-1. A "hummmm, mum, mum, mum".

Repeat all the exercises holding the hands on the lower ribs to feel the expansion. Repeat all the exercises placing the back of your hands on cheeks, lowering the jaw and slightly pouting the lips, with the elbows out to expand the rib cage.

Registration exercise

For men:
1. Use falsetto sounds on 5-4-3-2-1 scale all through the range.
2. Connect two groups of 5-4-3-2-1 scales: the first one falsetto; the next one beginning easy with the full voice.

For women:
1. Siren up and down.
2. Make puppy sounds high up on an "NG" sound.
3. Do octave jump exercises from the bottom to the next register.
4. Practice bringing the head voice down.

Remember, it is essential that the palate is raised in the passagio and the larynx lowered. Remember, the palate is raised and flexible, the larynx down but not depressed. Less is more.

For men and women:
1. Fioritre exercises and scales. Use any scale exercises to cover the full vocal range. Examples:
   - 1 123 345 567 789 987 765 543 321
   - 12345432 12345432 12345678987654321
   - 12345432 12345432 12345678998789878 987654321
   - 1 123 345 6789 10 11 11 10 99877654321
2. Staccato exercises (men and women) on 1-3-5-8-5-3-1 covering the full vocal range.
3. Use all consonants and vowels in combination in the previous exercises, e.g., "doo, boo, zoo", etc.
4. Use words in the above mentioned exercises such as "bidi, buzzy, bee, suzie,

zoo", etc.

5. Use sentences in the previous exercises and pitch sets. Use your imagination to create interesting sentences on pitch patterns. Examples: "Show me my name" to create the Bernouli effect; "Oh come see me for tea", etc.

Remember, analyze the need, design the exercise, habituate the free singing habit all throughout the vocal range. Use the sentences you created and speak and sing them in different voice qualities and intensities, always listening to the free flow phonation, not bearing down on the vocal folds, not gripping with the breath.

Subtext training sound qualities and acting

1. Give each song a given number of emotional qualities, such as love, hate, anger, longing, etc. Change arbitrarily from one emotion to another. Remember, we have to sing "in" to get the message across, which will travel out.
2. Use gibberish to describe the emotions in the song and act it out.
3. Speak the text in the original language. Speak the translation as an actor. Say what the text means in your own words. Remember, the speaking voice is part of the voice. Speak in a free, healthy, resonant way. Habituate this habit in your normal life.
4. Speak a sentence from the song or aria; then sing it.
5. Listen to the accompaniment of the piece and relate an experience that happened to you that triggers similar emotions as in the composition.

Self-esteem

Begin every lesson performance by saying:

1. I am (your name).
2. I am a singer.
3. I will sing (name of composition) by (name of composer and dates) for you.
4. Speak the text.
5. Tell us what the song means to you.
6. Synergize all elements and sing. Enjoy!

Conclusion

When we sing, we do not listen to ourselves. We pay attention to the word meaning and connecting the text and the music to our emotions. We cannot think about every moving part of the voice. We have experienced and habituated the fundamentals during the exercises, now it is time for free flight. Sing with a lot of energy and freedom. Most of all, sing with passion.

Voice Update.
M. Pais Clemente, editor.

Formants in singers

Ronald C. Scherer
Wilbur James Gould Voice Research Center, The Denver Center for the Performing Arts, Denver, Colorado, USA

Abstract. This overview paper discusses certain topics of resonance in performers with an emphasis on classical singing. Topics include general acoustic "rules", formant tuning, the singer's formant, voice classification, and vocal covering.

Key words: formants, larynx, resonance, singer's formant, singing, voice.

Introduction

Quality and intensity in vocal performance are more than an aspect of entertainment. Behind performance sound lie secrets of efficient physiology and effective acoustics, as well as cultural and personal artistic creativity. The study of performance sound leads to reconsiderations of what target vocal and vocal tract behaviors might be adopted for the most effective communication.

This report is a selective overview of performance resonance. Topics to be covered include formant tuning, the singer's formant, voice classification, and vocal covering.

The source of sound in phonation is considered to be the glottal volume velocity or its derivative. It is produced by the flow-induced mechanical action of the larynx and has some dependence on the acoustic pressures of the airways. The sound source as a time or frequency signal sent into the vocal tract can be highly varied. Partials or components of the source must exist if we want any resonance structure of the vocal tract to radiate those frequencies from the mouth, if we assume the usual acoustic theory.

Vocal tract length and constriction

Discussions of vocal tract resonance usually begin with the open-closed uniform tube. This is helpful because the glottis end of the vocal tract is nearly closed. As a uniform tube shortens, the formant frequencies increase. The formants themselves act to allow partials from the source to pass through the vocal tract if the partials are near the formant center frequencies. Thus, a person will have formant frequencies inherent to his or her vocal tract length. Also, vocal tract length can be voluntarily altered by

---

Address for correspondence: Ronald C. Scherer, Wilbur James Gould Voice Research Center, The Denver Center for the Performing Arts, 1245 Champa Street, Denver, CO 80204, USA. Tel.: +1-303-446-4833. Fax: +1-303-893-3206.

raising or lowering the larynx and protruding or spreading the lips, thus providing some limited control of formant frequencies through vocal tract length adjustment.

The formant values are highly dependent on the shape of the vocal tract. Both sung and speech sounds must conform to rules governing formant frequency values:

1. Vocal tract lengthening lowers all formant values.
2. A pharyngeal constriction raises the first formant and lowers the second formant, as in the production of /a/.
3. A constriction near the front of the mouth lowers F1 and raises F2, as in /i/.
4. Formant frequencies decrease with lip rounding and increase with lip spreading, similar to the first rule, as is /u/.
5. The first formant increases as jaw opening increases, to be discussed later. Titze [1] gives physical acoustic reasoning for these effects.

Formant tuning

Formant tuning occurs when a partial of the glottal source has the same or nearly the same frequency as one of the vocal tract formant center frequencies. When this occurs, that source partial will be radiated with relatively greater intensity. If the fundamental frequency is above the first formant value, however, there may be a clear mismatch of partials and formants, resulting in poor vowel integrity and relatively low intensity. As Sundberg [2,3] has shown, female singers can remedy this problem by modifying the first formant frequency by raising it with a greater jaw opening to bring the first formant in line with the fundamental frequency. Notice that in sung music, the fundamental is prescribed, but the formants can be manipulated. Data from [3] show that jaw opening for a soprano singing different vowels at different pitches increases by approximately 10–15 mm over the range of 250–700 Hz for most vowels (but not for /a/). The first formant and fundamental frequency match preserves intensity and a desired (acceptable) quality in classical singing.

Does formant tuning take place in performance voices other than the soprano's? Raphael and Scherer [4] studied the training techniques named "Call" by Arthur Lessac. This technique emphasizes quality and physical sensation, and de-emphasizes vowel specificity. The primary difference between the Speech and Call techniques is the amplitude of the second partial, which differs by about 16 dB in the most trained subject. The implication is that the subject tunes or matches the first formant with a source partial more for the Call than for the Speech techniques. This experiment suggests that formant tuning is at least a part of the training of some actors, if not an intent of quality enhancement during performance.

Sopranos utilize F1 formant tuning, and so may actors. Do tenors use formant tuning for high pitch singing? Data from Titze et al. [5] suggest that at high pitches tenors will raise F1, but not tune it to a voicing partial. For some vowels, however, they may tune F2 to the second or third partial. For example, for the vowel /i/, F1 increased and F2 decreased when the spoken formants were compared to the sung formants. F1 did not match with any partial, and the F1 movement even appeared to avoid the partials by going midway between them for /i, e, a, u/. But there was a movement to match F2 with the second partial for /u/ and with the third partial for /i/ and /e/. It is curious that F2 for /a/ and /o/ moved midway between partials two and three. These results may suggest that tenors attempt F2 tuning for high vowels. Since F2 is strongly related to vowel identification, tenors may attempt to preserve vowel identity as pitch rises, as well as a characteristic quality that would be destroyed by close formant tuning to F1, the strongest vocal tract formant. Spectra for male classical singers often are seen to be flat with approximately equal intensity in F1, F2 and the F3 region.

Carlsson and Sundberg [6] studied an extreme form of formant tuning. They played synthesized chromatic scales to conservatory students where the scales included F1 and F2 formant matches to partials for each note. These scales with formant-partial matches were compared to a scale with constant F1 and F2 values. The scales with constant F1 and F2 values were by far preferred. This study suggests that formant tuning in general is not a preferred device. Any gain in overall intensity would be overwhelmed by undesirable timbre discontinuities.

Singer's formant

Formant tuning concerns F1 and F2 primarily. The singer's formant concerns a significant boost in the F3 and F4 frequency region between about 2,500 and 3,500 Hz. As shown by Sundberg [3], the singer's formant for a male classical singer can have a spectral value of approximately 15 dB above the corresponding orchestra spectral value. The creation of the singer's formant can arise from the movement of F4 closer to F3, thereby boosting the vocal tract spectrum in the region, relative to F1 and F2 amplitudes.

We studied the spectra of voice modification of a mezzo-soprano [7]. She sang a scale without changing her vocal tract shape to preserve the vowel integrity, and then with changing her vocal tract shape to preserve the desired classical voice quality and intensity. In the unmodified version at the highest pitch of the scale, 740 Hz, the first and second partial of the voice for her intended /^/ vowel were strong and very close to the expected speaking formant values. There was a de-emphasis of energy between 2,000 and 4,000 Hz, and a prominence between 4,000 and 6,000. In contrast, in the modified production, the first partial or the fundamental frequency was relatively strong, and was accompanied by a relatively broad spectral area with an intense peak at approximately 3,400 Hz. There was a significant de-emphasis of the second formant. Thus, the modified production included both the strong representation of the fundamental and the singer's formant, and that was about all.

Do actors use the singer's formant, that is, an enhancement of the third formant region? It would seem evident from listening to the stentorian sounds of some actors in their loud voicings. We asked whether when students in our National Theatre Conservatory increased the presence of their third formant region, if their vocal quality was rated higher [8]. In the preliminary study, 32 students were recorded twice within an academic year producing 10 /a/'s in their best stage voice. Their voice qualities were rated on a 1–10 scale with 3 being "normal" and 10 being "exceptionally good". Mutual agreement was reached by both a voice coach and a voice scientist. One male and one female were randomly chosen from each rating category from 3 to 9. The results indicated a general trend for F3 to increase as the voice quality rating increases. The men produced an F1–F3 intensity difference of about 20 dB for the low quality ratings, but about 10 dB or less for the higher ratings. The relation was stronger for the males. An interesting finding was that, for the men across the 10 /a/ tokens, the standard deviation of the F3 level values decreased strongly as the voice quality rose. These results suggest that the presence of F3 for male actors may tend to increase with better voice quality, and is more consistent from a technique point of view.

What is the source of the singer's formant? This is a highly significant question because its implied association with the vocal tract, carrying power of the voice, and often a greater clarity and quality acceptance of the voice, suggests that it provides desirable communication enhancement and highly efficient production without added laryngeal and respiratory efforts.

Sundberg proposed [3,9] that larynx lowering to widen the hypopharynx, and laryngeal ventricle widening, might relate to the enhancement of the singer's formant on the basis of a laryngeal acoustic tube orientation. The primary logic was the acoustic isolation of the larynx tube so that its own resonance could ring through, regardless of the vowel. If the larynx tube is modeled as a cylinder with a length of 2 to 3 cm, the approximate length of the larynx tube, the independent resonance is in the singer's formant region. The opening of the larynx tube was prescribed to be smaller than the laryngopharynx by approximately a factor of six. There have been a number of video examples of the anterior-posterior motion of the epiglottis and arytenoid cartilages to create the relatively smaller larynx tube exit (e.g., Yanagisawa et al. [10]).

Wilson's 1972 dissertation [11] at Indiana University studied laryngeal and hypopharyngeal airways in singers, using radiography. Different vowels, pitches and intensities were sung. The suggestion by Yanagisawa et al. that there is more constriction for louder sounds was generally supported. This subject showed reduced A–P distance for the loud productions, in general. These characteristics did not hold, however, for some subjects.

Further consideration of the generality of the early criteria suggestions by Sundberg has come from a study by Detweiler [12]. She studied a tenor and two baritones using magnetic resonance imaging and video laryngoscopy. The subjects sang in vocal fry, wherein the ventricular folds touched the true folds, obliterating the ventricle, and found that the singer's formant was as strong as in their normal classical singing. She also tested the 6:1 area ratio concept and found that her singers produced about a 3:1 area ratio while producing a strong singer's formant. We can conclude that further refinement of our knowledge of the origin of the singer's formant is needed.

The acoustic isolation by larynx tube manipulation may refer to a highly refined control of three specific regions within a few millimeters of each other – the vocal folds and intrinsic muscles, the aryepiglottic structures, and the hypopharynx.

Vocal classification

Classifying the singing voice into bass, baritone, and so forth, as well as creating useful subclassifications, is important for practical performance literature purposes as well as for vocal health purposes. Cleveland [13] found that the voice classifications of eight professional singers were highly related to the center of each subject's vocal range, thus relating voice classification for men to the physiologic properties of the vocal folds – the higher the placement of the singing range, the higher the voice classification. Cleveland also showed that the center of the pitch range corresponded to the average of the first four formant frequency values, thus indicating a relation between laryngeal pitch properties and vocal tract resonance properties. In addition, he showed that the voice classifications were highly correlated with the value of the specific formant frequencies, especially F3 and F4.

Dmitriev and Kiselev [14] suggested that the specific classification of voice from bass to high soprano correspond to two aspects: the frequency of the high prominent formant area, which we will consider to be the singer's formant, as well as to the length of the vocal tract. This suggests the first acoustic rule discussed – the longer the vocal tract, the lower the formants, and here then, the lower the voice classification.

Berdtsson and Sundberg [15] performed an interesting classification study using singing synthesis. A panel of six singing teachers heard descending triads. There were two important results. First, as the singer's formant frequency rose, the teachers rated the voice with a higher voice classification, even when F1 and F2 were held constant. And secondly, if the triad was raised in its octave but without changing the singer's formant, the teachers tended also to raise the voice classification.

Thus, there is evidence to support the notions that voice classification into primary categories depends upon pitch range, average formant values, and even the frequency of the singer's formant alone.

Vocal covering

Lastly we will mention the most recent study on vocal covering, a topic with a long history. Hertegard et al. [16] studied 11 professional male singers (bass, baritone and tenor) who sang both normal open and covered productions on the vowel /ae/ on a passagio pitch. The first formant was lowered consistently in the covered sound compared to the open sound. Also, for the limited available data, the second formant was higher in covered than in open singing. The effect for both was 100 Hz or more. The interesting associated findings with these formant results were that there were tendencies to raise the soft palate, widen the pharynx, widen the laryngeal ventricles, and increase the transglottal peak-to-peak flow in the covered compared to open singing. Of significance is the anecdotal statement by the singers that this manipulation was necessary so as not to strain the voice above the passagio.

We can now add additional "rules" and observations regarding singing and vocal tract formants. F3 is dependent on the size of the cavity immediately behind the incisors (F3 is lower when the cavity increases) [6]. Please refer to [3]. F4 may be strongly dependent on the shape of the laryngeal tube [7]. Narrowing the frequency distance between F3 and F4 boosts the singer's formant amplitude [8]. Pitch-dependent formant tuning above 500 Hz for females preserves intensity and classical performance quality [9]. Pitch-dependent formant tuning may aid the intensity and quality (or the training) of the actor's voice [10]. Formant tuning of F1 and F2 in singing is not a general goal in Western classical training and performance, partly because of quality preference, although this needs further exploration, especially regarding tuning the second formant [11]. The singer's formant can be present in both male and female singers and actors, but is less consistently apparent in sopranos [12]. The singer's formant may be strongly associated with larynx tube configuration, but further modelling is necessary [13]. Voice classification (bass to soprano) depends upon the person's pitch range and formant frequency values, and can be estimated based on the singer's formant frequency itself [14], and covered singing appears to involve a lowered F1 and potentially a raised F2 [15], and in general a more elevated soft palate, a wider pharynx and laryngeal ventricles, and an increased peak-to-peak AC glottal flow.

If vocal efficiency of source and vocal tract filter is to be well established, the study of trained performers is obligatory. The selected studies reviewed here (e.g., [17]) help us to better conceptualize potential efficiency enhancement for the nonperformer through observation of resonance behaviors in the trained vocal performer.

Acknowledgements

Gratitude is extended to Chwen-Geng Guo, Christopher Linker and Paula Saraceno for their help in preparing this manuscript and the manuscript for the corresponding talk at the 1st World Voice Congress in Oporto, Portugal. Copies of that talk, with figures, can be obtained by writing to the author at 1245 Champa Street, Denver, Colorado 80204, USA. This paper and its presentation were supported by Grant P60 DC00976 from the National Institutes of Health.

References

1. Titze IR. Principles of Voice Production. Englewood Cliffs: Prentice Hall, 1994
2. Sundberg J. The acoustics of the singing voice. J Sci Am 1977;3:82–91.
3. Sundberg J. The Science of the Singing Voice. Dekalb, IL: The Northern Illinois University Press, 1987.
4. Raphael BN, Scherer RC. Voice modifications of stage actors: Acoustic analyses. J Voice 1987;1:83–87.
5. Titze IR, Mapes S, Story B. Acoustics of the tenor high voice. J Acoust Soc Am 1994;95:1133–1142.
6. Carlsson G, Sundberg J. Formant frequency tuning in singing. J Voice 1992;6:256–250.
7. Scherer RC, Church T, Root RS. Contrasting speech and singing – performance demonstration. J Acoust Soc Am 1993;94(3)Pt.2:1871J(A).
8. Scherer RC, Maes K, Horii Y. Voice quality of the actor in training: acoustic correlates (in preparation).

9. Sundberg J. Articulatory interpretation of the “singing formant”. J Acoust Soc Am 1974;55:838–844.
10. Yanagisawa E, Estill J, Kmucha S. Contribution of aryepiglottic constriction to “ringing” voice quality. Video tape, Yale Unviersity School of Medicine, New Haven.
11. Wilson JG. Variations of the laryngo-pharynx in singing. NATS Bull 1976;12:22–24; based on the 1972 dissertation from Indiana University School of Music.
12. Detweiler RF. An investigation of the larngeal system as the resonance source of the singer's formant. J Voice 1994;8:303–313.
13. Cleveland TF. Acoustic properties of voice timbre types and their influence on voice classification. J Acout Soc Am 1977;61:1622–1629.
14. Dmitriev L, Kiselev A. Relationship between the formant structure of different types of singing voices and the dimension of the superglottal cavaties. J Folia Phoniatr 1979;31:238–241.
15. Berndtsson G, Sundberg J. Perceptual significance of the center frequency of singer’s formant. STL-QPSR 1994;4:95–105.
16. Hertegard S, Gauffin J, Sundberg J. Open and covered singing as studies by means of fiberoptics, inverse filtering, and spectral analysis. J Voice 1990;4:220–230.
17. Bloothooft G, Plomp R. The sound level of the singer’s formant in professional singing. J Acoust Soc Am 1986;79:2028–2033.

Voice Update.
M. Pais Clemente, editor.

Heavy and light register, falsetto register, its history and use. Function and sensation of voice registers

Ank C. Reinders
The Hague, The Netherlands

Key words: chest register, falsetto registration, head register, Manuel Garcia, monody, terminology.

Introduction

Any tone we sing is generated by the vibrations of the vocal folds. If a singer sings a middle "a" on 440 Hz, his vocal folds touch each other 440 times/s. They are opening and closing all the time.

The singer can influence that procedure only by imagination, by "singing lightly" or "singing a heavier tone". So doing he can hold that open – or that closed – phase a split second longer.

Holding the open phase longer is referred to as light registration; keeping the closed phase longer is referred to as heavy registration.

Heavy registration of the voice may cause vibrations in the thorax, the so-called chest wall vibrations, but these vibrations, which the singer experiences and cherishes as his chest resonance, have no resonating function, no function in sound production. In fact, the vibrations are merely the mechanical response of the body to tones produced at a certain frequency. They have nothing to do with chest or head.

Some individual singers feel the high-pitched tones in their facial bone structure and then they assume that these vibrations have a resonating function. Thus, the expressions "head voice", "head resonance" and "head register" were created by our vocal ancestors. Similarly low-pitched tones can cause vibrations in the chest wall or in the breast bone, hence the terms "chest voice", "chest resonance" and finally "chest register".

The use of the "expanded breast" is part of the singer's breath behavior and has nothing to do with enlarged resonance.

In earlier days, when voice science was still in its infancy, one did not yet teach that registration of the voice depends on pitch (tension of the vocal folds), loudness (air pressure under the vocal folds, and airflow) and vowel (position of the articulators). That is why such personal explanations of chest- and head registers emerged from historical descriptions.

Address for correspondence: Dr Ank C. Reinders, Carel Reinerszkade 163, 2593 HP, The Hague, The Netherlands. Tel.: +31-070-382-4776.

The history of the terms

The history of the term "chest voice" can be traced in literature from the Middle Ages onwards. The first mention of the word is probably found in a treatise by Jerome De Moravia, a Dominican monk from Austria, living in a convent in Paris. His treatise dates from before 1260. He mentions different voices: "quaedam sunt pectoris, quaedam sunt gutturis, quaedam sunt ipsius capitis": voices produced in the chest, in the throat and in the head. He uses the terms which are still practiced in our modern, or let us say, less antiquated, studios.

De Moravia advocates isolated use of those different voices, which is similar to the rules that Conrad von Zabern taught in the second half of the 15th century. Zabern was aware of some kind of registration:

> "One should know that one has to divide the voice in three parts: the low tones should be sung loudly, the middle tones should be sung mezzo forte, and the high tones in a soft voice...although the human being possesses only one trachea where these three voices are produced. So let the change from one to the other voice be realized slowly".

It has always been known that the human voice has two possibilities of registration, the lower register was clearly felt in the chest, but the nature of the high voice was not clear. Was it generated in the throat or in the head, in the sinuses or even outside the skull? The terminology got confused; the lower region is still called chest by many singers but the name of the loft region, (i.e., singing in light registration) remains questionable.

The birth of monody

The new musical style, the monodic style of the early 17th century (a reaction to the polyphonic, mostly liturgical music of the preceding centuries), pointed to the birth of "opera"; this was a new concept, in which the solo voice had to be developed; the singer was on his way to becoming a soloist, and with that a singing technique for the solo voice became necessary.

This technique was different then to what it is now; until late into the 17th century the only demands were that the voice be lovely, civilized and smooth. How to manage the voice was not told. Thus started the dawn of monodic singing, of opera in 1600.

The most important tract on this new music dates from 1602 and was written by Giulio Caccini who referred to "voce di petto" or "voce piena e naturale" which means full voice, and "voce di testa" which means head voice. Actually he meant falsetto, head voice being another nonexisting phenomenon.

There is really no one valuable description of a head voice registration nor any description of physiological transitions to it. Garcia stated explicitly in 1840 that his falsetto and head voice were one register, one registration, one mode.

The only place where singers do "resonate" is in the vocal tract, for that is the way the soundwaves travel from the vocal folds to the lips and the nasal passages.

Falsetto registration, chest registration

The word falsetto has always been used in parallel to head voice in the voice-literature; the use of falsetto registration was accepted until the middle of the 19th century, the time when vocal registration changed drastically as will be pointed out later. The great teacher Tosi[1] complained about inconsistent and confusing use of the terms falsetto and head voice. He accused foreigners (i.e., anyone not of Italian origin) of creating the terminological mess-up.

For a long time the use of chest voice in singing was an exception for female singers. There is a description of the singing of Vittoria Tesi[2], which tells us that she was: "a contralto with masculine strength" evidently singing in a heavy registration; maybe she was the first belter ever described! She preferred to sing male roles, which was not exceptional in her days, she loved to sing bass airs transposed only one octave up.

The use of falsetto registration was a prerequisite for the male voice to sing high parts in early polyphonic music, it was asked for in the early opera as well, where castrati set the standard for the light and warbling use of the voice, even of those who were not castrated.

Falsetto was accepted until the first half of the 19th century but there are many recordings made in the first decades of the 20th century where the most beautiful falsetto tones are produced by famous singers.

It is incredible to see how many authors dare say that falsetto is only used for comical effects.

New vocal devices

In the 19th century the voice, again, had to follow new musical ideas of composers. The beginning of "Grand Opéra" changed vocal devices to adapt the voice to the new style, the style of "Grand Opéra", introduced by composers like Berlioz, Bellini, Donizetti and which was established in the works of Verdi and Wagner. Opera acquired a different face; there were new aspects to deal with as there were longer lines, an increase of articulative gesture which made words more expressive, and an increase of volume or carrying power.

The adjustment was made by lowering the larynx as in yawning and by protruding the lips. A new term was introduced: "To cover the voice". This new position replaced the smiling mouth-position of the castrati.

---

[1]Pier Francesco Tosi: Opnioni de' cantori antichi e moderni, 1723.

[2]Described by Quants in 1719 as a "contralto with masculine strength" (quotation from "The Great Singers" by Henry Pleasants.

Manuel Garcia's definition of a register

In 1840 Manuel Garcia presented his "Mémoire sur la voix humaine" at the "Académie Royale des Sciences" in Paris. In Garcia's tradition, which was a Spanish-Italian tradition, the question of the vocal registers was the heart of the matter, the base for all vocal education.

He described them as follows: "By the word register we mean a series of succeeding sounds of equal quality on a scale from low to high, produced by the application of the same mechanical principle, the nature of which differs basically from another series of succeeding sounds of equal quality produced by another mechanical principle".

The modification of the mode of vocal fold vibration may be regarded as a operational definition of voice register[3].

Garcia named the two modes of registration "chest" and "falsetto-head", the latter being described as one and only one mode.

A most puzzling remark by Manuel Garcia (1847)[4] is that chest voice is the essential base of the human voice in male and female singers. It was Garcia's opinion that women can (not "must") reach c^5 in chest voice (c^2 in Helmholtz counting). This fact, the extended heavy register to which Garcia refers, is taken into account in teaching the belting voice of today's pop singers. I think that we do not agree with the use of chest voice as high as c^5 in operatic singing of the female voice.

Garcia named the male top-octave, which is the female middle octave, falsetto (which from a point of vocal fold behavior, is correct), but he created confusion by calling the female top range "head voice". We still suffer from this confusion.

That is the reason why I advocate an easier and more consistent terminology: modal registration which can be heavy or light, and a separate register with its own vibratory pattern: falsetto.

Summary

A historical overview of the use and terminology of registers in the singing voice: Singers always translated the vibratory sensations in their thoracal or facial bone structures as resonances; it will not be easy to get rid of the terms "chest resonance" and "head resonance", which are better replaced by "heavy" and "light register"

Conclusion

We can conclude by saying that heavy registration has always been used in all kinds of singing. Falsetto was used in all kinds of eastern music and in classical western

---

[3]W.R. Zemlin, Speech and Hearing Science, p. 193, New Jersey 1968.

[4]M. Garcia : "Traité Complet de l'Art du Chant" Paris, 1847.

music until the 20th century, and then it went out of fashion. Falsetto came back in the voice of today's male alti, and it is manifesting itself more and more in nonclassical western music such as we can hear in many pop singers.

References

1. Garcia M. Mémoire sur la voix humaine, 1855. In: Contributions of Voice Register in Singing. Houston, 1980.
2. Garcia M. Traité Complete de l'Art du Chant. Paris, 1847.
3. Zemlin WR. Speech and Hearing Science. New Jersey, 1986.
4. Vennard W, Hirano M, Ohala J. Chest Head and Falsetto. Jacksonville, FL, 1970.
5. Sundberg J. The Science of the Singing Voice. Illinois, 1978.

Voice Update.
M. Pais Clemente, editor.

Basic vocal survival skills

Lucille Schutmaat Rubin
Professionally Speaking, New York, USA

Abstract. "Basic Vocal Survival Skills" is an experiential workshop for professional voice users, specialists, scientists, MDs, trainers, pathologists and performers. The workshop covers four areas: 1) centering the breath, 2) giving up the glottal hold, 3) releasing sound, and 4) using an effective pitch level. The purpose of the workshop is to provide vocal skills to voice users and specialists who share common needs.

Key words: speaking and acting voice workshop,voice workshop, vocal survival skills.

Basic vocal skills are necessary for the voice to "survive" the demands placed on professional voice users. These users include performers, actors, singers, speakers, commodity traders, clergy, auctioneers, teachers, and voice-over professionals. Vocal "survival" to the voice professional means something different to each user: to an executive it means "not losing my voice"; an actress, "being able to do eight shows a week"; a teacher, "avoiding vocal fatigue"; a voice-over professional, "maintaining a clear tone". The four skills explored in the survival workshop address four common voice problems: chest breathing, glottal holding and attack patterns, use of inappropriate muscles for vocal tasks, and speaking in nonoptimum pitch range.

The four basic vocal survival skills countering these problems are: centering the breath, giving up the glottal hold, releasing sound, and using an optimum pitch range. Mastering these skills contributes to vocal endurance, flow phonation, clear tone, and ease in projection. The participants, by identifying the appropriate muscles to accomplish a vocal task, learn how to avoid vocal misuse and to find optimal behaviors.

The first skill, centering the breath, is best experienced in a supine position on the floor. Once relaxed, the participant assumes a "one-half bridge" position: feet on the floor, knees pointed to the ceiling, pelvis lifted, and weight balanced between the legs and shoulders. There should be no weight on the head or neck. The participants are encouraged to allow the breath to drop in and flow out of their bodies while observing the movement of their "centers". The "center" is sometimes defined as that area located directly above and below the navel. Once this is experienced, the participants assume other positions to reinforce the feeling of the breath dropping low

---

Address for correspondence: Lucille Schutmaat Rubin PhD, Executive Director, Professionally Speaking, 119 West 57th Street, Suite 820, New York, NY 10019, USA. Tel.: +1-212-245-5944. Fax: +1-212-307-5072.

into the body. Additional tasks are added, for example:
1) connecting the breath to sound,
2) extending the length of the breath while speaking, and
3) developing flexibility in speaking patterns.

The participants are encouraged to create a relaxed internal environment that contributes to the natural process of breathing. Pulling air in and pushing air out is discouraged. Allowing the breath to move the body is encouraged at this stage of the workshop training.

The second skill, giving up the glottal hold, is explored through aerobic and weight lifting exercises. Exercises include push-ups, abdominal "crunches", and working with free weights on selected muscle groups. Working out their bodies encourages the participants to identify their holding patterns at the phonatory level. The use of earplugs is helpful in identifying the locking, freezing or holding patterns because earplugs amplify the sound of the breath flow. Holding the vocal folds in a closed position before exhaling or speaking is a common misuse pattern; once identified, participants can more readily monitor and alter the airflow. Exercises focus on experiencing a smooth, uninterrupted flow of air and voice through the throat.

The third skill, releasing sound, is designed to relax muscles that are not required in producing voice. Special attention is paid to the role of the jaw. Because performers and speakers frequently tend to engage the jaw while increasing volume levels or raising pitch levels, exercises are introduced to disengage jaw muscles in these activities. Other identified muscle tensions are discouraged through a series of exercises that address relaxation of the shoulders, neck, larynx, and throat. These exercises provide the participants with pleasurable sensations of muscle release and sound vibrations. At this stage of the workshop the focus is on releasing muscle tensions, phonating with ease, and enjoying the pleasure of sound vibrations.

The fourth skill, speaking in an optimum pitch range, helps participants find the area in their pitch range that provides maximum volume with minimum effort. A series of exercises include exploring the "head voice", playing with falsetto, and hearing the ring in the voice. Because many voice users frequently adopt pitch levels that are difficult for their vocal folds to produce, the training focuses on what feels easy, provides volume without effort, and produces a ring. The new pitch range is explored in text work with participants cupping their ears to listen for vocal ring. Blending resonators is also stressed as a way to identify optimum pitch range.

The workshop concludes with an opportunity for participants to apply their new vocal skills to text. The text used in this workshop is Shakespeare's Sonnet 23. During this sharing time participants can hear changes in their own voices and in the voices of others. The workshop also affirms the importance of experiencing and processing the voice skills if one wants to use them or teach them to others.

Centering the breath, giving up the glottal hold, releasing sound and using an optimum pitch range encourage the healthy use of the voice. After mastering these survival skills, voice users are ready for advanced voice training and better prepared to meet the demanding vocal tasks of their profession.

References

1. Barlow W. The Alexander Technique. New York: Alfred A. Knopf, Inc., 1973.
2. Berry C. Your Voice and How to Use it. London: Virgin Books, 1994.
3. Linklater K. Freeing the Natural Voice. New York: Drama Book Specialists, 1976.
4. Machlin E. Speech for the Stage. New York: Theatre Arts Books, 1966.
5. McCallion M. The Voice Book. New York: Theatre Arts Books, 1988.
6. Sataloff RT. Professional Voice: The Science and Art of Clinical Care. New York: Raven Press, 1991.
7. Saxon L, Schneider C. Vocal Exercise Physiology. San Diego: Singular Publishing Group, Inc., 1995.
8. Rodenburg P. The Right to Speak. London: Methuen Drama, 1992.
9. Rubin LS (ed). Movement for the Actor. New York: Drama Book Specialist, 1980.
10. Rubin LS. The Voice Handbook. New York: Printed by the author, 1994.
11. Skinner E. Speak With Distinction. New York: Applause Theatre Book Publishers, 1990.
12. Spreads C. Ways to Better Breathing. Great Neck, NY: Felix Morrow Publisher, 1986.

Future developments in voice science and care

Voice Update.
M. Pais Clemente, editor.

Contemporary voice issues and development of voice care

Minoru Hirano
Department of Otolaryngology – Head and Neck Surgery, Kurume University, Kurume, Japan

Key words: hemilaryngectomy, international consensus of voice test, sulcus vocalis, teamwork, voice care, voice issue.

Introduction

The topic Dr Clemente, the president of this congress, assigned to me is a huge one. It is difficult to cover all issues within the allotted time. Therefore I will concentrate on some selected issues here. Contemporary voice issues can be classified into, at least, three major categories: scientific issues for future research, clinical issues in evaluating and treating voice patients, and organizational and socioeconomic issues for improvements of voice care.

As for the scientific issues, three major issues, "molecular biology and genetics of voice disorders", "neurophysiology of phonation" and "computers and voice science" were beautifully presented by Drs Ludlow, Davis and Titze, respectively, in this session. Therefore I am not going to go into scientific issues here.

Clinical issues

There are several clinical issues awaiting improvements and advances: international standardization or consensus for clinical voice examinations; treatment for sulcus vocalis, vocal fold scar, presbyphonia and spasmodic dysphonia; reconstruction of normal voice following hemilaryngectomy; and voice rehabilitation for laryngectomized clients.

International standardization for clinical voice examinations

In the field of otology and audiology, several clinical hearing tests have been standardized internationally. As a result, one can compare the hearing function of different patients examined at different places and/or on different occasions and, also, one can monitor the results of treatment in a reliable manner.

As for vocal function, various techniques have been used by many clinicians, but none of them has yet been standardized on an international basis. Fortunately, there

---

Address for correspondence: Minoru Hirano MD, Department of Otolaryngology – Head and Neck Surgery, Kurume University, Kurume, Japan.

have been a number of valuable efforts towards standardization.

The Voice Committee, Japan Society of Logopedics and Phoniatrics, started working on this issue in 1975 and published a tentative guideline book in 1979, and later a revised version in 1994. The Voice Committee, Union of European Phoniatricians started in 1983. I do not know the details of their results but I do know that they have been working extensively. The Voice Committee, International Association of Logopedics and Phoniatrics (IALP) was established in 1986 and members have since worked hard towards the international standardization or consensus for clinical voice examinations.

Results of the activities of the Voice Committee, IALP were published in two publications; one is an official report at the 1989 International Congress published in the Folia Phoniatrica. The title was: "Objective evaluation of human voice. Clinical Aspects" [1]. The other publication appeared in one of the 1992 issues of the Journal of Voice. This was the proceedings of the voice committee workshop, presenting 12 papers [2–13]. There have been some other domestic and international activities which aim at standardization of voice tests.

I believe many voice clinicians in the world basically do have some agreements on the importance, clinical value and limitation of the perceptual voice evaluation, maximum phonation time, laryngovideostroboscopy, airflow measurement, measurement of F0 and SPL range of phonation or voice range profile. Some voice clinicians are also using the acoustic analysis of voice signal including measurements of jitter, shimmer, and signal-to-noise ratio, electromyography and electroglottography.

I believe we are very close to having some international consensus on these examinations, and I do hope we have it in the very near future.

Treatment for sulcus vocalis

The next issue is the treatment for sulcus vocalis. Several techniques, including intrafold injection, medialization surgeries, sulcusectomy [14], removal following wound-plasty with fibrin glue [15], slicing mucosa technique [16], and relaxation surgery of the vocal fold have been employed. They occasionally improve the voice but do not assure a normal postoperative voice.

The major pathophysiological aspects of sulcus are a deformity of vocal fold edge, an increase in stiffness of the vibrating structure, and glottic incompetence. The ideal treatment should be able to correct these problems. Figure 1 shows an ideal treatment. The deformed, stiff tissue around the sulcus is replaced with normal mucosa. The issue is how to achieve this. I hope some young, brilliant laryngologists develop a new technique.

Treatment of vocal fold scar

Treatment of vocal fold scar is another difficult problem. There are no existing effective techniques. I think future directions will be to develop techniques to replace

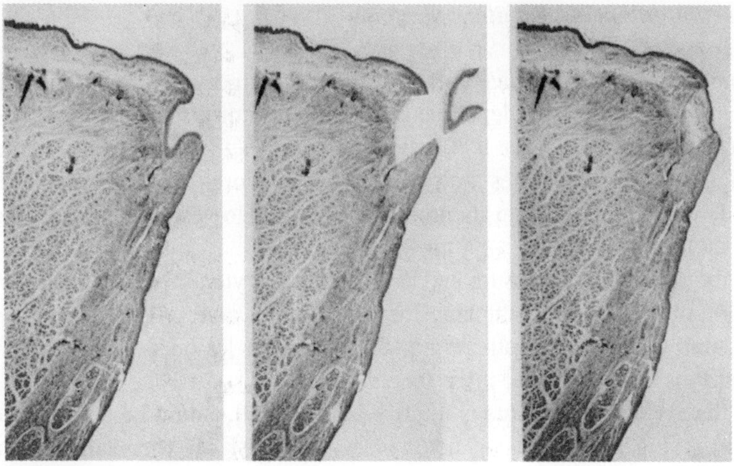

Fig. 1. Ideal surgery for sulcus vocalis.

the scar tissue with normal pliable mucosa or techniques to soften scar tissue with some medicines or some physical energy.

Treatment of presbyphonia

Treatment of presbyphonia, or aging of voice, is another clinical issue. We do not have any very effective modalities. This is a great contrast to spectacles for presbyopia.

The major pathogenetic aspects of presbyphonia are aging of the neural control of phonation, aging of the muscles of the voice organ, and aging of the vibrating structure. Therefore, the problems of presbyphonia are basically the same as those of aging of other motor activities. There might be no complete solution.

Treatment of spasmodic dysphonia

The next clinical issue is the treatment of spasmodic dysphonia.

Since 1976 when Dedo reported recurrent laryngeal nerve section [17], many surgical techniques have been developed and reported. Many discussions for and against surgical treatments have been made over nearly 2 decades.

Late in the 1980s, botulinum toxin (Botox) was first injected in the thyroarytenoid muscle of patients with spasmodic dysphonia. Since then, many reports of the effects of Botox on spasmodic dysphonia have been published and they all agree that Botox does improve voice but the effect only lasts about 2–9 months.

Development of treatments better than the existing surgeries and Botox awaits some new ideas.

Reconstruction following hemilaryngectomy

Reconstruction of normal voice following hemilaryngectomy is another challenge. Many techniques have been developed, but they do not result in normal voice.

The best possible technique is, I believe, to construct a flat wall at the midsaggital plane (Fig. 2). The wall does not vibrate but it works as a counterwall for the unaffected vocal fold, assuring its normal vibration. However, this principle is often not achievable.

When the anterior commissure and the ipsilateral arytenoid cartilage are preserved, construction of a flat wall at the anterior glottis is not a very difficult task (Fig. 3A). However, this condition is rather rare. Such a small lesion is usually treated with radiotherapy or endolaryngeal laser surgery.

When the arytenoid cartilage is removed, a flat wall should be constructed for the entire glottis (Fig. 3B). This is not a very easy task. If the wall is located too medially, the airway is too narrow resulting in breathing difficulty. If the wall is situated away from the midsaggital plane, the voice is not normal but hoarse.

In the majority of the cases for hemilaryngectomy, the anterior commissure and arytenoid cartilage have to be removed (Fig. 3C). If a flat wall is constructed along the entire length of the glottis, the airway is too narrow, causing breathing difficulty. Ideally, a flat wall should be constructed at the anterior glottis while the posterior glottis has more space as shown in the right bottom figure of Fig. 3C. At present, we do not have a technique which assures this postsurgical condition.

Voice reconstruction for the laryngectomized client

Another challenging clinical issue is voice reconstruction for laryngectomized clients. Since Dr Verkerke gave an ambitious presentation on this topic, I will not be going into it.

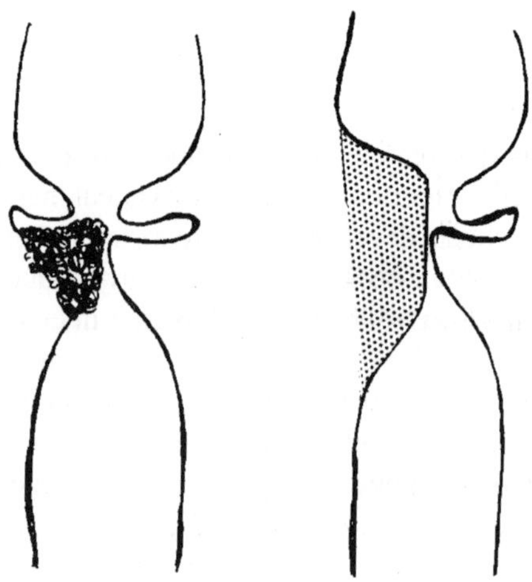

Fig. 2. Principle of surgical reconstruction following hemilaryngectomy.

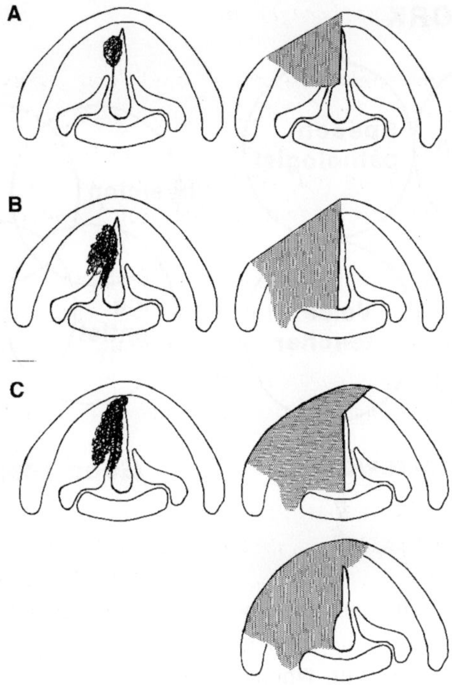

Fig. 3. Reconstruction following hemilaryngectomy. **A**: Case in which anterior commissure and arytenoid cartilage are preserved. **B**: Case in which arytenoid cartilage is removed. **C**: Case in which anterior commissure and arytenoid cartilage are removed.

Development of voice care

Finally, I would like to touch upon organizational and socioeconomic issues, in particular, development of voice care. We have to admit that voice care is poor in most parts of the world, especially in many developing countries. In such places, voice does not seem to be an important issue in health care. Even in well-developed countries, the voice care system has not been fully developed.

Voice care calls for an interdisciplinary teamwork. The voice team has to consist of at least four groups of specialists: physicians, i.e., laryngologists and/or phoniatricians, speech pathologists, voice scientists, and voice teachers. At present, we lack qualified specialists in most parts of the world. Nevertheless, good teams do exist in some lucky places.

Good teamwork cannot necessarily be made by simply putting different specialists next to each other as shown in the left portion of Fig. 4. A typical pattern with this setting is: a patient is first seen, for example, by the physician. The physician refers the patient to the other specialists and each specialist sees the patient independently and sends the patient back to the original physician with some information and opinion. I do not believe this is teamwork.

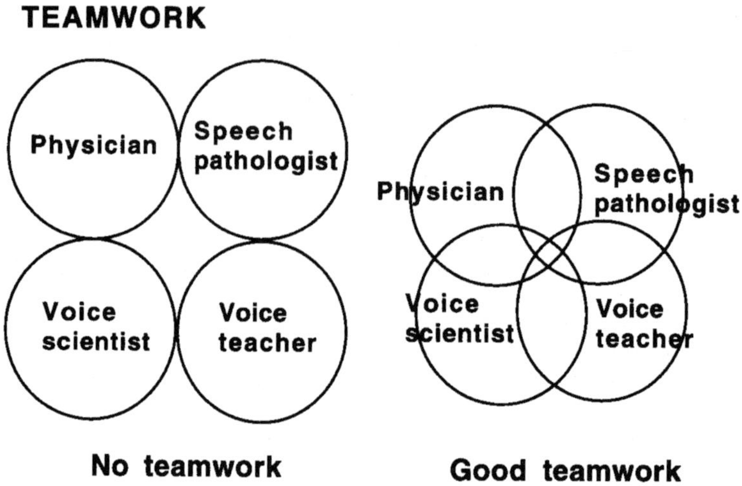

Fig. 4. Teamwork for voice care.

Good teamwork is schematically shown in the right half of Fig. 4. There are interactions among the specialists involved in this case. They may see the patient independently at some stage but, whenever necessary, they see the patient together, discuss and determine the tests to be employed, evaluate and interpret the test results together, discuss and determine the treatment plan together, make follow-up examinations interactively, etc.

The development of voice care first calls for education and training of well-qualified specialists, including laryngologists, phoniatricians, speech pathologists, voice scientists, voice teachers, etc. In order to have voice specialists of good quality and sufficient number for each country, they have to be well treated in terms of the economic and social status.

Secondly, a clinical voice center should be placed in each region of a country. Good teamwork should be presented to the patients. The voice center should be located in or closely affiliated with a medical center. Voice patients occasionally need to have the services of other medical specialties, including neurologists, psychiatrists, chest physicians, internists, endocrinologists, obstetricians, chest surgeons, etc.

I do hope this 1st World Voice Congress give some strong motivation and impact upon developments of voice care in the world.

References

1. Hirano M. Objective evaluation of the human voice: Clinical aspects. J Folia Phoniatr 1989;41:89–144.
2. Bless DM, Baken RJ. Introduction: Assessment of voice. J Voice 1992;6:95–97.
3. Baken RJ. Electroglottography. J Voice 1992;6:98–110.
4. Fritzel B. Inverse filtering. J Voice 1992;6:111–114.
5. Laver J, Hiller S, Beck JM. Acoustic waveform perturbations and voice disorders. J Voice

1992;6:115–126.

6. Schutte HK. Integrated aerodynamic measurements. J Voice 1992;6:127–134.
7. Titze IR. Vocal efficiency. J Voice 1992;6:135–138.
8. Faure MA, Muller A. Stroboscopy. J Voice 1992;6:139–148.
9. Wendler J. Stroboscopy. J Voice 1992;6:149–154.
10. Fex S. Perceptual evaluation. J Voice 1992;6:155–158.
11. Kotby MN, Fadly E, Madkour O, Barakah M, Khidr A, Alloush T, Saleh M. Electromyography and neurography in neurolaryngology. J Voice 1992;6:159–187.
12. Sonninen A, Hurme P. On the terminology of voice research. J Voice 1992;6:188–193.
13. Bless DM, Baken RJ, Hacki T, Fritzell B, Laver J, Schutte H, Hirano M, Loebell E, Titze I, Faure MA, Muller A, Wendler J, Fex S, Kotby MN, Brewer D, Sonninen A, Hurme P. International Association of Logopedics and Phoniatrics (IALP) Voice Committee discussion of assessment topics. J Voice 1992;6:194–210.
14. Hirano M. Phonosurgery. Basic and clinical investigations. J Otologia (Fukuoka) 1975;(Suppl 1):239–442.
15. Bouchayer M, Cornut G. In: Phonosurgery for Benign Vocal Fold Lesions. An Interactive Video Textbook. London: Olympic Printers Ltd., 1994.
16. Pontes P, Behlau M, Tosi O. Computer acoustical analysis of treatment of sulcus vocalis. J Folia Phoniatr 1989;41:204–205.
17. Dedo HH. Recurrent laryngeal nerve section for spastic dysphonia. J Ann Otol Rhinol Laryngol 1976;85:451–459.

1996 Elsevier Science B.V.
Voice Update.
M. Pais Clemente, editor.

The relevance of molecular biology to voice and voice disorders

Christy L. Ludlow, Julie Barkmeier, Julia Edgar and Ranjinidevi Ambalavanar
Voice and Speech Section, National Institute on Deafness and Other Communication Disorders, Bethesda, Maryland, USA

Abstract. Our focus is to explore how the expansion of knowledge and techniques in molecular biology have potential for advancing our understanding of voice and voice disorders. Questions can be posed pertinent to the control of laryngeal development: the progenitor cell systems, patterns of laryngeal development and development of the neural control systems. Of greater importance to most voice disorders, however, are the mechanisms controlling laryngeal function throughout the life span and following injury. Topics for investigation include: the control of cell growth, differentiation, and cell death during development and thereafter; neurotropic factors affecting innervation and reinnervation; neuromuscular plasticity resulting from injury or activity; central plasticity and cell excitability following inflammation, stimulation or injury to peripheral afferents; detection of proto-oncogene expression following neuronal activity to determine the functional neuronal pathways; neurotransmitter systems controlling laryngeal function; and immunologic responses to inflammation.

Key words: neurobiology, neuroplasticity, neurotoxicity, neurotransmission.

Introduction

The power of the new techniques and knowledge available in molecular biology and genetics will help those working in the voice and voice disorders fields better understand the mechanisms controlling laryngeal development, tissue changes following injury, and the pathophysiology and possible causes for many voice disorders. A revolution has taken place in the biomedical sciences with the rapid expansion of new knowledge of cellular mechanisms. The genetic code continuously controls adaptation and use throughout the life span. The transcription of the genetic code contained within the DNA into the many forms of RNA and the subsequent translation of RNA for the formation of proteins is the continued basis for the control of function and adaptation to change. Our future understanding of voice disorders will depend upon our understanding the regulation of these mechanisms and their response to changes in activity, function and injury. As demonstrated by Sataloff in his recent review of the genetics of voice, there are no familial voice disorders [1]. Although several familial disorders affect body systems which impact on the larynx and voice, there are none that are specific to voice production. However, because genetic mechanisms control all bodily mechanisms, these are of relevance to the voice and voice disorders. This paper will provide: 1) a few illustrative examples of how

Address for correspondence: Christy L. Ludlow PhD, 10 Center Drive MSC 1416, Bethesda, MD 20892-1416. Fax: +1-301-480-0803. E-mail: Ludlow@vss.nidcd.nih.gov molecular mechanisms and their control are relevant to voice function and voice disorders; and 2) references for the interested reader.

Development

To understand the development of the larynx, the mechanisms of embryogenesis must first be understood. The development of an embryo from a blastula is contingent on cell proliferation, migration, morphogenesis, differentiation, and programmed cell death (apoptosis). Initially, cells proliferate at a rapid rate and have the potential to become any type of cell. Intrinsic factors such as cell-type-specific patterns of gene expression are regulated by a variety of molecular mechanisms, leading to translation of proteins which determine cell fate and function. As the embryo generates sheets of epithelial cells, these sheets change shape to create new structures. Cell differentiation is genetically regulated; for example, a progenitor cell is limited to a specific cell type by gene activation [2].

Extrinsic systems (induction) can also affect how a cell develops. That is, if tissue from one region is transplanted, it can develop according to the region to which is has been transplanted rather than its origin [3]. Cells may also migrate to new positions where they differentiate into various cell types. The extracellular matrix, composed of a variety of materials including collagen, fibronectin, and laminin, provides the directional cues for cell migration. The transforming growth factor (TGF-ß), a superfamily of proteins, has been identified as a key player in growth and differentiation [4] and shares a common structural motif with nerve growth factor (NGF) and platelet-derived growth factor (PDGF). Extrinsic influences also include hormonal modulation, and cell-to-cell interactions. An interaction of intrinsic and extrinsic factors determine a cell's ultimate fate [5,6]. Abnormalities during embryogenesis are not likely to be specific to the voice but rather affect multiple body systems.

Apoptosis

Programmed cell death or apoptosis is a normal physiological process that eliminates unwanted, functionally abnormal, or harmful cells [7]. This process occurs during both embryonic development and throughout adult life. Apoptosis can eliminate an entire structure during development, such as a tadpole tail, or it can shape tissues such as eliminating webbing between fingers and toes, and cause diffuse loss of cells during organ development. Apoptosis differs from necrosis (pathological cell death) in that there is no inflammatory reaction, no damage to neighboring cells, and no scar tissue formation [8].

Cell death involves targeting affected cells, loss of cell contact with neighboring cells, gene activation, chromatin condensation resulting in DNA fragmentation, condensation of intracellular proteins and loss of cytoplasmic volume, cell shrinkage, membrane ruffling and blebbing, and cell fragmentation with neighboring cells and macrophages phagocytosing the cell fragments [9].

Cell death and cell survival are controlled by combined intracellular and extracellular signals. Imbalance between these signals in the developing embryo may result in deformities such as laryngeal atresias and laryngeal webs [10]. Cancer provides another example of cell death gone awry. Amyotrophic lateral sclerosis and Parkinson's disease are examples of inappropriate cell death in the nervous system. Inappropriately expressed genes may be responsible for cell death in these disease processes [11].

Specific genes initiate the cell death sequence, others conduct the actual killing while others serve to prevent cell death. Nerve growth factor is an example of a protein-regulating growth both during development and for the restitution of function following injury [12]. Processes of cell growth, determination, and apoptosis continue throughout the life span. With the exception of the nervous system, the body is under constant rejuvenation. In addition, the immune system creates new cells to combat illness in the body which must also be eliminated when their job is done [13,14].

Laryngeal development

The origin of the larynx occurs within the first 8 weeks [15,16]. The notochord, an axial structure, first emerges at day 17. From the notochord, the neural ectoderm emerges dorsally, the umbilical vesicle ventrally, and the floor plate of the neural tube. Neural crest cells accumulate between the neural tube and the somites. The surrounding somites give rise to the vertebral column and the musculature of the same segment.

The intrinsic laryngeal muscles and some parts of the tenth cranial nerve emerge from somites one and two [17–22]. The extrinsic laryngeal muscles and other portions of the tenth cranial nerve originate from somites 2–5. Only indirect evidence suggests that laryngeal cartilage, muscle and nervous tissues arise from the 4th–6th pharyngeal arches. Hox genes have been linked to the specification of axial structures in the hindbrain and branchial arches, involving the respiratory and craniofacial development [23].

Laryngeal development is first evident at 4 weeks with the formation of a median groove between the fourth and sixth pharyngeal arches elongating caudally. The development of the opening within the glottis by the 8th week is critical. The epithelial lamina provides the division for the glottis. It will eventually disappear leaving the opening for the airway. In general, the periods of greatest risk for malformations occurring are during embryogenesis for all structures including the larynx. Most of the severe laryngeal anomalies such as the atresias arise from the failure of the larynx to open at the 8th week [22].

Between 33–37 days, the superior laryngeal nerve (SLN) and the recurrent laryngeal nerve (RLN) appear in the laryngeal area and by 57 days, an adult-like pattern of motor innervation is evident. Axon growth cones are the nerve growth structures which navigate, often over long distances, to find and synapse with target cells. Growth cones follow, and are attracted or opposed by other cell types or neurotransmitters. These can grow as fast as 140 μm/h [24]. They interact with multiple types of cell surface molecules as well as extracellular matrices in guiding their growth as well as recognizing and making connections with target cells [5].

Cell growth is achieved by constant remodeling of the cytoskeleton or cellular structures; various adhesion proteins and integrins abound in the growth cone membrane to accomplish this process. Cell survival is contingent on reaching the target they innervate. The neurotrophic theory suggests that target cells are the source of certain substances that direct the axon such as nerve growth factor (NGF) [25]. When the axon reaches the target it differentiates from a growing structure to a secreting structure as a consequence of contact with the target [26]. It forms a synapse, thus altering the cell phenotype. In peripheral nerve development, axon outgrowth and synaptogenesis occur and are followed by elimination of improper or unnecessary connections.

Some laryngeal innervation abnormalities can appear early in development or later in life. Specific to the larynx, progressive motor neuron cell death is recognized as a rare autosomal dominant trait found in humans [27] and occurs as an autosomal dominant trait in Bouvier des Flanders and Husky-type dogs [28]. This may differ from the polyneuropathy, a possible autosomal recessive trait, affecting laryngeal adduction in Dalmations [29]. Peripheral neuropathies found in horses, may be preferential involvement of the distal parts of the RLN [29,30]. One study in humans suggested linkage with HLA and GLO, genetic markers indicating that the locus for this disorder in humans may be chromosome 6 [27]. Future molecular biological studies should provide information about the mechanisms responsible for cell death affecting the motor neurons and/or nerve fibers.

Reinnervation

Developmental patterns of nerve growth are important because reinnervation processes following injury may recapitulate these developmental processes to some degree. The molecular factors that promote and guide nerve growth cones may also regulate reinnervation [31]. It is known, for example, that the accuracy of reinnervation will depend upon the degree to which the surrounding tissues have not been altered.

For reinnervation to occur, the motoneuron must grow and establish connections with muscle fibers again. Following axotomy, the proximal axon dedifferentiates and returns to the nerve growth cone state. Branches of up to five “daughter” axons come off the injured axon proximal stump. Cytoskeletal elements are transported into the “daughter” axons, promoting their subsequent growth. Ultimately, only one reconnection will be made. Myelination of the sprouts is the result of connection of the axon with Schwann cells which provide guidance towards the original site and formation of the basal lamina.

Schwann cells proliferate along with the macrophages to clean up the site reducing the gap between the reinnervation site and the end of the proximal axon. They produce various neurotrophic factors as well as cytokines. They also express neural cell adhesion molecules which promote reinnervation and continue the process of myelination. Success in reinnervation is more likely to occur if the basement membrane is intact and the growing axon can use the same Schwann cell as the previous axon [32].

Muscle adaptation

Recent advances in neurobiology have demonstrated that the nerves and muscles are much more adaptive than was previously thought. With changes in nerve firing rates, muscle fibers undergo complete functional and biochemical transformation [33]. The functional characteristics may be altered, first with changes in the biochemical properties of the muscle fibers, and with changes in their contractile characteristics coming later. Muscle cells also change in the response to tension loads placed upon them. Therefore, thyroplasty and arytenoid adduction procedures may produce both functional and biochemical changes in muscle cells as long as the muscle continues to be innervated.

Neuromuscular junctions also adapt. Following botulinum toxin type A injection, endplates die due to the inactivation of the intracellular protein required for the presynaptic release of acetylcholine [34]. Recent new information on the botulinum neurotoxins has demonstrated the different modes of action of the various forms of botulinum toxin on proteins either within the synaptic vesicle membranes (types B, D and F) [35] or within synaptic membrane proteins (type A) [36]. Reinnervation involves the growth of nerve collaterals some of which form synapses and survive [37–40]. Collateral nerve sprouting could change the recruitment of muscle fibers for movement, if motor units develop a larger territory of muscle fibers [31]. With injury and aging, nerve terminal sprouting may also occur, resulting in less-specific muscle fiber activation for fine movement control. This sprouting could reduce fine muscle control for speech and singing.

Neurotransmitter systems

Multiple neurotransmitters and neuropeptides interact with specific receptors to produce complex processes within cells. Once a receptor is activated, second messenger systems produce biochemical changes throughout the cell [41]. If any part of the entire system is altered, function may be severely compromised. Neurotransmission therefore is the target of many therapeutic drugs to correct abnormalities in the nervous system.

By using antibodies, neuropeptides, neurotransmitters and neuromodulators involved in laryngeal function can be identified. For example, substance P, calcitonin gene-related peptide (CGRP), vasoactive intestinal peptide (VIP), and neuropeptide Y (NPY) have been localized in the feline, canine, rat and human larynges [42–46]. Regional differences in the distribution of peptidergic nerve fibers may be important in protective laryngeal mechanisms, local blood flow and exocrine secretion [47,48]. Neuropeptides are also associated with the autonomic nervous system and may act as mediators in the pathogenesis of laryngeal edema [42,47].

Many peptides have been detected in the cell bodies in nodose ganglia and in the nuclei of the solitary tract. The intrinsic role of NMDA glutamate receptors in synaptic transmission of the NTS has been shown by physiological and pharmacological experiments [49]. NTS serves as the first relay for the sensory information from the cardiovascular, respiratory and gastrointestinal systems. Further study will identify the specific neurochemical characteristics of NTS neurons involved in sensory processing from the larynx.

These neurotransmitters and second messenger neuromodulators can also serve as trophic agents for the establishment of neuronal circuitry during development and the rearrangement of synapses following changes in sensory experience or injury [12]. Studies of cells in slices have allowed investigators to examine long-term potentiation of synaptic connections between cells [50]. As Hebb [51] originally proposed, molecular studies are confirming how synaptic connections are altered by frequent simultaneous firing of two convergent neurons providing the basis for adaptation and change. These neuronal changes may be the basis for adaptation of laryngeal control for the development of new speech and singing skills.

Immediate early genes

Molecular tools are now available for the study of cellular mechanisms that link neuronal excitation to gene expression. A number of genes encode transcription factors that represent a link between an extracellular stimulus and changes in gene expression induced in cells as a result of stimulation. Increases in transcription of cellular immediate early genes occur within 5 min of the application of a stimulus to a cell and can terminate within 30 min [41].

Investigations have focused on the expression of a nuclear phosphoprotein, called Fos which is encoded by the proto-oncogene, c-fos [41]. Fos is rapidly induced in neurons by transsynaptic stimulation and membrane electrical activity [52]. By using an antibody to detect the Fos-protein individual neurons stimulated as a result of laryngeal stimulation can be detected [53]. This technique can be used to identify neuronal activity involved in behavior.

Neuroimaging

Parallel studies are being conducted in humans using functional neuroimaging techniques to examine the role of different brain regions in voice function for speech and singing. Positron emission tomography using ^{15}O-labelled water can average blood flow in different brain regions during behavior over 1-min intervals [54]. The role of primarily cortical systems for voice production in humans is striking. Voice use for untrained singing involves greater right hemisphere involvement while conversational speech primarily involves left hemisphere activation [55].

Functional magnetic resonance imaging, a newer technique, is less invasive and allows for the study of changes in blood flow within much shorter epochs, of a few seconds [32]. Future techniques will allow for the detection of molecules representing neurotransmission during behavioral intervals so that molecular activity can be contrasted for various voice tasks.

Neural plasticity

A considerable degree of cortical plasticity can occur in adult animals following either the loss of sensory input or motor training [56,57]. Cortical neurons previously controlling one motor region can assume new functions after motor training [58]. Cortical representation can be enlarged with motor training. Such plasticity, however, could also be detrimental when there is temporary loss of sensory input or motor behavior following injury [59]. As molecular mechanisms support considerable adaptation to change or use, both peripherally and centrally, they are also involved in immediate and long-term effects of injury and inflammation [60].

Peripheral injury: central effects

A peripheral injury and inflammation will produce immediate local responses affecting cell homeostasis. The release of cellular breakdown products such as interleukin-1 and other cytokines, can cause the release of nerve growth factor from skin fibroblasts. Immune-competent mast cells and basophils have nerve growth factor receptors and are stimulated to release serotonin and histamine which sensitizes nocioceptors [13]. At the spinal cord or brain stem levels, the action of peptides as well as glutamate receptors can produce increased sensitivity to sensory stimuli [60].

The various inflammatory cells mediate their responses by releasing or generating chemical compounds or by recruiting other cells to do the same. These chemical mediators participating in inflammation are also capable of damaging tissues and interfering with the functioning of the organs [61,62]. In fact, one of the major excitatory amino acids, glutamate, is present in many sensory systems including the nucleus tractus solitarius [63]. Increased release of glutamate can cause neurotoxicity if amplification is continued in central neurons due to prolonged nociceptive stimulation [60,64]. The levels of early gene products, such as Fos, are increased following prolonged peripheral stimulation suggesting an adaptive hyperexcitability in central neurons following peripheral injury which may eventually lead to cell death.

Cytokines

Finally, the immune system is finely tuned to produce a proliferation of "T" cells which can be cytotoxic. These cells are activated to produce the cytokines, which are extremely potent, soluble mediators peptides or glycoproteins that regulate local homeostasis and recruit external systems. Although cytokines may have action in normal physiological events these polypeptides are released by activated immune cells during infection and inflammation. When there is tissue trauma or systemic insult, cytokines may enter the circulation and result in a threat to systemic or local tissue homeostasis by affecting the regulation of the blood brain barrier. Many cytokines and their receptors are widely distributed in the central and peripheral nervous systems [65,66]. During the inflammatory response, cytokines are involved in the neurogenic component of inflammation and can influence many neurotransmitters and second messenger systems, affecting the defense and repair of both neuronal and nonneuronal tissue [61,62,67]. The cytokines have diverse effects on many aspects of neuronal function in the central and peripheral nervous system and have been implicated in a variety of neurological disorders including multiple sclerosis. It is possible that inflammatory mediators underlie some of the laryngeal disorders of unknown etiology either by acting centrally in the brain regions controlling laryngeal function or peripherally on the nerves and other laryngeal tissues. A better understanding of the mediators of inflammation operating in the larynx and the relevant brain regions may help to clarify the pathogenesis of these diseases and to devise more efficacious therapy.

This review has only mentioned some of the immediately apparent applications of molecular biology for providing new knowledge concerning laryngeal development, adaptation for use and response to injury. With the application of this rapidly growing new knowledge to our fields, many more avenues for increasing our understanding of voice and voice disorders will emerge.

References

1. Sataloff RT. Genetics of the voice. J Voice 1995;9:16–19.
2. Shostak S. Embryos and development. In: Embryology, an Introduction to Developmental Biology. Harpert Collins Publishers, Inc., 1991;7–32.
3. Purves D, Lichtman JW. Pattern and positional information. In: Principles of Neural Development. Sinauer Associates, Inc., 1985.
4. Wall NA, Hogan BLM. TGF-b related genes in development. J Curr Opin Genet Devel 1994;4:517–522.
5. Cypher C, Letourneau PC. Growth cone motility. J Curr Opin Cell Biol 1992;4:4–7.
6. Shostak S. Pattern formation in the blastula. In: Embrology, an Introduction to Developmental Biology. Harpert Collins Publishers, Inc., 1991;415–447.
7. Stellar H. Mechanisms and genes of cellular suicide. J Science 1995;267:1445–1462.
8. Bright JJ, Khar A. Apoptosis: programmed cell death in health and disease. J Bio Rep 1994;14:67–81.
9. Hengartner MO, Horvitz HR. Programmed cell death in *Caenorhabditis elegans*. J Curr Opin Genet Devel 1994;4:581–586.
10. Zaw-Tun HI. Development of congenital laryngeal atresias and clefts. J Ann Otol Rhinol Laryngol 1988;97:353–358.
11. Thompson CB. Apoptosis in the pathogenesis and treatment of disease. J Science 1995;267:1456–1462.
12. Russell DS. Neurotrophins: Mechanisms of action. J Neuroscientist 1995;1:3–6.
13. Mendell LM. Neurotrophic factors and the specification of neural function. J Neurosci 1995;1:26–34.
14. Nagata S, Goldstein P. The Fas death factor. J Science 1995;267:1449–1455.
15. Müller F, O'Rahilly R, Tucker JA. The human larynx at the end of the embroyonic period proper. J Acta Otolaryngol 1981;91:323–336.
16. Müller F, O'Rahilly R, Tucker JA. The human larynx at the end of the embroyonic period proper. II. The laryngeal cavity and the innervation of its lining. J Ann Otol Rhinol Laryngol 1985;94:607–617.
17. Hast MH. Early development of the human laryngeal muscles. J Ann Otol Rhinol Laryngol 1972;81:524–531.
18. Noden DM. Cell movements and control of patterned tissue assembly during craniofacial

development. J Cranio Gen Dev Biol 1991;11:192–213.

19. Tucker JA, Tucker GF. Some aspects of fetal laryngeal development. J Ann Otol Rhinol Laryngol 1978;87:636–644.
20. Vermeersch H, Kluyskens P. Embroyology of the larynx. J Acta Otorhinolaryngol Belg 1983;37:900–906.
21. Wilson DB. Embryonic development of the head and neck: Part 2, the branchial region. J Head Neck Surg 1979;2:59–66.
22. Zaw-Tun HI, Burdi AR. Reexamination of the origin and early development of the human larynx. J Acta Anat 1985;122:163–184.
23. Krumlauf R. Mouse *Hox* genetic functions. J Curr Opin Genet Devel 1993;3:621–625.
24. Stirling RV, Dunlop SA. The dance of the growth cones – where to next? J TINS 1995;18:111–115.
25. Purves D, Lichtman JW. Neuronal health during development. In: Principles of Neural Development. Sinauer Associates, 1985;135–143.
26. Vrbova G, Gordon T, Jones R. Development of motoneurons. In: Nerve-Muscle Interaction, 2nd edn. London: Chapman & Hall, 1995;30.
27. Mace M, Williamson E, Worgan D. Autosomal dominantly inherited adductor laryngeal paralysis – a new syndrome with a suggestions of linkage to HLA. J Clin Gen 1978;14:265–270.
28. O'Brien JA, Hendriks J. Inherited laryngeal paralysis. Analysis in the Husky Cross. J Vet Quart 1986;8:301–302.
29. Braund KG, Shores A, Cochrane S, Forrester D, Kwiecien JM, Steiss JE. Laryngeal paralysis-polyneuropathy complex in young Dalmatians. Am J Vet Res 1994;55:534–542.
30. Cahill JI, Goulden BE. Further evidence for a central nervous system component in equine laryngeal hemiplegia. N Z Vet J 1989;37:89–90.
31. Vrbova G, Gordon T, Jones R. Nerve regeneration and muscle reinnervation. In: Nerve-Muscle Interaction, 2nd edn. London: Chapman & Hall, 1995;199–204.
32. Prichard JW. The nuclear magnetic resonance revolution in basic and clinical neuroscience. J Neurosci 1995;1:84–94.
33. Vrbova G, Gordon T, Jones R. Plasticity of muscles and their motor units. In: Nerve-Muscle Interaction, 2nd edn. London: Chapman & Hall, 1995;109–136.
34. Borodic GE, Ferrant RJ, Pearce LB, Alderson K. Pharmacology and histology of the therapeutic application of botulinum toxin. In: Jankovic J, Hallett M (eds) Therapy With Botulinum Toxin. New York: Marcel Dekker, Inc., 1994;119–157.
35. Montecucco C, Schiavo G. Tetanus and botulism neurotoxins: a new group of zinc proteases. J Trends Biochem Sci 1993;18:324–327.
36. Blasi J, Chapman ER, Link E et al. Botulinum neurotoxin A selectively cleaves the synaptic protein SNAP-25. J Nature 1993;365:160–163.
37. Borodic GE, Ferrante R. Effects of repeated botulinum toxin injections on orbicularis oculi muscle. J Clin Neuro-opthalmol 1992;12:121–127.
38. Alderson K, Holds JB, Anderson RL. Botulinum-induced alteration of nerve-muscle interactions in the human orbicularis oculi following treatment for blepharospasm. J Neurol 1991;41:1800–1805.
39. Holds JB, Alderson K, Fogg SG, Anderson RL. Motor nerve sprouting in human orbicularis muscle after botulinum A injection. J Invest Opthalmol Vis Sci 1990;31:964–967.
40. Harris CP, Alderson K, Nebeker J, Holds JB, Anderson RL. Histologic features of human orbicularis oculi treated with botulinum A toxin. J Arch Ophthalmol 1991;109:393–395.
41. Morgan JI, Curran T. The immediate-early gene response and neuronal death and regeneration. J Neurosci 1995;1:68–75.
42. Basterra J, Dilly P, Perez M, Chumbley C. Vasoactive intestinal peptide and neuropeptide Y as possible mediators in laryngeal oedema. An immunoflourescence study. J Acta Otol Rhinol Laryngol Belg 1989;43:99–104.
43. Domeiji S, Dahlqvist A, Forsgren S. Regional differences in the distribution of nerve fibres showing substances P and calcitonin gene-related peptide-like immunoreactivity in the rat larynx. J Acta Embryol 1991;183:49–56.

44. Domeiji S, Dahlqvist A, Forsgren S. Studies on colocalization of neuropeptide Y, vasoactive intestinal polypeptide, catecholamine synthesizing enzymes and acetylcholinesterase in the larynx of the rat. J Cell Tis Res 1991;263:495–505.
45. Hauser-Kronberger C, Albegger K, Saria A, Hacker GW. Regulatory peptides in the human larynx and recurrent laryngeal nerves. J Acta Otolaryngol (Stockh) 1993;113:409–413.
46. Tanaka Y, Yoshida Y, Hirano M, Morimoto M, Kanaseki T. Distribution of SP- and CGRP-immunoreactivity in the cat's larynx. J Laryngol Otol 1993;107:522–526.
47. Lundberg JM, Saria A. Capsaisin-sensitive vagal neurons inolved in control of vascular permeability in rat trachea. J Acta Physiol Scand 1982;115:521–523.
48. Masuko S, Kawasoe M, Chiba T, Shin T. Target specific projections of intrinsic ganglionic neurons with different chemical codes in the canine larynx. J Neurosci Res 1991;9:270–278.
49. Champagnat J. Transmitter/peptide interactions in NTS neuronal circuits. In: Barraco IRA (ed) Nucleus of the Solitary Tract. CRC Press, 1994;215–224.
50. Malenka RC. LTP and LTD: Dynamic and interactive processes of synaptic plasticity. J Neurosci 1995;1:35–41.
51. Hebb DO. The Organization of Behavior. New York: John Wiley & Sons, 1949.
52. Hunt SP, Pini A, Evan G. Induction of c-fos-like protein in spinal cord neurons following sensory stimulation. J Nature 1987;328:623–624.
53. Tanaka Y, Yoshida Y, Hirano M. Expression of Fos-protein activated by tactile stimulation on the laryngeal vestibulum in the cat's lower brain stem. J Laryngol Otol 1995;109:39–44.
54. Raichle ME. Exploring the mind with dynamic imaging. J Sem Neurosci 1990;2:307–315.
55. Braun AR, Ludlow CL, Varga M, Stager S, Schulz G. Correlates of speech and language production in humans studied with H_2O^{15} positron emission tomography. J Soc Neurosci Abstr 1993;19:1493.
56. Kaas JH, Merzenich MM, Killackey HP. The reorganization of somatosensory cortex following peripheral nerve damage in adult and developing animals. J Ann Rev Neurosci 1983;6:325–356.
57. Brasil-Neto JP, Valls-Solé J, Pascual-Leone A, et al. Rapid modulation of human cortical motor outputs following ischaemic nerve block. J Brain 1993;116:511–525.
58. Sanes JN, Wang J, Donoghue JP. Immediate and delayed changes of rat motor cortical output representation with new forelimb configurations. J Cereb Cortex 1992;2:141–152.
59. Merzenich MM, Recanzone G, Jenkins WM, Allard TT, Nudo RJ. Cortical representational plasticity. In: Rakic P, Singer W (eds) Neurobiology of Neocortex. New York: John Wiley & Sons, 1988;41–67.
60. Coderre TJ, Katz J, Vaccarino AL, Melzack R. Contribution of central neuroplasticity to pathological pain: review of clinical and experimental evidence. J Pain 1993;52:259–285.
61. Pousset F. Cytokines and the brain. J Eur Cytokine Netw 1992;4:57–61.
62. Pousset F. Cytokines as mediators in the central nervous system. J Biomed Pharmacother 1994;48:425–431.
63. Henry JL, Sessle BJ. Effects of glutamate, substance P, and eledoisin-related peptide on solitary tract neurons involved in respiration and respiratory reflexes. J Neurosci 1985;14:863–873.
64. Urban L, Thompson SWN, Dray A. Modulation of spinal excitability: cooperation between neurokinin and excitatory amino acid neurotransmitters. J TINS 1994;17:432–438.
65. Bartfai T, Schultzberg M. Cytokines in neural cell types. J Neurochem Int 1993;22:435–444.
66. Hopkins SJ, Rothwell NJ. Cytokines and the nervous system I: expression and recognition. J TINS 1995;18:83–88.
67. Rothwell NJ, Hopkins SJ. Cytokines and the nervous system II: actions and mechanisms of action. J TINS 1995;18:130–136.

Voice Update.
M. Pais Clemente, editor.

Development of a totally implantable artificial larynx

Gijsbertus J. Verkerke[1], Aalze Veenstra[1], Martin P. de Vries[1], Harm K. Schutte[2], Henk J. Busscher[3,4], Ingo F. Herrmann[5], Henny C. Van der Mei[4] and Gerhard Rakhorst[1]

[1]Centre for Biomedical Technology and [2]Department of Medical Physiology, Faculty of Medicine, University of Groningen, Groningen, The Netherlands; [3]Scientific and Applied Surface Advice BV (Sasa BV), Thesinge, The Netherlands; [4]University of Groningen, Faculty of Medicine, Materia Technica, Groningen, The Netherlands; and [5]European Hospital, ENT-Department, Rome, Italy

Abstract. *Background.* The consequences of a life-saving laryngectomy are still very distressing. The Eureka project "Artificial Larynx" aims at realization of an implantable artificial larynx to eliminate all drawbacks.

Methods. The artificial larynx will consist of artificial vocal folds of adjustable pitch and variable frequency during speech, an artificial epiglottis controlled by muscles, a valve mechanism to switch between breathing and speaking, and a tissue connector to connect the artificial larynx to the trachea.

Results. The valve mechanism has been designed and built and it can already be used as a tracheostoma valve. For the voice-producing element we intend to use mechanical and electrical vibrating principles. Potential principles are selected and will be built as prototype. A tissue connector with a porous surface has been designed. Research will focus on optimal materials for soft tissue ingrowth. To prevent bacterial and fungal adhesion to the artificial larynx the adhesion process to silicone rubber shunt valves has been analyzed. Bacterial colonization is followed by more harmful yeast strains. The materials resistance to this adhesion process will be developed.

Conclusions. Numerous problems have to be solved. Each solution, however, can be applied already to improve the existing rehabilitation process of laryngectomized patients.

Key words: artificial larynx, artificial organs, laryngectomy, voice rehabilitation, voice prosthesis.

Introduction

For patients with a laryngeal tumor, a laryngectomy is a life-saving operation. Using the common reconstruction technique [1,2] the trachea is led outside to an opening in the neck (tracheostoma), thus separating the airway and digestive tract. After a tracheoesophageal puncture, speech is restored by inserting a shunt valve in the created fistula. When the patient wants to speak, the tracheal opening has to be closed with the thumb or a finger, forcing air through the shunt valve into the upper part of the esophagus. When expired air flows through the cricopharyngeal muscle, vibrations will be created that make speech possible. The shunt valve prevents leakage from the esophagus and stenosis of the fistula. There is a possibility to avoid manual closure of the tracheostoma by using a valved tracheostoma prosthesis. This device has a

Address for correspondence: G.J. Verkerke, University of Groningen, Faculty of Medicine, Centre for Biomedical Technology, Oostersingel 59, 9713 EZ Groningen, The Netherlands.

valve that will close when the patient produces a sudden spurt of airflow. The consequences of this operation, however, are still very distressing. The main disadvantages of this treatment are:

- The stoma is always visible and embarrassing to the patient.
- The speech quality is often very poor [3,4]. Frequency is low and can hardly be varied during speech.
- Because the airway does not pass the nasal airways anymore, the ability to smell is lost.
- Cold or dry air may irritate the trachea causing coughing.
- A tracheostoma valve needs manual adaptation to allow coughing. This takes time and is impractical.
- Air leakage between tracheostoma valve and tracheostoma might occur, resulting in unpleasant noises and less air capacity for speech.
- Leakage between shunt valve and the surrounding soft tissue occur.
- The shunt valve has a limited life ranging from weeks to months [2]. Due to *Candida* and bacterial adhesion the shunt valve has to be changed frequently.

All drawbacks could be eliminated if it was possible to develop an implantable artificial larynx that restored all lost functions. The quality of life of these patients would improve tremendously. Therefore, in 1992 the project "Artificial Larynx" was started at the University of Groningen in The Netherlands as a cooperation of medical experts and technical experts. The aim of the project was to develop a totally implantable artificial larynx for laryngectomized patients.

Materials and Methods

In the artificial larynx (Fig. 1), the airway between trachea and pharynx will be restored. There will be no need for an opening in the neck, so patients will be able

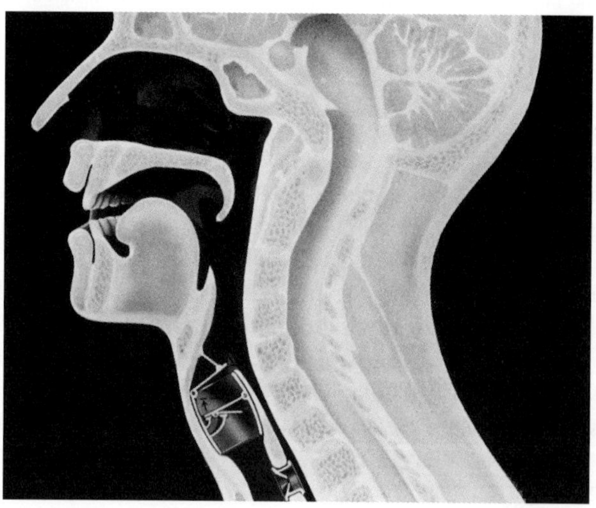

Fig. 1. Artist's impression of the artificial larynx.

to breathe again through their nose or mouth and regain their sense of smell. The trachea will no longer be exposed to the irritating effects of cold and dry air.

As with the natural larynx, the artificial one will be covered by a mobile epiglottis to stop food and fluid from entering the airway when swallowing. We intend to use muscles involved in the swallowing process to control the artificial epiglottis. There will be a shunt valve below the larynx carrying artificial vocal folds of adjustable pitch to offer an individual voice frequency to each patient. A permanent connection between the artificial larynx and surrounding soft tissue provided by a tissue connector will prevent leakage. A valve mechanism (comparable to a tracheostoma valve) will make it possible to switch between breathing and speaking.

To realize all these ideas, it was necessary to add several other groups with additional medical and technical expertise to the Groningen research team. Nowadays, the project is carried out by 11 research institutes and five industries from The Netherlands, Italy and Germany:

- Centre for Biomedical Technology, University of Groningen, Groningen, The Netherlands.
- Faculty of Chemical Technology, University of Twente, Enschede, The Netherlands.
- Faculty of Mechanical Engineering, University of Twente, Enschede, The Netherlands.
- Academic Hospital of the Free University, ENT-department, Amsterdam, The Netherlands.
- Academic Hospital Nijmegen, ENT-department, Nijmegen, The Netherlands.
- Medin Instruments, Groningen, The Netherlands.
- SASA, Scientific and Applied Surface Advice BV, Thesinge, The Netherlands.
- ESKA Medical GmbH, Lübeck, Germany.
- European Hospital, ENT-department, Rome, Italy.
- European Research Institute, Rome, Italy.
- University of La Sapienza Roma, IV ENT Clinic, Rome, Italy.
- University of Udine, ENT-department, Udine, Italy.
- Techniconsult s.r.l., Rome, Italy.
- SIST, Societa' Italiana Stampaggio Termoplastici, Rome, Italy.

Results

To date the following results have been obtained:

Valve mechanism

Prototypes of valve mechanisms to choose between breathing and speaking have been designed and built. This part of the artificial larynx consists of two valves, the first one is a speech valve, the second one is a cough valve. The speech valve is necessary to choose between speaking and breathing. The valve will be open during normal breathing: inspiration and expiration is possible.

The valve will be closed by forced expiration. The expired air is lead through a voice-producing element. That is another part of the project, namely the development of artificial vocal folds that produce a sound identical to the sound of the vocal folds. After each spoken sentence, inspiration opens the speech valve again, which enables normal breathing.

A second valve, the cough valve, is placed in the artificial larynx. This valve opens when during coughing the intratracheal pressure becomes too high. The valve will close on inhalation.

When both valves, the speech valve and the cough valve, are incorporated in one prosthesis, the prosthesis can be used separately from the total artificial larynx, namely as a tracheostoma valve.

A prototype of this new tracheostoma valve has been built. It consists of a housing with two serial valves. The first valve (speech valve) rotates by strong expiration towards a frame to occlude the outlet. When the intratracheal pressure becomes too high, both the frame and speech valve (functioning as a cough valve) will open. Magnets keep the valves in both closed and open positions. With two levers the magnetic forces for speech and cough valve can be adjusted to individual needs.

This tracheostoma valve that allows hands-free speaking and hands-free coughing have been tested in vitro [5] by measuring airflow resistance and the adjustment of the speech valve. We found that the properties of the speech valve of the new tracheostoma valve are comparable to the properties of an existing tracheostoma valve, the ESKA-Herrmann tracheostoma valve [6] (ESKA, Lübeck, Germany). The adjustment of the cough valve also seemed to be good.

The cough valve did not open at pressures comparable to the intratracheal pressure during phonation [7]. It only opened when the pressure was higher.

Preliminary in vivo experiments performed by professor Herrmann in Rome, indeed showed that the adjustment of both valves and the airflow resistance were good. Patients were enthusiastic, even although the prototype showed some imperfections. Further development will be done in close cooperation with the ESKA company in Germany, participant of the Artificial Larynx project.

Artificial vocal folds

The voice-producing element should create an amplitude spectrum comparable to that of the vocal folds. Because the human ear is not sensitive to phase differences between the harmonics, there is no need to look at the glottal wave in the time domain. For the voice-producing element we intend to use mechanical [8] and electrical vibrating principles. Mechanical principles have the advantage that they can use air pressure in the lungs as an energy source. Electrical principles need an external electrical power supply. Potential mechanical principles are:

- The siren. This consists of two plates with sleeves in it. One is fixed to the housing, the other is provided with vanes and will rotate driven by expired air. The disadvantage is the fact that the rotating mechanism is very sensitive to moisture.

- A membrane with incisions. If expired, air flows through the sleeves and the membrane starts to vibrate. Research is focused on finding the right number of incisions and the right thickness of the membrane.
- A reed. Expired air flowing along the reed makes the reed start to vibrate. To produce a sound with a sufficient low fundamental frequency (for male patients) the dimensions will be rather large. In vitro tests with a reed in a Groningen button have been carried out and showed hopeful results. The measured amplitude spectrum resembles the desired range rather well. A first in vivo experiment, performed by Professor Herrmann in Rome, showed that it is possible to speak with such a device and to adjust the fundamental frequency to the individual need. It appeared to be possible to give a woman her female voice back.

Three electrical solutions for voice production are also possibly good options: the electrodynamic and electromagnetic loudspeaker and the piezo-bimorf principle that functions like a bimetal. The dimensions, the energy supply and the control of the sound frequency are the main difficulties in the research.

Tissue connector

To connect the artificial larynx to the trachea, a tissue connector has been designed. The basic principle is that soft tissue will grow into the porous surface of the tissue connector. For initial stabilization a marlex mesh is used. The artificial larynx can be coupled with the tissue connector. Animal experiments with the tissue connector are being run to enable selection of the best biomaterial and optimal pore structure.

To date, soft tissue ingrowth could not be accomplished, although we have tried several materials like silicone rubber coated with polylactate, porous PMMA, and polyurethane with different pore sizes. Our next effort will be the use of titanium. In literature promising results are mentioned.

Materials research to prevent microbial adhesion

Research is focused on bacterial and fungal adhesion to silicone rubber shunt valves because this will also be a theme for the artificial larynx. To be able to select proper materials, it is necessary to understand the adhesion process of the microorganisms. Therefore a study was started to identify the adhesion process. Explanted Groningen buttons showed brown deposits identified as mixed biofilms consisting of yeasts and bacteria. Ingrowing yeast cells have been observed with a sharp edge between yeast colony and the silicone rubber (Fig. 2). So yeast cells are mainly responsible for the failure of shunt valves; how they attack the silicone rubber, mechanically or chemically, is not certain, but the sharp edge between yeast colony and silicone rubber suggest a chemical attack mechanism.

To follow the adhesion process in time a second study was started [9]. A 65-year-old male patient volunteered for this study. After 1, 2, 4, 8, 31 and 61 days he removed his shunt valve and replaced it with a new one. A range of different bacterial and yeast strains could be isolated from the explanted shunt valves. The

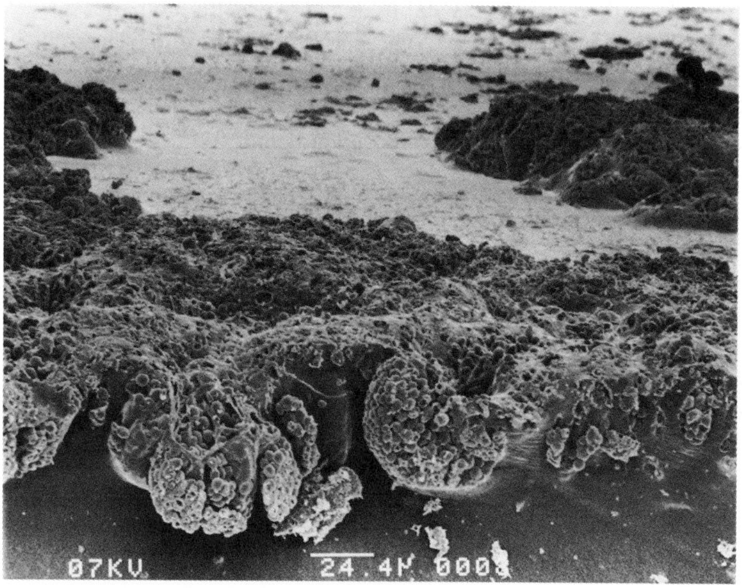

Fig. 2. Ingrowing yeast cells in a silicone rubber shunt valve.

yeast strains have been identified as *Candida albicans* and *Candida tropicalis*. The hydrophilic *C. albicans* was only isolated from the early explants (i.e., shorter than 8 days), the hydrophobic *C. tropicalis* was isolated from late explants. It is difficult to understand the dominance of hydrophilic *C. albicans* in the early stages of colonization on the hydrophobic silicone rubber. To resolve this obvious contradiction it has been argued that colonization by *C. albicans* is supported by a conditioning film possibly produced by pioneering, adherent hydrophobic bacteria. This colonization succession of bacteria and yeasts was observed before in denture stomatitis.

In conclusion, it is suggested that bacterial colonization is a prerequisite for the adhesion of more harmful yeast strains. *C. tropicalis* is tentatively identified as the main causative organism for the failure of the prosthesis, as this organism was only isolated from late explants. This hypothesis was recently supported by in vitro experiments, where it became possible to simulate the complete attack mechanism. The next step is to find new or modified materials and better resistance against the bacterial and yeast colonization.

Discussion

We are only at the beginning of the development of a total implantable artificial larynx. A lot of work has to be done, but we hope that parts of the artificial larynx can be applied separately within short notice to improve the quality of life of laryngectomized patients.

Acknowledgements

This project EU-72310 is funded by a EUREKA research grant from the department of Economic Affairs of the Dutch Government.

References

1. Herrmann IF, Amatsu M (eds). Speech restoration via voice prostheses. Berlin: Springer-Verlag, 1986.
2. Mahieu HF. Voice and speech rehabilitation following laryngectomy. PhD thesis, University of Groningen, Groningen, 1988.
3. Pabon JPH. Objective acoustic voice-quality parameters in the computer phonetogram. J Voice 1991;5:203–216.
4. de Graaf T, Nieboer GLJ, Schutte HK. Aerodynamic and phonetic properties of voice production with the Groningen button. In: Kas M, Reuland E, Vet C (eds) Language and Cognition 1. Year book 1991 of the Research Group for Linguistic Theory and Knowledge Representation of the University of Groningen. Groningen: Universiteitsdrukkerij, 1991;91–97.
5. Verkerke GJ, Veenstra A, Schutte HK, Herrmann IF, Rakhorst G. Design and test of a hands-free tracheostoma valve to improve the rehabilitation process after laryngectomy. Int J Art Organ 1994;17:175–182.
6. Herrmann IF, Koss W. Experience with the ESKA-Herrmann tracheostoma valve. In: Herrmann IF (ed) Speech Restoration via Voice Prostheses. Berlin: Springer-Verlag, 1986;184–186.
7. van Lith-Bijl JT, Mahieu HF, Patel P, Zijlstra RJ. Clinical experience with the low-resistance Groningen button. Eur Arch Otorhinolaryngol 1992;249:354–357.
8. Pelorson X, Hirschberg A, Auregan Y, Bailliet H. Fluid dynamics aspects of voiced sound production: a modified two mass model. In: Proceedings of SMACC 93. Stockholm: Pub. Royal Swedish Academy of Music, 1994;79:234–239.
9. Neu TR, de Boer CE, Verkerke GJ, Schutte HK, Rakhorst G, van der Mei HC, Busscher HJ. Biofilm development in time on a silicone voice prosthesis – a case study. Microbial Ecol Health Disease 1994;7:27–33.

Free papers, workshops and poster presentations

Voice Update.
M. Pais Clemente, editor.

Reliability and relevance of differentiated perceptual evaluation of pathological voice quality

P.H. Dejonckere[1], M. Remacle[2] and E. Fresnel-Elbaz[3]
[1]The Institute of Phoniatrics, Utrecht University, Utrecht, The Netherlands; [2]ORL et Chirurgie Cervico-Faciale, Cliniques Universitaires de Mont-Godinne, Université Catholique de Louvain, Belgium; and [3]ORL et Chirurgie Cervico-Faciale, Fondation A. de Rothschild, Paris, France

Abstract. The perceptual GRBAS scale for deviant voice quality, completed with an "I" (instability: fluctuation of voice quality) parameter was tested in three different institutes on a total of 504 voice patients. Each voice was evaluated separately by two professionals, and each patient was classified in one (out of seven) diagnostic category. The interrater correlation is highest for G (grade) (r reaching 0.8 after training); G is mainly correlated with B and R, which do not correlate with each other. Statistically different averaged GIRBAS profiles can be demonstrated for the seven principal categories of etiological diagnoses. The GIRBAS scale seems to be – with known limitations – a valuable instrument for clinical practice.

Key words: perceptual scaling, voice quality, voice.

Introduction

A standardized perceptually based description of deviant voice quality is of importance for clinical purposes (comparisons, efficacy of treatment) as well as for research in voice disorders (correlations with acoustic and physiological measurements). The five-parameter scale (called "GRBAS") proposed by the Japan Society of Logopedics and Phoniatrics [1] has become the most widely used scale, although it is still scarcely used in a systematic way. Previous research on a limited number of voices [2] showed that, on the base of intrarater (low), interrater (low) and intervoice (high) variances, the GRBAS scale parameters appear as quite reliable and of clinical relevance. Further experience with the scale, and comparison studies with acoustic parameters pointed out that it is necessary to account, when scaling a pathologic voice, also for the variability of the quality from one moment to another. So, we introduced an additional parameter: "I" (instability) which is independent of the quality level. For phonetic reasons, "I" is placed in the scale between "G" and "R". The revised GIRBAS protocol now had to be tested with a large number of different voices, and in different institutes. An important question was also whether the interrater agreement can be improved by training.

Address for correspondence: P.H. Dejonckere, The Institute of Phoniatrics, Utrecht University, P.O. Box 85500, N1-3508 GA, The Netherlands.

Material and Methods

Figure 1 shows the rating protocol, with the six visual analog scales with reference marks (no deviance: 0; slight deviance: 1; moderate deviance: 2; severe deviance: 3).

G (Grade): the overall degree of deviance of the voice. I (Instability): the abnormal variation over time in any vocal parameter of voice. R (Roughness): the voice quality related to the impression of irregular glottal pulses, of a low-frequency noise component, of harshness or vocal fry. It is proposed to consider not only random fluctuations of the glottal pulses, with a wide Fo-range, but also abnormal Fo-patterns as diplophonia. B (Breathiness): the voice quality related to the audible turbulent noise generated at the glottal level by air leakage. A (Asthenicity): auditive impression of weakness or powerlessness in spontaneous phonation. Hypofunctional, hypokinetic voicing. S (Strain): auditive impression of excessive effort of tension associated with spontaneous phonation. Hyperfunctional, hyperkinetic voicing (which is not necessarily correlated with loud voicing). (N.B., as strain and asthenicity are antagonistic, only one of the two scales can be scored for one single patient.)

A total of 504 voice patients (196 males, 308 females) were examined in a time period of about 18 months in three different institutes (France, Belgium and The Netherlands). Each voice was perceptually rated separately by two experienced clinicians: a laryngologist/phoniatrician and a speech therapist. Further, a clinical diagnosis had to be selected in a list of 39 items, after complete examination,

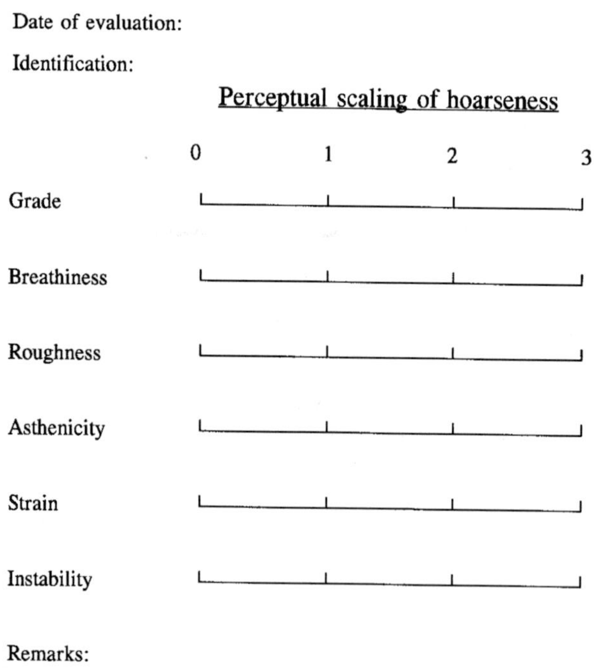

Fig. 1. Perceptual GIRBAS scale for voice quality.

especially with videolaryngostroboscopy. Afterwards, diagnoses were grouped in seven main categories: 1) functional, 2) vocal fold nodules, 3) benign vocal fold lesions, 4) chronic laryngitis, 5) paralysis, 6) malignancy, and 7) central neurogenic. Age, time elapsed since the beginning of the voice symptoms, and anterior voice treatment (yes/no) were also noted. The training effect was investigated by comparing, in two institutes, the early group of patients with the later group.

Results

Interrater correlation (n = 504)

	r	
G	0.76	p < 0.000
R	0.57	p < 0.000
B	0.68	p < 0.000
AS	0.41	p < 0.000
I	0.47	p < 0.000

Inter-parameter correlation matrix

	G	I	R	B	/AS/
G	1				
I	0.49	1			
R	0.64	0.57	1		
B	0.66	0.29	0.19	1	
/AS/	0.51	0.43	0.44	0.30	1

One-way analysis of variance: comparison of GIRBAS profiles

Between:

Diagnoses	:	p <.000
Institutes	:	p <.001 (ns if x Diagnosis)
Sexes	:	p <.000 (ns if x Diagnosis)
Treatment (Y/N)	:	ns

Training effect: the ratings of two institutes (I1 and I2) are considered separately for the earlier (a) and later (b) group of patients. A significant improvement in interrater agreement is noticed for G.

		r	
G	I 1a + I 2a	0.70	$p < 0.05$
	I 1b + I 2b	0.81	
R	I 1a + I 2a	0.55	
	I 1b + I 2b	0.58	
B	I 1a + I 2a	0.67	
	I 1b + I 2b	0.70	
AS	I 1a + I 2a	0.39	
	I 1b + I 2b	0.43	
I	I 1a + I 2a	0.46	
	I 1b + I 2b	0.47	

(I 1a: n = 54; I 1b: n = 171; I 2a: n = 192: I 2b: n = 68)

Conclusions

The interrater correlation is highest for G (grade) (r reaching 0.8 after training), and lowest for AS (strain/asthenicity) (r = 0.41). G is mainly correlated with B and R. B and R do not correlate with each other. Statistically different ($p < 0.01$) averaged GIRBAS profiles can be demonstrated for the seven principal categories of etiological diagnoses.

There is no significant interinstitute difference between averaged GIRBAS-profiles for these seven principal diagnostic categories.

Training significantly improves the interrater concordance. The GIRBAS scale seems to be — with known limitations — a valuable instrument for clinical practice. Further correlation studies with objective measures will possibly strengthen this conclusion.

References

1. Hirano M. Clinical Examination of Voice. New York: Springer Verlag, 1981.
2. Dejonckere PH, Obbens C, de Moor GM, Wieneke GH. Perceptual evaluation of dysphonia: reliability and relevance. J Folia Phoniat 1993;45:76–83.

Voice Update.
M. Pais Clemente, editor.

Normal strobovideolaryngoscopy: variability in healthy singers

Maria Emilia Elias[1], Robert Thayer Sataloff[2], Deborah C. Rosen[1], Reinhardt J. Heuer[1] and Joseph R. Spiegel[2]

[1]*American Institute for Voice and Ear Research, Philadelphia, Pennsylvania; and* [2]*Deparment of Otolaryngology, Thomas Jefferson University, Philadelphia, Pennsylvania, USA*

Abstract. Strobovideolaryngoscopy has proven essential to accurate diagnosis of voice disorders. Clinical interpretation of stroboscopic images usually follows a standard assessment protocol. Features analyzed typically include symmetry of amplitude, symmetry of phase, regularity of periodicity, amplitudes and waveforms of individual vocal folds, presence or absence of adynamic segments, and other features. Speed and smoothness of abduction and adduction are also assessed. In order for stroboscopic data to be used meaningfully in a clinical setting, it is essential for the laryngologist to recognize the range of normal variability of these parameters. This may be particularly important when trying to establish diagnoses for subtle voice disorders in professional voice users [1]. This study investigates strobovideolaryngoscopic findings in a population of normal professional singers without voice complaints. "Abnormal" strobovideolaryngoscopic findings occur in this asymptomatic population of "volunteers". They might have been misinterpreted as causing voice complaints if seen for the first time when the singer sought medical care for a voice problem. Physicians must be aware of the range of vibratory behavior that may be found among normal subjects, and must be cautious when interpreting strobovideolaryngoscopic findings. This study also highlights the importance of obtaining "normal" baseline strobovideolaryngoscopic evaluations on professional voice users.

Key words: baseline assessment, strobovideolaryngoscopy, variability.

Strobovideolaryngoscopy has become an essential and practical technique for clinical examination of the larynx in any patient with vocal complaints. It has proven essential to an accurate diagnosis of voice disorders because it provides valuable information concerning the anatomy and function of the vocal folds, including slow-motion evaluation of the mucosal layer of the leading edge, and data on vocal function of the normal and disordered larynx. This review of strobovideolaryngoscopy performed upon 65 healthy asymptomatic professional singers revealed an incidence of 58% "abnormal" findings. Our protocol for strobovideolaryngoscopy and its clinical rationale has been extensively described previously [2–5].

Materials and Methods

Sixty-five strobovideolaryngoscopic examinations were performed on the same

Address for correspondence: Maria Emilia Elias, The Voice Foundation, 1721 Pine Street, Philadelphia, PA 19103, USA. Tel.: +1-215-735-7999. Fax: +1-215-735-9293.

number of healthy singers from the Academy of Vocal Arts (AVA) in Philadelphia, PA, USA during a period of 7 years (1985–1993). The Academy of Vocal Arts is an advanced operatic conservatory. The subjects ranged in age from 22 to 35 years, with a mean age of 26 years. They had an average of 8 years of singing training. All examinations were performed by the senior author (RTS). None of the students described voice complaints or listed voice-related health problems during the completion of an extensive history questionnaire [1]. All stroboscopic examinations were conducted with the patient seated. The observations were accomplished using a Bruel and Kjaer (model 9414) stroboscope. More recent examinations using the Kay Elemetrics stroboscope are not included in this report. An Olympus ENF-P3 or ENF-L3 flexible nasolaryngoscope was used in all cases followed by observations with a rigid Wolf 90° or Nagashima telescope. Simultaneous synchronized electroglottography was performed, and the EGG waveform was superimposed on the screen with the laryngeal images. Speech and nonspeech tasks during the strobovideolaryngoscopic examination include phonation of the patient's name at a comfortable pitch to observe habitual speech behavior. They are performed at various frequencies and intensities. Sniffing and whistling offer an opportunity to observe abductory and adductory vocal fold behavior in the absence of supraglottic function effects. Glissando singing maneuvers provide an initial observation of vocal fold flexibility and pitch range, and assessment of superior laryngeal nerve function. Rapid repetition of short syllabic utterances evokes vocal fold behavior during conditions of muscle fatigue and may reveal neuromuscular abnormalities. Phonation of /i/ at various pitch and loudness levels provides a vocal sample for observation of glottic competence, vibratory patterns and mucosal wave. In professional singers, it is especially critical to visualize the larynx and supraglottic vocal tract during singing tasks utilizing familiar repertoire [5].

The relevant observable characteristics of the vibratory pattern include: symmetry of movement of the vocal folds, periodicity or regularity of successive vibrations, glottal closure, amplitude (horizontal excursion) of the vocal folds, color and consistency of laryngeal tissues and the vocal folds themselves, presence and amplitude of the mucosal wave, existence of nonvibratory portions of the vocal folds, and additional observations relative to the presence of lesions and their apparent effect on vibratory behavior [6–8].

Results

During the 65 examinations, (six) different "abnormal" entities were identified, although the students denied voice complaints during verbal histories or in a detailed questionnaire designed to review and identify vocal symptoms in professional voice users. Table 1 displays the abnormalities identified during the examinations. Forty-two percent of the subjects demonstrated signs of gastroesophageal reflux laryngitis characterized by varying degrees of erythema and/or edema of the arytenoid cartilages and posterior portion of the larynx with no signs of "cobblestoning" or granuloma. Two students (3%) had bilateral, very small "pinpoint" nodules without impairment

Table 1.

	n	Incidence in %
Reflux laryngitis	27	42%
Nodules	2	3%
Cyst	2	3%
Varicosity	2	3%
Asymmetry	4	6%
Weakness	1	1.5%
Total	38	(58.5%)
Normal	27	41.5%
Abnormal	11	17%
Reflux	27	41.5%
Total	38	(58.5%)

of glottic closure. Both also had reflux. Two examinations (3%) revealed vocal fold cysts, and one also had reflux. The first had a small reactive mass in the vibratory margin of the opposite vocal fold, and the other showed only contact swelling in the opposite site. Two singers (3%) had varicose vasculature without evidence of prior hemorrhage. Four subjects had prominent asymmetry of the horizontal (lateromedial) excursion of the vocal folds. One subject showed weakness, incomplete glottic closure, smaller amplitude of vibration, and decreased longitudinal tension/stretching of the right vocal fold. These were due to previously undiagnosed superior laryngeal nerve paresis. In total, 58% of subjects with no symptoms had abnormalities. If reflux is excluded, 17% had abnormal findings. Table 2 demonstrates the incidence of findings by sex of the subjects.

Discussion

Strobovideolaryngoscopy is an important diagnostic procedure allowing the visualization of vibratory behavior of vocal folds. Interpretation must be based on a

Table 2. Incidence of abnormal findings by sex.

	Male (n = 29)	(Female n = 36)
Reflux laryngitis	12	15
Nodules	0	2
Cyst	0	2
Varicosity	0	2
Asymmetry	1	3
Weakness	1	0
	14	24
Total	38 (58%)	

solid understanding of laryngeal anatomy and physiology, as well as their possible normal variability. These aspects have been discussed in other literature and will not be repeated in detail [2,4,6].

A full understanding of the technical aspects of stroboscopy is also essential to accurate interpretation. This subject also will not be reviewed in detail. However, a few basic principles are worthy of emphasis. Stroboscopy goes beyond the limitations of the human eye during laryngeal examination. The naked eye perceives no more than five distinct images per second which remain on the retina for 0.2 s each after exposure. With the use of pulsed light, illuminated points are visually fused to provide an averaged vibratory pattern over successive cycles. During speech phonation, the vocal folds generally vibrate at between 100–300 cycles/s, and may reach more than 1,000 Hz during singing. The stroboscope flashes a light at a rate equal to or approximating the vibrating rate of vocal folds. When the rate is slightly different, cycles are illuminated at different phases, and the effect is a slow-motion vibration permitting detailed examination. If the pulse is equal in rate to vocal fold vibration, the vocal folds appear to stand still since they are illuminated at the same phase of successive vibratory cycles. Hence, strobovideolaryngoscopy provides simulated slow motion, rather than true slow motion. However, for practical clinical purposes, this allows perfectly adequate physical examination of the vibratory margin.

Although some degree of variability was noted in the examination of these singers, the abnormal entities had no impact on vocal performance as assessed by the subjects, and it is reasonable to postulate that their neuromuscular vocal training allowed compensation for the observable abnormalities.

Reflux laryngitis is common among singers, perhaps secondary to increased intra-abdominal pressure required for proper breath management, behavioral patterns common to performance demands, and the stress of a performance career. Many singers deny symptoms. However, careful questioning often reveals the presence of multiple gastroesophageal reflux effects such as frequent throat clearing, excessive phlegm, frequent sore throats, and others.

Vocal fold asymmetry and/or weakness observed during strobovideolaryngoscopy requires other diagnostic testing (such as laboratory testing and laryngeal EMG) to determine whether they are pathologic or normal variance. For example, superior laryngeal nerve paresis may cause asymmetry, but occasionally, there are minor motion asymmetries in the presence of electromyographically normal nerves. These are felt to represent normal variations.

Small benign masses (cysts, nodules, polyps), as well as vocal fold varicosities can be present without voice complaints which are evident to the singer. Strobovideolaryngoscopy assumes great importance as a follow-up procedure to monitor the status of such lesions and to visualize changes that may be associated with alterations in voice quality and/or vocal production.

It is clear that normal larynges span a broad distribution of structure and function. This study also reveals that variations from expected to normal laryngeal behavior may be present even in trained professional singers. Consequently, especially in this group of demanding voice professionals, it is extremely important for physicians to obtain a baseline assessment of laryngeal function. This should include at least strobovideolaryngoscopy. The authors also routinely recommend objective voice analysis and high quality voice recordings. Such baseline data permits accurate diagnosis of the causes of voice dysfunction in voice professionals whose baseline laryngeal behavior may be unusual, asymmetric, or frankly pathologic despite the absence of symptoms. It is essential for laryngologists to recognize the fact that normal voice may occur even in the presence of "abnormal" laryngeal findings, and to take this fact into account before determining causality in any individual with voice complaints.

Acknowledgements

Published with permission of The Voice Foundation, Philadelphia, Pennsylvania, USA.

References

1. Sataloff RT, Spiegel JR, Carroll LM et al. Strobovideolaryngoscopy in professional voice users: Results and clinical value. J Voice 1988;2(4):359–364.
2. Sataloff RT. Professional Voice: The Science and Art of Clinical Care. New York: Raven Press, 1991.
3. Sataloff RT, Spiegel JR, Hawkshaw MJ. Strobovideolaryngoscopy: Results and clinical value. Ann Otol Rhinol Laryngol 1991;100(9):725–727.
4. Sataloff RT. The human voice. Sci Am 1992;267(6):108–115.
5. Sataloff RT. The professional voice: physical examination. J Voice 1987;1(2):191–201.
6. Sataloff RT, Gould WJ. Voice Surgery. St. Louis: C.V. Mosby Co., 1993.
7. Bless D, Hirano M. Videostroboscopic Examination of the Larynx. San Diego: Singular Publishing Group, Inc., 1993.
8. Hirano M. Clinical Examination of Voice. New York: Springer-Verlag, 1981.

Voice Update.
M. Pais Clemente, editor.

Analysis of the vocal score in lyrical singers

G. Motta, U. Cesari, S. Motta, N. Straziuso and R. Canessa
University of Naples, Institute of Otolaryngology and Phoniatrics, Naples, Italy

Abstract. The authors take into consideration the necessity of an accurate study of the vocal score before evaluating the vocal effort needed for the interpretation of a lyrical role. To achieve this, they examined the scores of two operas, studying the following parameters:
— vocal extension,
— notes under and above the stave, and
— notes sung together with the choir.
Then, with a sound spectrograph set directly in a lyric theatre they evaluated the orchestral tuning of such operas. The results indicated a clear identification of the vocal requirements for each role and gave the opportunity to reveal how the theoretical data are linked to the correct observation of the orchestral tuning.

Key words: singing voice, vocal demand, vocal score, voice extension.

Introduction

An accurate evaluation of vocal activity during the interpretation of a lyrical role requires all the factors of the vocal score that may affect the voice efficiency of the singer. During the last few years, some authors [1—3] have proposed to evaluate the score for delimitation of the extension necessary for the role to be interpreted. The vocal effort for a lyrical role, on the other hand, may be affected by some other factors related not only to the characteristics of the vocal score but also to the tuning of the orchestra and to the number of the instruments necessary for the performance of the opera, that may be indicative for the vocal strain.

The aim of the study was:

— To evaluate features and details of the vocal score by drawing the different level of difficulties that the singer may come across in the interpretation of an opera.
— To study the factors that may affect the choice of the most adequate repertoire for a singer.

Material and Methods

In order to achieve this, two operas were examined, both representative of two different musical styles. La Traviata (Verdi) and Sonnambula (Bellini), performed during 1994 in the S. Carlo Theatre of Naples.

The following factors were studied:

— the extension of the role (including notes under and above the stave);

Address for correspondence: Dr G. Motta, Via Petrarca 141/M, 1-80121 Napoli, Italy.

- number of notes in concertato;
- number of instruments composing the orchestra;
- number of tones to be sung in pianissimo (pp) and in fortissimo (ff); and
- orchestral tuning, known as "La", taken by means of a spectrograph (Speech Station) during the beginning of each opera from the first oboe and the first violin.

Results

The study of the vocal score for La Traviata and Sonnambula are reported in the Tables 1 and 2, respectively.

Discussion

The analytical examination of the vocal score gave the opportunity to obtain useful information to evaluate the vocal demand. Previous experiences were referred [1] to, but only the vocal extension has been considered: other factors, such as number of pianissimos and fortissimos, composition of the orchestra, or number of notes in concertato are not yet reported in the literature.

Such parameters undoubtedly give a more precise identification of the vocal effort

Table 1. Vocal score, the number of instruments and the orchestral tuning in La Traviata.

La Traviata (G. Verdi)		Number of instruments: 72		Orchestral tuning: 450 Hz for the 1st, 2nd and 3rd act		
Roles	Extension	Notes above the stave	Notes below the stave	Notes in concertato	Notes in pianissimo	Notes in fortissimo
Violetta (soprano)	Do3 – Mi4	168	1	24	20	12
Alfredo (tenor)	Re2 – Do4	60	0	15	11	13
Germont (bariton)	Re2 – Solb4	11	11	11	11	11

Table 2. Vocal score, the number of instruments and the orchestral tuning in Sonnanbula.

Sonnambula (V. Bellini)		Number of instruments: 68		Orchestral tuning: 450 Hz for the 1st act and 450 Hz for the 2nd		
Roles	Extension	Notes above the stave	Notes below the stave	Notes in concertato	Notes in pianissimo	Notes in fortissimo
Amina (soprano)	Do3 – Re5	233	1	2	4	5
Elvino (tenor)	Mi2 – Do4	300	0	7	5	5
Lisa (soprano)	Mi3 – Do4	109	0	11	11	0

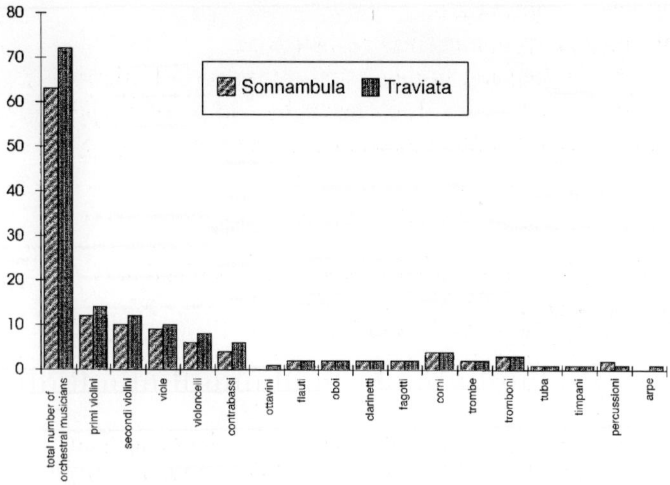

Fig. 1. Graphic representation of the orchestral composition in La Traviata and in Sonnambula.

necessary for a lyrical interpretation.

Evaluation of the characters: Violetta, the soprano of La Traviata, needs the same extension as Amina, the soprano of Sonnambula (differing only by a semitone), but many more pianissimos (20 vs. 4) and fortissimos (12 vs. 5) and notes in concertato (24 vs. 2) are necessary. So, Violetta seems to be a more difficult role. On the other hand Amina must sing many more notes above the stave (233 vs. 168 of Violetta): this character needs a well trained voice for high tones. Another character of Sonnambula, Lisa, is written for a soprano, but just five fortissimos are necessary,

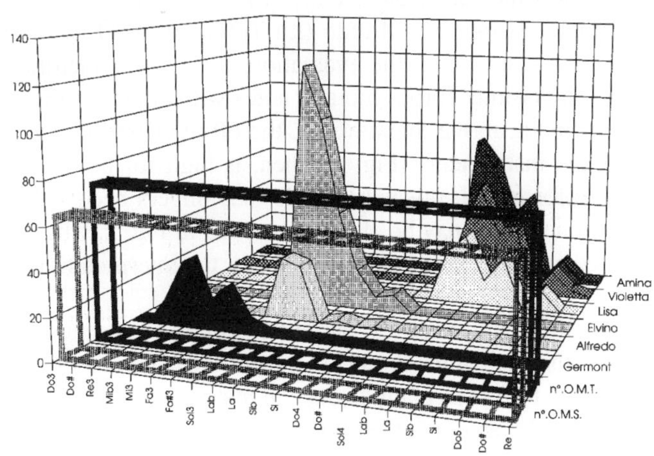

Fig. 2. Graphic representation of the vocal extension and notes above the stave for each role and the orchestral walls for both operas. n°.O.M.S. = number of musicians for Sonnanbula; n°.O.M.T. = number for musicians for La Traviata.

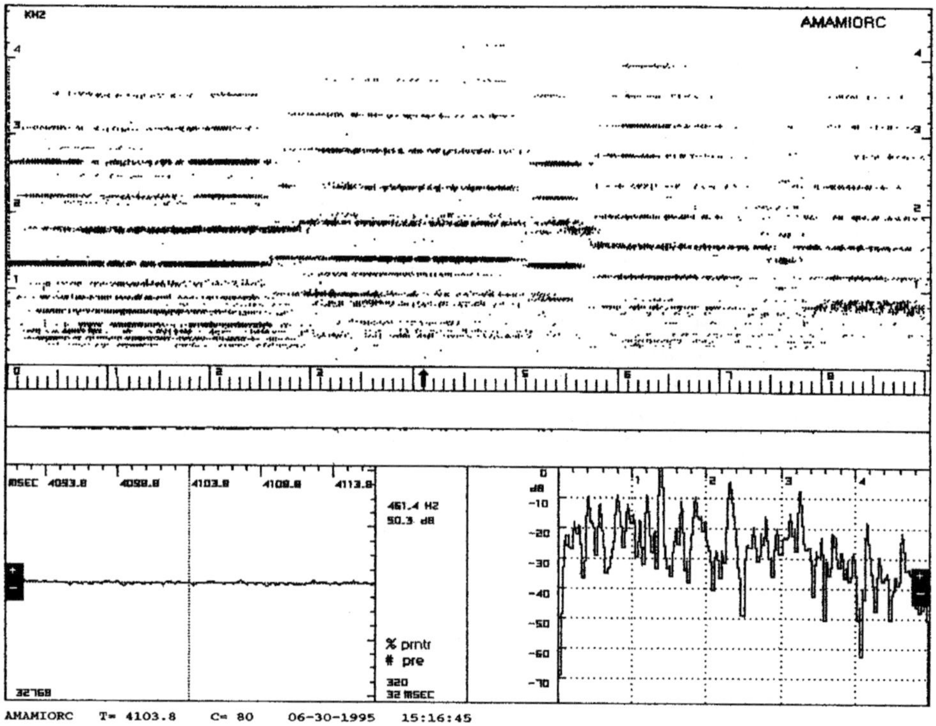

Fig. 3. Spectrum analysis of the orchestral sound during La Traviata: the tuning is at 450 Hz.

neither pianissimo nor tones under the stave nor concertato with the choir are required. So, the extension is still the same, but the effort is clearly less for this role.

Observing the male characters, Alfredo (La Traviata) and Elvino (Sonnambula) have the same extension, however, the evaluation of the other factors show that the former needs more pianissimo, fortissimo and notes with choir; on the other hand the latter must sing 300 notes above the stave vs. the 60 of Alfredo.

The number of the instruments (Fig. 1), then, is high for both operas examined and is representative for a high intensity hurdle that singers need to pass.

The above-mentioned data may be clearly observed in Fig. 2, where the orchestral walls are represented and the extension necessary for the interpretation of all the roles examined.

Orchestral tune: this data requires particular attention, because many singers normally report that the conductor does not respect the value of tune at 432 Hz for La3 as Verdi proposed. In fact in many European theatres, more than in the USA, the "La" is usually at 450 Hz, as confirmed during the present research (Fig. 3).

In this way, the original notes reported in the score are not respected and the whole extension is set to higher frequencies. Observing our spectrograms, it is also remarkable that the high intensity of the orchestra masks the singing formant (Fig. 4).

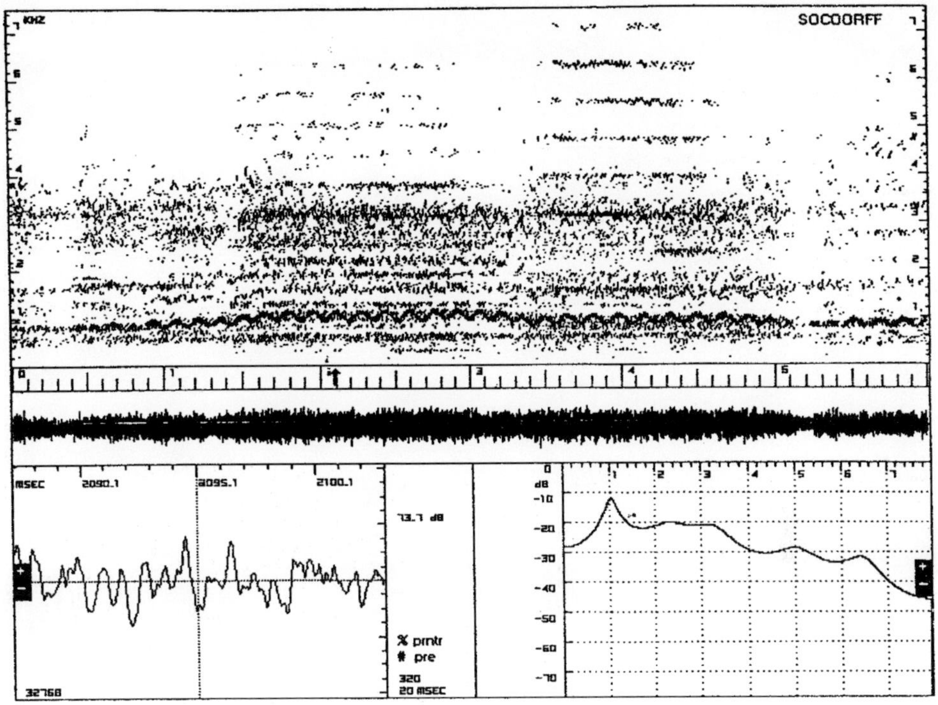

Fig. 4. Spectrum analysis performed in the theatre during La Traviata: the orchestral sound covers the voice spectrum. The LPC indicates a reduction of the singing formant.

Conclusion

The obtained data point out all the features of a lyrical role, and may create the presupposition for a future "archive" of all the characters that may be consulted by the singers for a deep knowledge of the vocal effort that they are going to deal with.

Furthermore, the direct evaluation of the tune during the playing of an opera may give documentary evidence to the wrong conduction (too high) of the orchestra and settle the disputes between the singers and the conductor.

References

1. Coleman RF. Performance demands and the performer's vocal capabilities. J Voice 1987;1(3).
2. Thurmer S. The tessiturogram. J Voice 1988;2(4).
3. Fussi F, Magnani S. Fonetografia e tessiturografia nella voce artistica. J Acta Phon Lat 1990;12: 403–408.
4. Cesari U, Motta S, Canessa R, Straziuso N. Confronto tra tessitura e canto lirico: considerazioni teoriche e rilievi strumentali. Comm. XXVIII Congr. Soc Italiana Foniatria Logopedia Montesilvano, 7–9 Aprile, 1994.

Voice Update.
M. Pais Clemente, editor.

Lasertherapy in T1 — T2 and T3 laryngeal glottic tumors

G. Motta, E. Esposito and B. Cassiano
Faculty of Medicine, "Federico II", Naples, Italy

Introduction

The therapeutic procedures practiced in the treatment of glottic cancers, classified T1, T2 and T3 for the TNM/UICC of 1987, are the subject of many studies by laryngologists [1—12] and radiotherapists alike [13—15]. The need of obtaining not only a good oncologic result (in terms of survival rate) but also a phonetic one, respecting possibly the function of the voice instrument (so improving the quality of life), have led through the years to the succession of new therapeutic purposes respecting these two aims.

To define the subject better we believe it is necessary to distinguish the monolateral tumors (T1a — T2a) from bilateral ones (T1b — T2b) either related to anatomical or prognostic factors [2,5,6]. In fact, for monolateral tumors there are no real differences in the literature in terms of survival among the results obtained with radiotherapy [13—15] and those obtained with surgical, either traditional [1,2,8] or endoscopic techniques [5,7,10—12]. On the contrary, for the bilateral tumors and especially for the commissural ones, nowadays there are still some disagreements between the supporters of traditional surgery [1,2], the supporters of endoscopic surgery using CO_2 laser [5,6,10] and the radiotherapists [13].

Since 1982 we have underlined the importance of the CO_2 laser in the treatment of the commissural cancers. The aim of our study is to share the experience we have derived at the Ear, Nose and Throat Department of the University Federico II of Naples in endoscopic treatment using CO_2 laser for cases of glottic cancers T1—T2 N0 M0, and in selected T3 N0 M0.

Patients and Methods

From 1981 to 1995 we have treated, by CO_2 laser, 516 cases of glottic cancers classified T1, T2 and T3; more precisely:
- 321 T1 cases (194 T1a and 127 T1b);
- 158 T2 cases (104 T2a and 54 T2b); and
- 37 T3 cases.

Concerning the histological type, every patient presented with a squamous carcinoma.

Address for correspondence: Dr Erik Esposito, ENT Department, Faculty of Medicine, Frederico II, Naples, Italy. Tel.: +39-81-5781927/360-274807. Fax: +39-81-5467447.

Relating to the extension of the tumoral process and to the surgical operation performed, our cases can be classified into five groups:

1. T1a: cancer limited to one vocal cord: 194 patients underwent simple cordectomy.
2. T2a: monolateral cancer involving the ventricle and the false vocal cord: 104 cases underwent extended cordectomy.
3. T1b: mono- or bilateral glottic cancer involving the anterior commissure: 127 cases underwent bilateral cordectomy.
4. T2b: mono- or bilateral cancer involving anterior commissure extended to the hypo- or supraglottic region: 54 cases underwent bilateral extended cordectomy.
5. T3: these are patients carefully selected in which the fixation of emilarynx was due to: a) the volume of the tumor extending into the laryngeal lumen; and b) the infiltration into the paraglottic space.

We performed every operation following precise surgical techniques, which enabled us to ensure a complete excision of the tumor with adequate margins of normal surrounding tissue and to avoid intratumoral maneuvers.

The complete excision of the tumor has often been made following the plan of dissection performed under the inner thyroid perichondrium; to those patients in which cancer was strictly confined and seemed to be superficial, we proceeded with limited excision that respected the lateral thyro-arytenoid muscle and the inner perichondrium of the thyroid cartilage.

The surgical specimen has to undergo intraoperatory histological examination to confirm the radicalness of the excision; in those cases where there are some doubts due to the necrosis provoked by the laser, it is necessary to perform some biopsies of the edges of the surgical wound that will undergo preoperatory histological examinations.

Results

The results after 5 years are shown in Table 1.

Postoperative course

Dysphagia is a rare event. Those patients without any postoperative complications were dismissed 24–72 h after the operation; in those cases where emphysema appeared (5%), the stay was prolonged for 7–15 days; those patients who had a hemorrhage (1.6%) were dismissed after 15–20 days.

Dysphonia will occur soon after the operation; but the voice will work better after 5–6 months.

Considerations

The results we obtained using the CO_2 laser in the treatment of the T1 and the T2 cancers in direct microlaryngoscopy are usually better than those reported in the literature referring to the traditional operations [1,2,8] and/or RT [13–15]. Our surgical results are similar to those of other authors and they respect the same

Table 1.

No. of cases	Disease-free survival (%)	Adjusted survival rate (%)	Observed survival rate (%)
T1a 197 cases	83	94.5	79
T2a 104 cases	66.5	77	67
T1b 127 cases	79.4	96.5	88.4
T2b 54 cases	67	90	82
T3 37 cases	43.8	67	55

principles of radicalness used in oncological surgery. Moreover, the use of the microscope offers further security about the complete excision.

The exposed data allow us to make two considerations:

1. Whether endoscopic surgery is able to obtain a similar percentage of recovery, even when the tumour involves the anterior commissure – T1b, T2b – as the traditional surgery and a higher percentage than radiotherapy.
2. Whether treatment of recurrences is more effective in cases where the surgical treatment fails than compared to radiotherapeutic treatment. In fact we can perform salvage surgery earlier without radiotherapeutic complications such as edema, fibrosis and radionecrosis [10].

Furthermore, recurrences due to radiotherapy are often more undifferentiated with respect to the initial lesion.

In our opinion, CO_2 surgery, for its brevity and radicalness, is surely preferable to the physical therapy used to cure laryngeal cancers, and we want to point out how, related to the traditional surgery, endoscopic surgery offers the following advantages:

- the operations through natural tracts;
- reduced surgical trauma;
- possibility to avoid tracheotomy (this was performed only in 1% of our cases);
- respect of the integrity of the cartilage structure;
- short postoperative course and reduced social costs; and
- better functional results.

We have to underline, with regard to the previous statements, how the dysphonic manifestations due to surgical operation using the CO_2 laser seems to be more reduced than those due to the traditional operation [16] and the phonetic results in glottic tumors are better in the T1a cancers limited to the medial part of the vocal cord. In these, in fact, it is possible to spare the lateral thyroarytenoid muscle.

However, we have good results in every T1 cancer. In fact, in these cases, the growth of a new cord reducing the glottic space, and a good logopedic treatment lead to very good functional results. If necessary, a certain time after the operation, if there is no local recurrence, it is also possible to try an infiltration of the new cord with collagen, to obtain a further reduction of the glottic space [17].

In T2 glottic tumors and in transglottic tumors functional results depend on scars and on the compensatory mechanism.

In conclusion, in the early stages of the cancer, transoral microsurgical resection using the CO_2 laser as curative monotherapy is the preferred method. In fact, laser surgery can treat laryngeal tumors with block resection preserving the functional important laryngeal structures.

For the success of this surgery technique we have to recommend:

- careful selection of the patients;
- cooperation with a skilled pathologist; and
- meticulous follow-up examinations.

References

1. Calearo C, Staffieri A, Bignardi L. Risultati chirurgici a distanza nel cancro laringeo. Acta Othorinol Ital 1984;4:587–598.
2. De Campora E, Radici M. La commessura anteriore nell'evoluzione dei tumori del piano glottico: considerazioni classificative, prognostiche e terapeutiche. Acta Othorinol Ital 1994;14:143–155.
3. Kim Davis. Laser in Otorhinolaringology Head and Neck Surgery. Philadelphia: W.B. Saunders Co., 1990.
4. Yako GJ, Fabiani M. La Chirurgia con il laser a CO_2 in otorinolaringoiatria. Riv ORL Audfon 1982;3:343–364.
5. Motta G. Il trattamento dei tumori glottici in microlaringoscopia diretta in sospensione mediante l'impiego del laser a CO_2. Attualità in otorinolaringologia. Ed Scientif Valeas 1983;271–291.
6. Motta G. Il laser a CO_2 nella microchirurgia laringea. Acta Othorinol Ital 1984;49–68.
7. Motta G, Villari G, Esposito E, Cassiano B. Chirurgia endoscopica delle neoplasie glottiche. In: Chirurgia Funzionale della Laringe: stato attuale dell'arte. Relazione Ufficiale LXXX Congresso Nazionale SIO e Ch. CF, Pacini Ed. 1993 Pisa.
8. Piquet JJ, Darras JA. Les resultats du traitement des cancers glottiques. Rev Laryngol 1984;105:3.
9. Riddington Young J. Laser surgery for T1 glottic carcinoma: the arguments against. J Laryngol Otol 1983;97:243–246.
10. Steiner W. Esperienza sull'uso del laser in laringologia. Acta Othorinol Ital 1982;2:113–119.
11. Strong MS, Jako GJ. Laser surgery in the larynx. Ann Otol Rhinol Laryngol 1972;81:781.
12. Vaughan CW, Strong MS, Jako GJ. Laryngeal carcinoma: transoral treatment utilizing the CO_2 laser. Am J Surg 1978;136:490.
13. Kowalski LP, Batista MBP, Santos CR et al. Prognostic factors in glottic carcinoma clinical stage I and II treated by surgery or radiotherapy. Am J Otolaryngol 1993;14(2):122–127.
14. Nicolai P, Bovarini M, Bonfioli F, Bonetti B, Moretti R, Magno L, Antonelli AR. Le neoplasie T1a glottiche: esperienze di chirurgia e di radioterapia. Acta Othorinol Ital 1988;8:581–590.
15. Small W, Mittal BB, Brand WN et al. Role of radiation therapy in the management of carcinoma in situ of the larynx. Laryngoscope 1993;13 June.
16. De Vincentiis M, Ruoppolo G, Croce A, Romualdi P, Gallo A. Phoniatric results of chordectomy in patients treated with traditional and laser chordectomy. Il Valsalva 1990;3:147–154.
17. Remacle M, Clerin M, Dubois P, Ryckaert M, Bertrand B, Hamoir M. Exploration of glottic function before and after injection of collagen for rehabilitation of vocal cord. Paper presented at Meeting Belgian Soc. ENT, 1985.

Voice Update.
M. Pais Clemente, editor.

Analysis of a complex of 25 factors influencing the course of voice rehabilitation in laryngectomized patients

Antoni Pruszewicz
Department of Phoniatrics and Audiology, K. Marcinkowski University School of Medical Science, Poznań, Poland

Abstract. The investigations were performed on 160 subjects after laryngectomy, who were aged between 34–79 years, and selected at random out of a total number of 3,193 (2,991 males, 202 females) patients laryngectomized during the period 1946–1993.

In all the patients the complex of 25 factors affecting voice and speech rehabilitations was divided into three groups:

1) those present before surgical procedure,
2) those resulting from both surgical and irradiation treatment, and
3) those being the late consequence of laryngectomy.

Rehabilitation of voice and speech in laryngectomized patients does not depend on single, individual factors, but rather on a complex of factors existing before the operation and those as a consequence of treatment. All the analysed factors could be divided into essential (statistically significant) and secondary (statistically insignificant). The essential ones, when present in numbers of 3 or more, could make the acquisition of substitute voice and speech difficult or even impossible.

Key words: factors facilitating and hindering, laryngectomized, voice/speech rehabilitation.

The aim of the study was the analysis and evaluation of the complex of 25 factors influencing voice and speech rehabilitation in patients after total laryngectomy.

Material and Methods

The investigations were performed on 160 subjects, after laryngectomy, who were aged between 34–79 (mean 56.5, median 59) selected at random out of a total number of 3,193 (2,991 males, 202 females) laryngectomized during the period 1946–1993. The time from the operation to the moment of examinations varied from several months to 20 years. The examinations methods comprised: routine ENT and phoniatric examination, roentgenological examinations during voice production and deglutition (shape of hypopharynx, shape and localisation of pseudoglottis, recesses), measurement of oesophageal pressure (direct and indirect), hearing examination (pure tone and speech audiometry), and psychological examination (estimation of IQ and personality).

Address for correspondence: Antoni Pruszewicz, 6 Reymonta St., 62-041 Puszczykowo 3, Poland.

In the quality evaluation of the oesophageal voice and speech, the classification according to Pruszewicz based on subjective and objective parameters [1] was used, distinguishing the oesophageal speech as: very good, good, sufficient, pharyngeal, pseudowhisper buccopharyngeal and lack of any sound production (Table 1). In all the patients parameters used in the assessment of voice and speech after total laryngectomy were as follows: fluency of speech, amount of syllables produced after one filling of air to the substitute reservoir, co-ordination of voice and speech production with breathing, intensity (level) of tracheal inspiration noise, character of voice and speech (clear, hoarse, etc.) and their production (free, easy, pressed, hard), MPT and mean voice range, intelligibility in the surroundings, readiness to the onset of speech production, assessment of musical factors (rhythm, dynamics, melody), intelligibility of a one syllable test (balanced phonetically, structurally and semantically) by laymen, and sonographic analyses (Kay Electric devices). In some selected patients the EMG examination of cricopharyngeal muscles was performed [2]. The acquisition of voice and speech in analysed material is presented in Table 2. The results of the examinations were analysed in a statistical manner calculating the χ^2 and convergency coefficient.

In all the patients the complex of 25 factors affecting voice and speech rehabilitations was divided into three groups:

1. Those present before surgical procedure: age, sex, intelligence level, education, hearing, localisation of the ca. changes in the larynx, extension and advancement of the neoplastic process (TNM).
2. Those resulting from both surgical and irradiation treatment: a) extension of the operation: simple laryngectomy, laryngectomy and neck dissection, laryngectomy and hypopharynx or baseos linguae excision, XII cranial nerve paralysis,

Table 1. Possibilities of communication in patients after total laryngectomy.

Means of communication			Range
Substitute voice and speech	oesophageal	very good (I)	Voice and speech socially efficient
		good (II)	
		sufficient (III)	Limited word contact with the surrounding situation preserved
	pharyngeal	(IV)	
Lack of voice and articulated speech	pseudowhisper buccopharyngeal	(Va)	Due to consonant speech possible contact with the family and familiar surroundings
	lack of creating any sounds or whispers	(Vb)	Lack of verbal contact. Necessity of using writing, mimics and gestures

Table 2. Acquisition of voice and speech in analysed material.

Quality of voice and speech	I	II	III	IV	Va	Vb	Total
Number of patients	20	45	46	21	20	8	160
%	12.50	28.12	28.75	13.13	12.50	5.00	100.00
Total		132 – 82.50%			28 – 17.50%		

laryngectomy and removal of the os hyoideum; b) postoperative course: the oesophageal drain remaining, fistulae to hypopharynx or oesophagus; c) irradiation treatment.

3. Those as a consequence of laryngectomy: a) morphology of the vicarious voice organ: shape and level of the pseudoglottis creation, shape of the hypopharynx, recesses of the hypopharynx, function of the oesophagus; b) tension of the oesophageal mouth; c) state of the dentition; d) coexisting diseases; f) profession and employment after the operation; g) family and environment; and h) some psychical features of the laryngectomized.

Special attention was paid to the following factors: tumor localisation in the larynx, extent of the tumor, extent of the operation and irradiation therapy [3].

Results

Tumor localisation

Localisation of tumorous changes in the larynx was divided into three levels: supraglottal I, glottal II, subglottal III. From 160 patients only four revealed changes within one level, in the remaining ones the tumor included two or three levels. In the group of patients with very good oesophageal speech, the highest percentage of patients occurred in the tumor localisation on the second and third larynx level, lower on the first, second and third level, and the lowest on the first and second level of the larynx.

Extent of the tumor

Out of 88 (100%) patients from the second clinical progression stage (TNM), 85 (96.6%) mastered substitute speech, among those 45 (51.2%) achieving very good and good voice. In the group of 18 (100%) patients from the fourth stage of clinical progression, substitute speech was used by six (33.3%). The remaining 12 (66.6%) patients could not speak.

Extent of the operative procedure

Out of the 72 (100%) patients where the hyoid bone was preserved, only six (8.3%)

Table 3. Dependence of the substitute speech quality on the preservation or removal of the hyoid bone.

Hyoid bone	Speech quality						
	I	II	III	IV	Va	Vb	Total
Preserved	10 50%	28 62.1%	20 43.4%	8 38%	5 26%	1 12.5%	72 45.0%
Removed	10 50%	17 37.9%	26 56.6%	13 62%	15 75%	7 87.5%	88 55.0%
Total	20 100%	45 100%	46 100%	21 100%	20 100%	8 100%	160 100%

did not master substitute speech. The percentage in patients in whom the hyoid bone removed was 25%, so in the nonspeaking group the number of patients with hyoid bone removed was 3 times higher (Table 3). In the group of patients using oesophageal speech no significant influence of removing or preserving of the hyoid bone on speech quality was noticed. Among the patients with pharyngeal speech, those with the hyoid bone removed predominated.

In the majority of patients (51–81%) laryngectomy was performed together with resection of the cervical lymph nodes (Table 4). Nothing but laryngectomy was carried out in 57 (30%) patients, and extended laryngectomy in 22 (13%) patients. Among the patients with laryngectomy alone the percentage of those who mastered substitute speech was 95%, which was considerably higher than in patients after

Table 4. Dependence of the substitute speech quality on the extent of operative procedure.

Extent of operative procedure		Speech quality						
		I	II	III	IV	Va	Vb	Total
Laryngectomy alone		12 7.50%	14 8.75%	19 11.67%	9 5.63%	1 0.62%	2 1.25%	57 35.62%
Laryngectomy with resection of the deep lymph nodes	+	4 2.50%	10 6.25%	5 3.13%	3 1.88%	3 1.88%	2 1.25%	27 16.89%
	–	3 1.88%	17 10.62%	17 10.62%	4 2.50%	9 5.63%	4 2.50%	54 33.75%
Laryngectomy with:	resection of the hypopharynx	–	–	2 1.25%	2 1.25%	7 4.37%	–	11 6.87%
	resection of the radix linguae	–	1 0.62%	–	2 1.25%	–	–	3 1.87%
	op. m. Crilé a	1 0.62%	3 1.88%	3 1.88%	1 0.62%	–	–	8 5.00%

Note: +, metastases histologically confirmed. –, metastases in lymphatic glands of nec histologically unconfirmed.

laryngectomy with resection of the deep lymph nodes, where it was found to be 78%.

Among the patients after laryngectomy with resection of the hypopharynx, the percentage of patients who mastered substitute speech was lower and reached 37%.

The time of tube-drain remaining in the oesophagus affected the postoperative course indirectly. Out of the 28 (100%) patients who did not master substitute speech, 18 (64%) had the tube-drain removed after 30 days. Among the patients with oesophageal speech the highest percentage was found in the period of tube-drain remaining, up to 15 days (45.2%), and then it decreased gradually. The influence of pharyngeal fistulae on the speech acquisition was as follows: out of 160 patients pharyngeal fistula was found in 54 (37.7%). In eight subjects these closed in 20 days, in 46 subjects they remained over 20 days, and in six subjects they required operative closing. Among the patients with the fistula remaining over 20 days, 20% were using very good and good oesophageal speech, and 61% were nonspeaking. In patients without a fistula, 74% used very good and good oesophageal speech, and 39% did not speak.

Irradiation therapy before or after total laryngectomy

Generally there were 123 (77%) patients exposed to radiation – 27 (16.90%) before the operation, and 96 (60.96%) after the operation (Table 5). All the irradiated patients received the full doses of 7,000 rad. From 28 nonspeaking patients as many as 25 (89.2%) were radiated. In the group of patients speaking very well and well the percentage of those irradiated was 65%. From the total number of 37 (21.14%) patients not exposed to radiation there were only 8% nonspeaking and 92% speaking patients. In the group of patients who were X-rayed postoperatively, the percentages were 21 and 79%, respectively, whereas in those exposed before operation, percentages were 19 and 81%.

It evidently seems that there is no difference between speech mastering among patients radiated before and after operation. From our own data it was found that in patients exposed to radiation before operation the postoperative course is much longer, more often complicated with fistulae to the pharynx, and lymphostasis on the

Table 5. Dependence of substitute speech quality on X-ray therapy.

X-ray irradiation patients	I	II	III	IV	Va	Vb	Total
Speech qality before the operation	3 1.88%	6 3.76%	8 5%	5 3.13%	3 1.88%	2 1.25%	27 1.69%
Speech quality after the operation	11 6.86%	23 14.36%	29 18.12%	13 8.12%	15 9.37%	5 3.13%	96 60.96%
Unirradiated patients	6 3.76%	16 10%	9 5.63%	3 1.88%	2 1.25%	1 0.62%	37 21.14%
Total	20 12.50%	45 28.12%	46 28.75%	21 13.13%	20 12.5%	8 5%	160 100%

neck, thus making the onset later and duration of rehabilitation longer and more difficult. Lymphostasis and infiltrations on the anterior wall of the neck were found in 12 patients; nine were nonspeaking, and two were using sufficient oesophageal, and one, pharyngeal voice.

None of those symptoms were found in patients who mastered very good and good oesophageal speech. Another consequence of the irradiation therapy was the necessity of using the tracheal tube longer due to the tendency of tracheostomy narrowing. Long-term use of the tube post irradiation negatively influences the acquisition of substitute voice (bleeding, narrowing of tracheostomy, drying of the mucosa, encrustation). In patients after total laryngectomy who have been referred for postoperative irradiation, we started with the training of substitute voice as soon as possible in order to teach them the basic principles of rehabilitation before the onset of radioreaction which can cause reduction of pseudoglottis phonation abilities [4].

Discussion

Rehabilitation of voice and speech in laryngectomized patients does not depend on single, individual factors but rather on a complex of factors existing before the operation and those resulting from treatment (surgical and irradiation) [5,6]. All the analysed factors according to statistical analysis could be divided into essential (statistically significant convergence coefficient 0.7834–0.4196) and secondary (statistically insignificant).

The essential factors hindering the acquisition of substitute voice and speech were: 1) the pressure required to overcome the tension of the oesophageal mouth above 80 mmHg; 2) hearing defects in the speech frequencies (0.5–3 kHz) of 50–60 dB; 3) mental retardation higher than debility; 4) surgical procedure involving laryngectomy with pharyngectomy and a partial tongue base resection; 5) absence of teeth and dentures; 6) serious coexisting diseases of the circulatory, respiratory or alimentary system; 7) IV° clinical advancement of cancer process (TNM); 8) large atonic recesses of hypopharynx [7]; 9) ages above 70; 10) profuse tracheal secretion; 11) depression [8]; and 12) infiltrations and lymph stases in the neck.

The essential factors, when present in numbers of 3 or more, could make the acquisition of substitute voice and speech difficult or even impossible.

References

1. Pruszewicz A. Voice and speech quality classification in laryngectomized patients. Otolaryngol Pol 1975;29:487–491.
2. Pruszewicz A, Woźnica B, Kruk-Zagajewska A, Obrębowski A. Electromyography of cricopharyngeal muscles in patients with oesophageal speech. Acta Otolaryngol (Stockholm) 1992;112:366–369.
3. Pruszewicz A, Obrębowski A, Kraśny J. The effect of surgical factors, progression state and location of the neoplasms on voice and speech rehabilitation in laryngectomized patients. Otolaryngol Pol 1987;41:145–157.
4. Izdebski K, Fontanesi J, Ross JC, Hetzler D. The effects of irradiation on a laryngeal voice of totally laryngectomized patients. Int J Radiat Oncol Biol Phys 1988;14:1281–1286.
5. Hagen R. Voice rehabilitation after total laryngectomy in West Germany. Current state of the art.

HNO 1990;38:417–420.
6. DelGaudio JM, Fleming DJ, Esclamado RM et al. Hemilaryngectomy for glottic carcinoma after radiation therapy failure. Arch Otolaryngol 1994;120:959–963.
7. Pruszewicz A, Obrębowski A, Donat-Jasiak T, Szmeja A. Radiologic picture of the hypopharynx recesses after laryngectomy. J ORL 1972;34:296–302.
8. Pruszewicz A, Obrębowski A, Gąsiorek J, Gąsiorek M. Psychosocial conditions of laryngectomized patients. Bull d'Audiophon Ann Sc Univ Franche-Comté 1992;8:113–120.***

Voice Update.
M. Pais Clemente, editor.

A new concept of surgical voice restoration after total laryngectomy: the female voice

Ingo F. Herrmann[1], Sara A. Recio[1] and Jesus A. Guimera[2]
[1]*ENT-Department, European Hospital, Rome, Italy; and* [2]*Hospital Virgen de Aranzazu, San Sebastian, Spain*

Introduction

In 1979 E. Blom and M. Singer presented a new technique to restore the voice after total laryngectomy using a so-called "voice prosthesis". While puncturing, a shunt between the trachea and the upper digestive tract was made.

Stimulated by this idea, we developed, in 1980, a surgical technique for primary voice restoration, i.e., together with total laryngectomy, laryngopharyngectomy or laryngopharyngoesophagectomy using shunt valves (voice prosthesis). After a short period we saw that the acceptance and the results of the primary technique were better than the results of the secondary technique. Establishing the myotomy and the reconstruction of the pharynx after partial pharyngectomy using the skin-platysma-fascia-flap, we could noticeably improve the voice and deglutition quality.

However, female patients had severe problems in accepting their new voice, due to the fact that the female voice after total laryngectomy is of a low-pitched male voice frequency. Because of the fluency and strength of their "male" voice, many women refused to speak. The fluent "male" voice was worse for them than the esophageal voice.

Therefore, in 1988, our group started the experimental work for a new concept of voice production which allows us to create a female voice. In the first step, patients with hypotonic PE-segment helped us to obtain experience using a voice-producing element. We found that there is no voice production of the voice valve possible, if the expired air has to pass a mucosal voice-producing segment after the voice valve. In that case the function of the voice element is impeded by the mucosa.

Therefore, we developed a new concept of voice restoration:

- In 1995, the ESKA company started to produce voice valves with five different frequencies of the voice-producing element (between 150 and 400 Hz). After in vitro tests of the material of the voice-producing element and of a new shunt valve, we decided on the implantation of the voice valve.
- A new surgical technique was established.

Address for correspondence: Prof Ingo F. Herrmann, Servizio di Otorinolaringoiatria e Chirurgia Cervico-Facciale, European Hospital, via Portuguese N.696, 00149 Rome, Italy. Tel.: +6-65975-639,604. Fax: +6-65975716.

The surgical technique consists of four steps, which are different from the surgical technique we described earlier:

1. Blunt mobilization of the anterior and lateral wall of the trachea downwards to the carina.
2. A cranial traction of the trachea with the help of fascia lata. The fascia is fixed on the lateral tracheal wall and on the mandibula bilaterally (Fig. 4).
3. An ample pharynx is constructed using the skin-platysma-fascia-flap.
4. The shunt is created on the tracheal roof and the voice valve is inserted immediately.

This technique can be used as a primary or secondary technique.

Figure 1 shows the cranial movement of the trachea after blunt mobilization. The prepared skin-platysma-fascia-flap is sutured to the tongue base and laterally to the pharyngeal mucosa together with the constrictor muscle. The fascia forms the inner layer of the flap instead of mucosa.

Figure 2 shows that the fascia lata is prepared from both sides of the thigh. A hole is made in the mandibular branch using the drill for the fixation of the fascia. A nonepithelized shunt is then formed in the roof of the trachea and the corresponding pharyngeal wall.

Figure 3 shows how to close the tracheal roof after pulling through the fascia and where to fix the fascia. The tracheostoma is then formed.

Figure 4 shows that the pharynx suture as well as the tracheostoma is completed. This technique, which places the shunt on the top of the trachea, allows the use of the voice valve without disturbances.

Case report

A 43-year-old woman, who underwent two operations with partial laryngeal resection, was diagnosed with recurrent cancer T4 N0 M0 of the glottic area which was

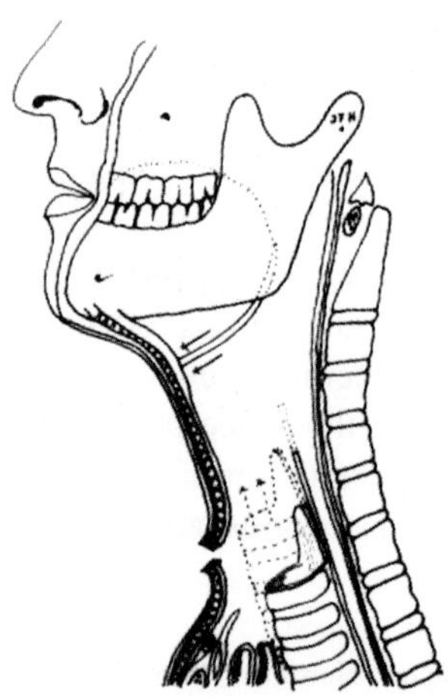

Fig. 1. Cranial movement of the trachea after blunt mobilization.

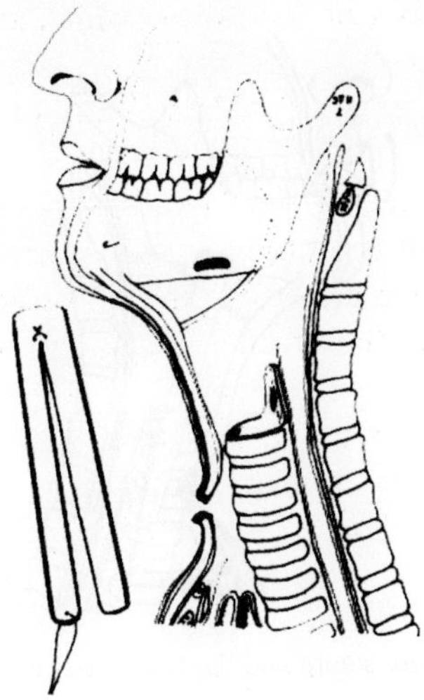

Fig. 2. The fascia lata is prepared from both sides of the thigh.

reaching the subglottic level. The scar formation of the skin was excised together with the tumor-affected larynx and two tracheal rings as a safety margin. A bilateral neck dissection was performed. The above-described technique for surgical voice restoration was used.

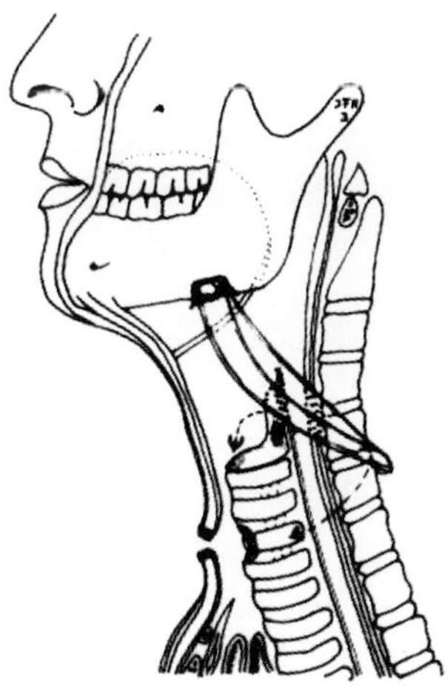

Fig. 3. The closure of the tracheal roof after pulling through the fascia and the fixing of the fascia.

Ten days after surgery the patient started to speak. We tested five different voice valves with different frequencies. The tests were done as an outpatient procedure. Including video documentation the test took 30 min. The patient herself made the

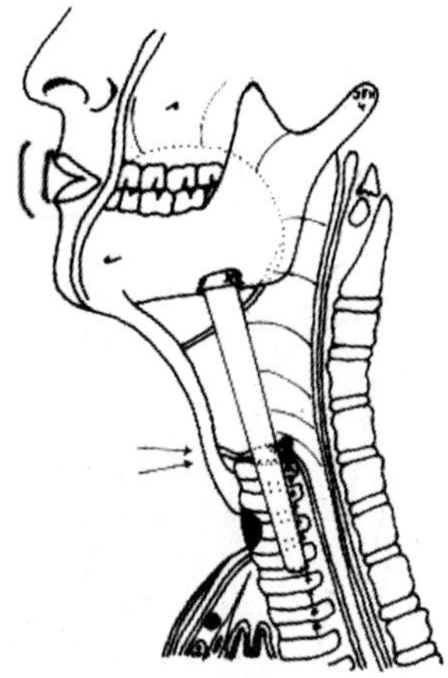

Fig. 4. The completion of the pharynx suture and the tracheostoma.

choice of her voice. Literally the patient said: "This voice is the most natural; it seems more similar to my former voice. I like this one."

References

1. Singer MI, Blom ED. An endoscopic technique for restoration of voice after laryngectomy. Ann Otol Rhinol Laryngol 1980;89:529–533.
2. Herrmann IF, Kley W. The Glottoplasty Proceedings of The XII World Congress of Otorhinolaryngology Head and Neck Surgery, Budapest. Surjan L, Bodo G (eds) 1981;191.
3. Herrmann IF. Die Pharynxrekonstruktion mit dem Platysma-Fascienlappen. Laryngol Rhinol Otol 1984;63:274–276.

Voice Update.
M. Pais Clemente, editor.

Prosthetic voice rehabilitation results

Özkul M. Doğan, Kaptaner Suat, Altar Bedri, Uğur Ömer and Tatar Alper
SSK Tepecik Educational Hospital ENT Clinic, Yenişehir-Izmir, Turkey

Abstract. Prosthetic voice rehabilitation of the totally laryngectomized patient has been the main goal of surgeons. There are different kinds of prosthesis. We compared Provox® and Blom-Singer® devices applied at our clinic. Provox® was used on 75 patients and Blom-Singer® on 15. The prostheses are inserted with a new set designed by us. The intelligibility of the prostheses is measured by using a mono- and double-syllabled word list. The recorded voices of the patients are given to young, normal hearing patients 50 dB above their thresholds. The intelligibility of Provox® was 72% with monosyllable, and 92% with double syllable, and 53 and 77% for Blom-Singer®. The mean device life for Provox® was 18 months, 5 for Blom-Singer®. Major complications were not seen with any prostheses. We advise Provox® with its self-retaining ability and longer device life.

Introduction

Total laryngectomy has been a real problem for patients, because of the loss of the voice since the first laryngectomy in 1873. The main goal of the surgeons was to create a method to maintain speech. Prosthetic rehabilitation is one of these methods. There are different kinds of prosthesis. Our goal was to compare some of these and advise the preferable one.

Materials and Methods

Seventy-five Provox® and 15 Blom-Singer® prostheses have been used at the ENT clinic of SSK Tepecik Educational Hospital, Izmir, Turkey since 1993. First, an insufflation test is performed and if it is negative we operate to make a myotomy. Most of the prostheses were adapted with a second operation using a new instrumental set designed at our clinic including a trochar, and a suction tube. We create a fistula first with a number 14 Nelaton tube and then adapt the Blom-Singer® 2 days later.

Voice exercises began 24 h after the prosthesis insertion. The voices of the patients were recorded using a phonetically balanced word list of Ege University composed of 20 mono- and 20 double-syllabled words (Table 1). These recordings were given to young, normal-hearing adults, 50 dB above their hearing thresholds and their mistakes or misunderstandings were recorded.

Results

The prostheses are adapted on patients whose adjuvant therapies are finished. The

Address for correspondence: M. Doğan Özkul, 1452 sok, 15/3 Alsancak-Izmir, Turkey.

Table 1. Word list of Ege University.

Monosyllable			Double syllable		
Düz	sağ	Hir	Sinir	Damla	Astar
Fok	Sam	Han	Tören	Yokuş	Gelin
Tep	Bel	Tiz	Funda	Dolap	Bağli
Tav	Bor	Şef	Aygit	Resim	Kavun
Sev	Sav	Fal	Bilek	Zehir	Kazan
Yut	Vur	Dev	Reçel	Müjde	Yemiş
Hür	Put		Kinci	Türbe	

patient's ages were within 38–70 for Provox® with 73 male and two female, and 34–69 for Blom-Singer®, all male. The insufflation test was negative for 21 patients in whom a myotomy was performed.

Two out of 90 patients were not able to use the prostheses. We had a liquid leakage problem with one patient and it diminished by itself. There was a granulation around the fistula in two patients. This was solved by fixing the prosthesis with 00 silk sutures. This suturing also solved the problem of disappearing of the prosthesis that was seen in two patients.

The intelligibility of Provox® was 72% with mono- and 92% with double-syllabled words. The values for Blom-Singer® were 53% with mono and 77% with double syllables.

The device life for Provox® lasted from 12 to 26 months, and 5 to 18 months for Blom-Singer®.

Discussion

The prostheses found in Izmir, Turkey were initially the Provox® and Blom-Singers®. We now have the Groningen prosthesis. We shall compare this one with the others soon. The insertion lasted 10–15 min. The only problem with Blom-Singer® is that you have to first create a fistula and then insert the prosthesis at a second stage. You can insert Provox® at the same time as tracheoesophageal puncture (TEP).

We preferred secondary prosthesis insertion because of the follow-up problems. We insert the prosthesis in those whose adjuvant therapies are finished, such as radiotherapy and in whom the insufflation test is positive. If it is negative, then a myotomy is performed. The main problem was narrowing of the tracheostoma. We prevented this by using a perforated silver cannula the perforation of which fits the TEP.

We prefer the patients to use their thumbs when speaking, because it is preferable and rentable than valves [1]. The valves are also too expensive. We had adhesion problems with the discs and also with the liquid silicone adhesives.

The device life was longer with Provox®. The longest period with Provox® is 26 months and 7 with Blom-Singer®. The need for taking Blom-Singer® prosthesis out to clean is the main problem of our patients because of their educational levels. We, and the patients, prefer Provox® for these reasons. The new instrumentation set is easy to use and prevents the damaging of the mucosa of the posterior hypopharynx during puncture [2]. The trochar opens a small puncture and the tube cleans the hypopharynx during the operation. We did not have any bacterial or fungal infection and pneumothorax [3]. We did not use any antibiotics. This is an outpatient procedure. The only disadvantage of Provox® is the length of the device. It is sometimes too short. Blom-Singer® has longer ones. The interesting thing is the patients cannot pronounce the Turkish "M" sound that is laryngeal with Provox® [4] and "G" with Blom-Singer®.

The intelligibility of the prostheses was acceptable as it is listed in the literature [5,6], but the voice with Provox® is more intelligible. This is proved by Mann-Whitney's U test ($p < 0.05$)

Conclusion

Provox® is preferred to Blom-Singer® because of its self-retaining ability, long device life, it can be easily used by patients, and its higher rate of intelligibility.

References

1. Blakley BW, Podraza BL. Acoustic and perceptual assessment of speech using a voice prostheses with valvular and manual occlusion. Otolaryngol Head Neck Surg 1987;97:552–554.
2. Andrews JC, Michel RA, Hanson DG et al. Major complication following tracheoesophageal puncture for voice rehabilitation. Laryngoscope 1987;97:562–565.
3. Palmer MD, Johnson AP, Ellioth TSJ. Microdial colonization of Blom-Singer® prosthesis in postlaryngectomy patients. Laryngoscope 1993;103:910–912.
4. Altar S, Özkul MD, Kaptaner S, Uğur Ö, Dinçer H. The intelligibility of the voice of Provox®. The proceedings of the XV World Congress of ORL, Head and Neck Surgery. Multiscience Pub Co., 1993;687–690.
5. Hilgers JM, Schouwenburg FS. A new low resistance self-retaining prosthesis (Provox® for voice rehabilitation after total laryngectomy. Laryngoscope 1990;100:1202–1207.
6. Tardy-Mitzell S, Andrews ML, Bowman SA. Acceptability and intelligibility of tracheoesophageal speech. Arch Otolaryngol 1985;111:213–215.

Voice Update.
M. Pais Clemente, editor.

Acoustic and morphological lesions of the larynx in alcoholics

G. Niedzielska[1] and A. Pruszewicz[2]

[1]*Department of Paediatric Otolaryngology, Phoniatrics and Audiology, Medical School of Lublin; and* [2]*Department of Phoniatrics and Audiology, University of Medical Sciences, Poznań, Poland*

Abstract. The objective of this paper was to diagnose organic injuries of the larynx and to make an acoustic evaluation of the voice in heavy drinkers. Also, experiments were carried out on the influence of ethanol on the laryngeal mucus in animals. Clinical tests were performed in 30 adult men addicted to alcohol. Acoustic tests referred to the voices of the men recorded on the tape recorder. For the experiments white Wistar rats were used. The animals were administered "ad libitum" 25% solution of ethanol during 4 months. After completing the experiment the mucus of the larynx was sampled for the histological and histochemical tests as well as for study under transmission electron microscope.

The tests confirmed injuries in the mucus membranes of the larynx that are typical for chronic infection. The acoustic tests proved changes within the basic frequency Fo. Also, a significant increase of jitter mean values, which signal harmonic structure deterioration and intonation worsening, were confirmed. The experiments proved lesions injuring the laryngeal mucus following the intoxication with ethanol. The lesions included hypertrophy of ephitelium with its exfoliation and inflammatory infiltrations. Lesions of cytological structures in laryngeal mucus were also noted.

Key words: acoustic evaluation, alcohol, morphology, voice.

Introduction

Chronic consumption of alcohol results in many-sided toxic effects with medical consequences. Extensive research points to a close relationship between overconsumption of alcohol and the increased risk of neoplasms being created in the upper respiratory tract and in the alimentary tract [1,2]. The lack of comprehensive studies on the influence of chronic intoxication with ethyl on the larynx made me start research on the subject.

Objective

The objective of the paper was the acoustic analysis of the voice of alcohol addicts as well as realization of experimental tests on the influence of ethanol on the laryngeal mucus in animals.

The clinical tests were carried out on 30 adult alcoholics. For the acoustic tests the voice of these individuals recorded on tape was used.

For the experiments the Wistar white rats were used.

The individuals and the animals under evaluation were divided into groups to

Address for correspondence: Prof Dr G. Niedzielska, Department of Paediatric Otolaryngology, Phoniatrics and Audiology, Medical School, Staszica 11, 20-081 Lublin, Poland.

determine the alcohol intoxication time influence on the quality of lesions:
1st group — 19 individuals addicted to alcohol for 1—10 years.
2nd group — 11 individuals addicted to alcohol for 11—20 years.
3rd group — 10 individuals of the control group not addicted to alcohol.

From the recorded verbal material some of the speech parameters characteristics for the evaluation of lesions in larynx were extracted. The mean value of basic frequency Fo, the range of Fo, the mean and maximum jitter values, i.e., the variability of the length of vocal folds' vibration period from one cycle to another, the harmonic structure of speech signal and different distribution of vowels periodicity, noise contents in individual bands of analysis as well as the character of intonation courses variability, were defined.

The acoustic evaluation of voice was performed with application of digital analysis of the spectral structure and time component of the signal, using the microcomputer system IBM/AT with adequate software.

The experiments included 30 white rats that were divided at random into two experimental groups and one control group. The experimental groups differed from each other in the duration of the experiment.

The animals from the first group were administered 25% ethanol solution "ad libitum" for 3 weeks; the animals from the 2nd group, for 4 months. The animals in the control group were drinking the same amounts of water in a similar way. After the experiment was completed, the laryngeal mucus was sampled for histologic and histochemical tests.

The results of the acoustic tests

The acoustic tests proved changes within the basic frequency range Fo.

The increased value of Fo minimum, mean and Fo maximum were noticed in comparison to the control groups. Similar results were obtained by Kunzel, Braun and Eysholdt [3]. The acoustic jitter analysis proved the increase of mean and maximal values in both groups (Fig. 1). The sonographic analysis confirmed the decrease of signal harmonic structure and more frequent interference of vowels periodicity duration by the wide-band noise in alcohol addicts. Melodic courses were hardly differentiated during intonation evaluation (Fig. 2). Also, a rapid and steep variability of the vocal cords' vibrations periods length was observed such as is found in pathology of the larynx.

The statistical analysis of the acoustic evaluation results confirmed a significant influence of the duration of alcohol addiction on the quality of changes. A statistical significance of the experimental group's results was noted in comparison to the control group, in all the evaluated values of Fo. An increase of jitter mean and maximal values, decrease of signal harmonic structure, reduction of the value of "clear" periodic courses, worsening of intonation and more frequent occurrence of continuous and step-like vibrations length variability were also noted. Long-lasting alcohol addiction significantly influenced a considerable increase of mean and maximal jitter values.

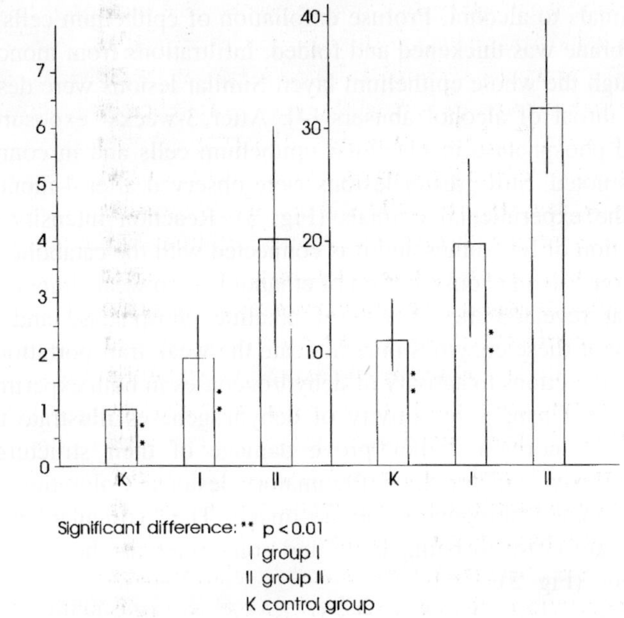

Fig. 1. Jitter values in the evaluated groups. (Note: in groups K and I, p < 0.01.)

The results of experiments

The evaluation proved morphological and histochemical lesions in the laryngeal mucus. The specimens colored H and E after 3 weeks of ethanol exposure demonstrate lesions in the form of squamous epithelium focal exfoliation, swelling and hypertrophy of glands. Much bigger lesions are observed after 4-months'

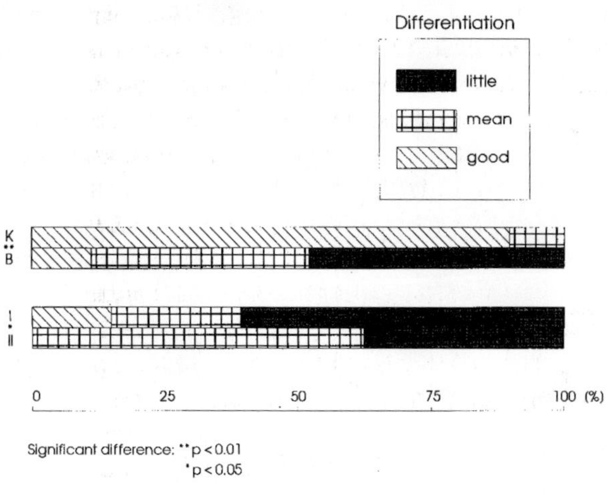

Fig. 2. Parameters of intonation in the evaluated groups.

exposure of animals to alcohol. Profuse exfoliation of epithelium cells was present. The basal membrane was thickened and folded. Infiltrations from mononuclear cells penetrated through the whole epithelium layer. Similar lesions were described in the esophagus and throat of alcohol abusers [4]. After 3-weeks' exposure to ethanol, increase of acid phosphatase in glandular epithelium cells and in connective tissue phagocytes was noted. Still greater lesions were observed after 4-months' exposure to alcohol of the experimental animals (Fig. 3). Reaction intensity supports the augmented function of lysosomes and it is connected with the catabolic and cytolytic processes [5]. Long-lasting consumption of ethanol lead to weakening of the intensity of reactions that revealed the activity of alkaline phosphatase and of ATP-ase. Reduced activity of these enzymes may indicate the weak transportation through the cell membranes. Reactions to activity of dehydrogenases in both experimental groups decreased (Fig. 4). Changes in activity of dehydrogenases illustrate the disturbed function of mitochondria and they prove damage of their structure within the epithelium. This may confirm the inflammatory lesions. Coloration according to Feulgen proved great heterogeneity of the image. The "vesicular" nuclei that are almost "empty" are close to being large and sometimes are heteromorphous with numerous nucleoli (Fig. 5).

Conclusions

1. Alcohol addiction is a syndrome that results in morphological lesions of the larynx which cause phonatory disorders.
2. The acoustic analysis of alcoholics' voices indicated a significant increase of basic frequency, the increase of mean and maximal jitter values, signal harmonic structure reduction, the increase of periodic courses occurrence with noise and

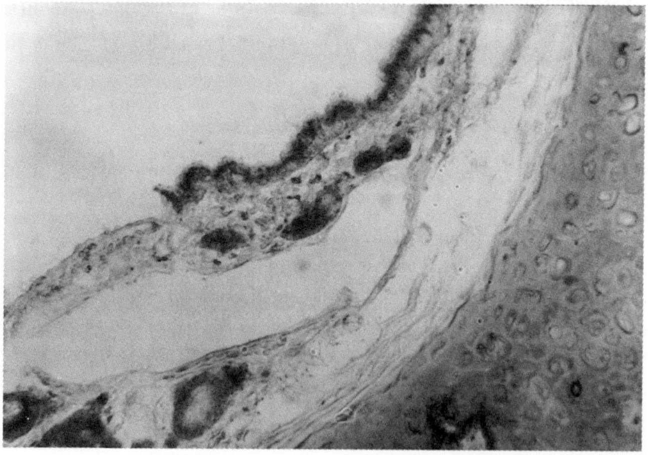

Fig. 3. Reaction to the acid phosphatase. The preparation of larynx from the experimental group of animals subjected to chronic alcoholic intoxication. Visible considerable changes in the laryngeal mucous membrane. Partially diffused reaction in the damaged epithelium, uniformity of mucous membrane fibrous structures. (Enlargement 300×)

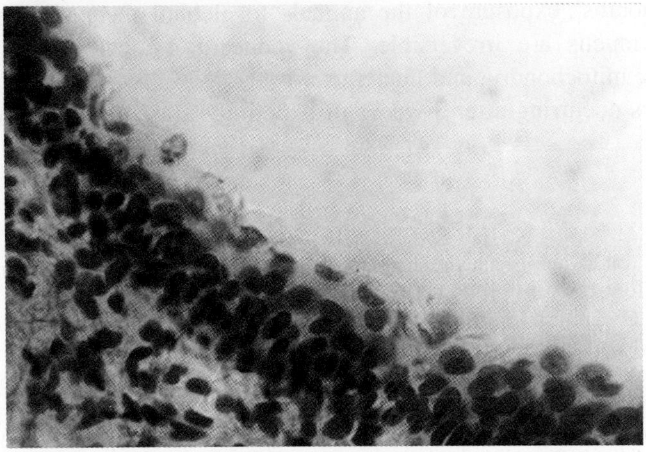

Fig. 4. Feulgen's method stain. Preparation from the experimental group animals after chronic alcoholic intoxication. Intensive stain of chromarine stroma. The shape of nuclei and their structure differ from the regular image; a considerable enlargement of nuclei is visible. (Enlargement 1,000×)

more frequent presence of vocal folds' vibrations period length variability. The above parameters are the exponent of existing organic and functional changes of the larynx that are marked by the enlarging of vocal fold mass.

3. Long-lasting alcohol addiction significantly influenced a considerable increase of the mean and maximal jitter values observed in the organic diseases of the larynx.
4. The experiments proved that ethanol administered orally to animals causes significant lesions of the laryngeal mucus.

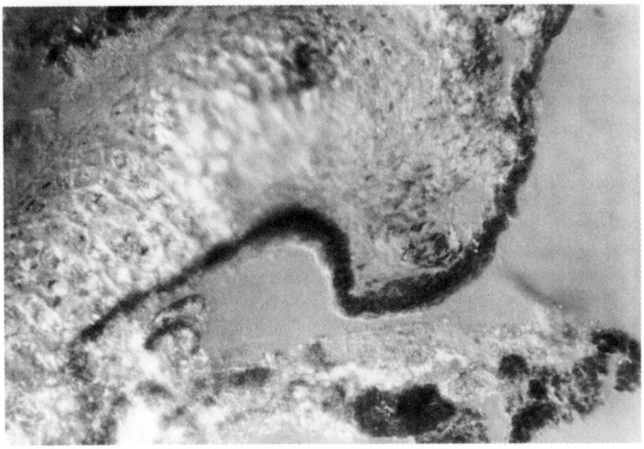

Fig. 5. Reaction to lactate dehydrogenase activity. The experimental group – chronic alcoholic intoxication. Focal decrease of lactate dehydrogenase activity is noticeable, the reaction is of microgranular character and is irregular in individual segments of the preserved epithelium.

5. After 4-months' exposure of the animals to alcohol the pathologic lesions of laryngeal mucus are irreversible. They concern the cytological structures – lysosomes, mitochondria and nuclei.
6. The lesions occurring after 3 weeks of experiments are of reversible character.

References

1. Hirabayashi H, Koshii K, Uno K, Chgaki H, Nakasone Y, Fuisawa T, Shono N, Hinohara T, Hirabayaski K. Laryngeal epithelial changes of effects of smoking and drinking. Auris Nasus Larynx 1990;17(2):105–114.
2. Niedzielska G. Einfluss von athylakohol auf das verhalten der schleimhaut des des rattenracharns. Gegenbaurs Morphol Jahrb (Leipzig) 1987;5:761.
3. Kunzel HJ, Braun A, Eysholdt U. Einfluss von Alkohol auf Sprache und Stimme. Heidelberg: Kriminalistic-Verlag, 1992.
4. Martini GA, Wisenbeck M. Beguenstigt alkohol die enstehung eines barret-syndrome (endo-brachyoesophagus). Dtstch Med Wochenschr 1974;99–434.
5. Ostrowski K, Kawiak J. Warszawa: Cytofizjologia PZWL. 1985.

Voice Update.
M. Pais Clemente, editor.

Recent findings on laryngeal microneuroanatomy

M. Pais Clemente[1], Rui Pratas[1] and Victor Cardoso[1,2]
[1]*Department of Otorhinolaryngology and* [2]*Institute of Anatomy, Oporto Medical School, Hospital São João, Oporto, Portugal*

Abstract. Recent studies have questioned the traditional, widely accepted description of laryngeal innervation. However, the conventional anatomic dissections and serial histological sections are inadequate to determine the exact nerve branching of laryngeal muscles.

The authors have processed 16 adult human larynges with a technique that clears soft tissue and counterstains the nerve supply. This technique allows detailed information about the neural branching patterns and neuromuscular compartments, in whole specimens, with all of the three-dimensional relationships remaining intact.

This work allows the identification of several connections between the recurrent laryngeal nerve (RLN) and the superior laryngeal nerve (SLN), the existence of neuromuscular compartments and the presence of the communicating nerve (CN).

Key words: communicating nerve, recurrent laryngeal nerve, superior laryngeal nerve.

Introduction

Many questions regarding laryngeal neuroanatomy remain almost completely unanswered. These include several cross-innervations from side to side in the larynx and between the superior laryngeal nerve (SLN) and recurrent laryngeal nerve (RLN) systems [1–3]. Nevertheless, a second source of motor innervation for the thyroarytenoid (TA) muscle, other than the RLN, has been suggested by clinical and experimental observations [4–7]. Early anatomists [8,9] noted small nerves connecting the cricothyroid (CT) and TA muscles. These observations, however, were disputed by later anatomists and subsequently forgotten.

The two available techniques for the study of laryngeal microanatomy, microdissection and serial histological sections, are inadequate [10]. Microdissection only allows identification of the more proximal nerve branches as they enter the muscle, and the serial reconstructions are time consuming and technically difficult.

To overcome these problems, the authors have processed 16 human larynges with a technique that clears soft tissue and counterstains the nerve supply. It allows detailed information about the neural branching patterns and neuromuscular compartments in whole specimens, with all of the three-dimensional relationships remaining intact.

This work, using this particular technique, will be of value in answering some of the controversial questions about laryngeal neurophysiology.

Address for correspondence: M. Pais Clemente MD, PhD, Instituto Português da Voz, Rua Caldas Xavier 38 - 6°E, 4150 Oporto, Portugal.

Materials and Methods

Sixteen adult human larynges were obtained from autopsies and processed following the techniques described by Sanders et al. [11] and Wu et al. [12], with modifications introduced by the authors:

1. Fixation: 10% unneutralized formaldehyde solution.
2. First dissection:
   a) The extralaryngeal tissues were dissected away from the whole larynx.
   b) Identification of the laryngeal gross anatomy.
   c) The thyroid and cricoid cartilages were dissected intact from all specimens.
3. Maceration: 3% potassium hydroxide solution + ultraviolet radiations.
4. Staining: Sihler's solution no. 2 (Ehrlich's hematoxylin + glycerin + 1% aqueous chloral hydrate).
5. Destaining: Sihler's solution no. 1 (glacial acetic acid + glycerin + 1% aqueous chloral hydrate).
6. Neutralization: 0.05% lithium carbonate solution.
7. Clearing: increasing concentrations of glycerin until 100% + thymol crystals.
8. Second dissection: using the microscope, the mucosa and connective tissues were removed to show the neural distribution.

Results

1. All 16 larynges were dissected away from the extrinsic muscles and the thyroid and cricoid cartilages. The external (ESLN) and internal (ISLN) superior laryngeal nerves and the RLN were isolated. At the same time, some intrinsic laryngeal muscles were identified: the posterior cricoarytenoid (PCA), interarytenoid (IA), CT, lateral cricoarytenoid (LCA) and TA muscles.
2. The RLN innervates a group of four muscles, which consist of PCA, IA, LCA and TA muscles:
   a) Following the ascending direction of the nerve, the PCA muscle was the first one to be innervated; two branches of the RLN were observed, one of them was directed to the combined vertical/oblique compartment (PCA muscle's lateral aspect) and the other to the horizontal compartment (PCA muscle's medial aspect). In 11 of the 16 specimens, those two branches arose separately off the main trunk of the RLN.
   b) The IA muscle was the second one to receive a branch of the RLN from both sides. Besides the innervation by the RLN, all the 16 IA muscles were also innervated by branches of both ISLN, forming a dense anastomotic plexus which was highly variable between specimens.
   c) The terminal branches of the RLN innervated the LCA and TA muscles.
3. The ESLN enters the superolateral surface of the CT muscle, where it divides into several branches.

   In 12 of the 32 hemilarynges, an individual branch of the ESLN passed through the CT muscle, travelled across the LCA muscle and entered the lateral surface of the TA muscle. This branch seems to be the communicating nerve (CN) described by some authors [8,12] (Fig. 1).

4. The ISLN and the RLN are connected by the Galen's anastomosis in all larynges.

Discussion

Staining technique

In this work we used a modified version of Sihler's technique which is very useful in mapping laryngeal microinnervation. It makes soft tissue translucent while counterstaining all nerves, which allows a clear view of nerve branching within the muscles.

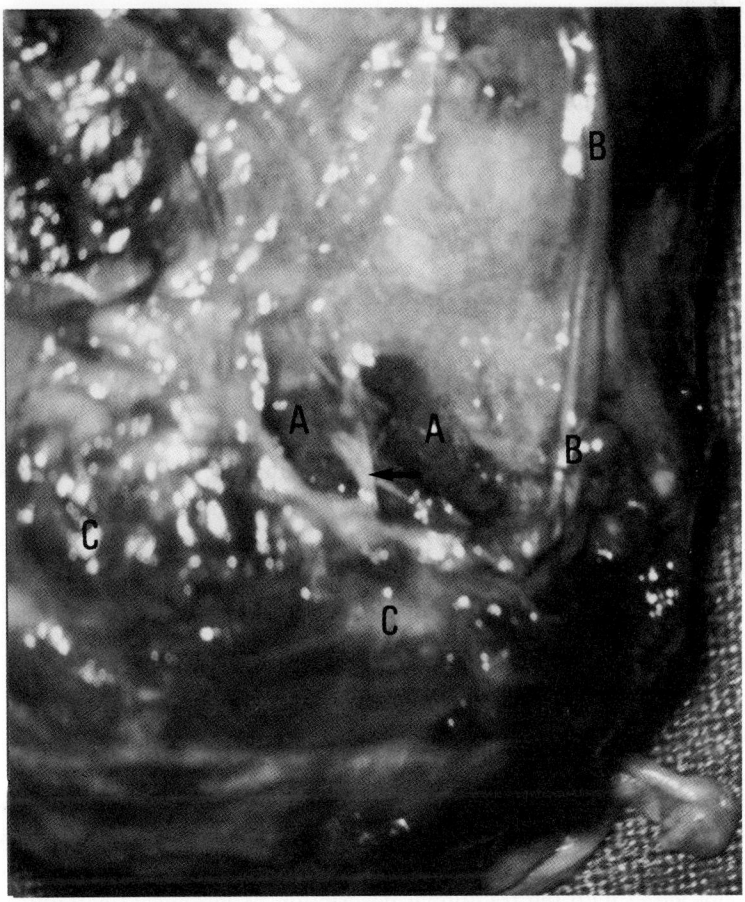

Fig. 1. Communicating nerve (arrow) supplying the thyroarytenoid muscle (A) (20×). B: External superior laryngeal nerve. C: Cricothyroid muscle.

Neuromuscular compartments

The classical description of PCA muscle innervation refers to a single branch that comes from RLN to innervate the entire muscle.

According to the results of this study, in 11 out of 16 specimens the nerve supply of the PCA muscle is separated into two main branches that arise directly from the RLN: the superior one supplies the horizontal compartment and the inferior innervates the lateral aspect of the PCA muscle (combined vertical/oblique compartment).

These findings suggest that the PCA muscle bellies are neuromuscular compartments with distinct functional roles during vocal cord movement. The lateral compartment may be primarily involved with vocal cord abduction during inspiration and the horizontal one may be responsible for stabilizing the arytenoid cartilage during phonation. These different functional roles may have important clinical implications, mainly related to reinnervation of the paralyzed PCA muscle.

SLN and RLN systems connections

Some of the most important findings in this study involve connections between the SLN and RLN systems. It is widely accepted that the RLN innervates the intrinsic laryngeal muscles while the SLN external branch innervates the cricothyroid muscle. Based on these results, multiple connections were found. The IA muscle has another innervation in addition to the RLN, by a variable number of ISLN branches that converge to form a complex intramuscular plexus. Another area of connection is in the region of the piriform fossa.

The potential connections between the RLN and SLN may have clinical significance in the understanding of the paralyzed vocal cord positions.

This matter has been controversial since the previous century. Semon [5] believed that the vocal cords go through various stages before reaching complete paralysis; the initial stages involve loss of the abductor function and, at a later stage, the adductor function is lost. Wagner and Grossman [5] stated that the position of the vocal cords depends on which of the main laryngeal nerves is paralyzed; isolated RLN paralysis results in a paramedian position of the vocal cords, while a combined RLN and SLN paralysis results in an intermediate position.

This study demonstrated that CN innervates the TA muscle in 12 of the 32 hemilarynges. The presence of motor fibers in the CN, that originate from the ESLN, might explain the controversial aspects of these two theories.

Conclusions

The evidence of neuromuscular compartments suggests that the same muscle may have different roles in laryngeal movements, namely on vocal fold mobility.

The multiple connections between the SLN and RLN systems demonstrated in this study do not agree with the traditional description of laryngeal anatomy, but might explain some of the controversial aspects of the paralyzed larynx and the difficulties in reinnervating the laryngeal muscles.

The presence of the CN, an additional supply to the TA muscle, may explain the different positions of the vocal cords when the laryngeal nerves are damaged.

Acknowledgements

The authors express their sincere appreciations to Prof M.A. Tavares and Dr N.T. Cunha for comments and suggestions, and to Mrs M.M. Pacheco for technical assistance.

References

1. Kobler JB, Benecchi EJ. Innervation of the larynx, pharynx, and upper esophageal sphincter of the rat. J Comp Neurol 1994;349:129–147.
2. Mu I, Biller HF. The intramuscular innervation of the human interarytenoid muscle. Laryngoscope 1994;104:33–38.
3. Sanders I, Biller HF. The innervation of the human posterior cricoarytenoid muscle: evidence for at least two neuromuscular compartments. Laryngoscope 1994;104:880–884.
4. Hiroto I, Tomita H. Electromyographic investigation of human vocal cord paralysis. Ann Otol Rhinol Laryngol 1968;77:296–304.
5. Semon J, Dedo HH. The paralyzed larynx: an electromyographic study in dogs and humans. Laryngoscope 1970;80:1455–1517.
6. Yamashita T, Oda M. Three cases with full recovery of the recurrent laryngeal nerve paralysis following thyroidectomy and electromyogram of the intrinsic laryngeal muscles. Otorhinolaryngol Clin 1964;57:366–373.
7. Tanaka S, Umeno H. Laryngeal behavior in unilateral superior laryngeal nerve paralysis. Ann Otol Rhinol Laryngol 1994;103:93–97.
8. Meng ZH, Li L. Observations on the anatomy of laryngeal nerves. Clin Med J 1976;56:177–180.
9. Lemere F. Innervation of the larynx. Am J Anat 1932;51:417–438.
10. Hugh I, Telman F. The human larynx. J Otolaryngol 1993;120:935–941.
11. Sanders I, Li Y. A technique for displaying the entire nerve branching pattern of a whole muscle: results in 10 canine posterior cricoarytenoid muscles. Laryngoscope 1993;103:141–148.
12. Wu BL, Mu L. The human communicating nerve. Arch Otolaryngol Head Neck Surg 1994;120: 1321–1328.

Voice Update.
M. Pais Clemente, editor.

Distribution of motor end-plates in intrinsic laryngeal muscles of the rat: a comparative study with man

M. Pais Clemente[1] and M. Lima Rodrigues[1,2]

[1]Department of Otorhinolaryngology and [2]Institute of Histology, Oporto Medical School, Hospital S. João, Oporto, Portugal

Abstract. Intramuscular injections of myoneural blocking agents (e.g., botulinum toxin) has shown to be quite effective in the treatment of some neurogenic dysphonias. In order to get a more successful treatment, it is important to know the motor end-plates distribution in the intrinsic laryngeal muscles. Some studies suggest that the pattern of the motor end-plates is not the same along the muscle fibers.

For this study, the rat was used as an animal model and human vocal folds were obtained from fresh larynges from the autopsy specimens. Histochemical techniques and light microscope seriated images were used to determine the distribution of neuromuscular junctions as well as to show their acetylcholinesterase activity.

In the rat, motor end-plates occurred in a transverse middle band in the thyroarytenoid muscle. Although motor end-plate arrangements were diffuse in man, there was a preferential area of higher concentration at the middle-third of the thyroarytenoid muscle.

In accordance with these preliminary findings we can postulate that intramuscular injections of myoneural blocking agents will probably give better results in the middle area of this muscle.

Key words: cricothyroid and posterior cricoarytenoid muscles, motor end-plate, thyroarytenoid.

Abbreviations: Iso-OMPA, tetramonoisopropylpyrophosphortetramide.

Introduction

Many questions remain unsolved with regard to the management of certain neurogenic dysphonias such as spasmodic dysphonia, for which no satisfactory treatment has yet been found. The intramuscular injection of drugs (e.g., botulinum toxin) producing selective muscular inactivation of its motor innervation has given acceptable results [1].

The knowledge of the distribution of neuromuscular junctions in intrinsic laryngeal muscles may therefore be important for appropriate treatment strategies [2].

It is known that in most mammalian species, skeletal muscles have a single motor end-plate at mid-distance from the insertion points of the muscle fibre. In a muscle composed of fibres of equal length, end-plates will thus be arranged in a transverse row making up the "motor region" [3,4].

Exceptions occur in the human lateral rectus muscle of the orbit [5] and orbicularis muscle of the eyelid [6], in which motor end-plates are disposed at variable distances

Address for correspondence: M. Pais Clemente MD, PhD, Instituto Português da Voz, Rua Caldas Xavier 38 - 6°E, 4150 Oporto, Portugal.

from the insertion zones, producing "multimotor end-plate" arrangements. This has also been observed in the predominantly tonic muscles of birds [6] and batrachia [7].

The "multimotor end-plates" were found in the human vocalis muscle [6] and a diffuse distribution rather than a single band or any other clustered configuration was observed in the thyroarytenoid muscle [8]. Other reports have described neuromuscular junctions scattered over an area occupying about two-thirds of the entire vocalis muscle, and similar findings have been obtained for the cricothyroid and lateral cricoarytenoid muscles of man [6].

In this work the distribution of neuromuscular junctions was studied in the intrinsic laryngeal muscles of the rat and in the thyroarytenoid muscle of man.

Material and Methods

Six female Wistar rats, 60–100 g in weight, aged 20–40 days (prior to calcification of thyroid cartilage) and six thyroarytenoid muscles from fresh larynges from autopsy specimens were used for this study.

The rats were anaesthetised with an intraperitoneal injection of 35% chloral hydrate.

Removal of the total larynx was performed by careful dissection under the operating microscope and placed immediately in buffered 10% formalin at pH 7.4 during 24 h at room temperature. The thyroarytenoid, cricothyroid (Fig. 1) and posterior cricoarytenoid muscles (Fig. 2) from the rat and the thyroarytenoid muscle from the human larynx were sectioned into 50 μm sections.

These sections were incubated in Koelle and Friedenwald's medium (thiocholine method) [9], with final staining in ammonium sulphide 5% and mounting in entellan (Fig. 3).

The maintenance of the proper pH of the reaction mixture, combined with the addition of a selective pseudocholinesterase inhibitor (Iso-OMPA), allowed for the specific staining of acetylcholinesterase activity only [2,10].

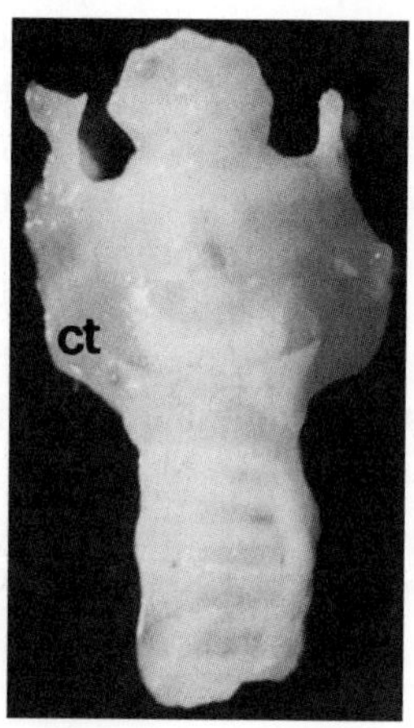

Fig. 1. Ct – Cricothyroid muscle of the rat (10×).

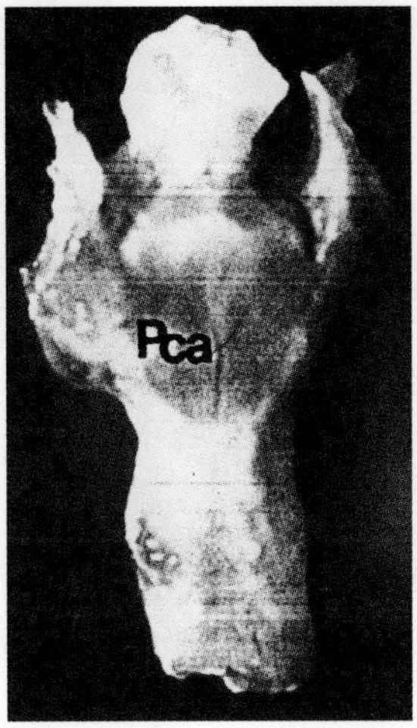

Fig. 2. PCa – Posterior cricoarytenoid muscle of the rat (10×).

Results

Concentrated areas of acetylcholinesterase activity revealed the presence of motor end-plates in the muscles studied.

In the thyroarytenoid (Fig. 4), cricothyroid (Fig. 5) and posterior cricoarytenoid muscles of the rat, end-plates exhibited the single motor end-plate arrangement in a transverse middle band.

In the thyroarytenoid muscle of man, although a somewhat diffuse distribution ccurred, motor end-plates prevailed at the middle zone of the muscle length (Fig. 6).

Discussion

The knowledge about the distribution of motor end-plates in intrinsic muscles of the

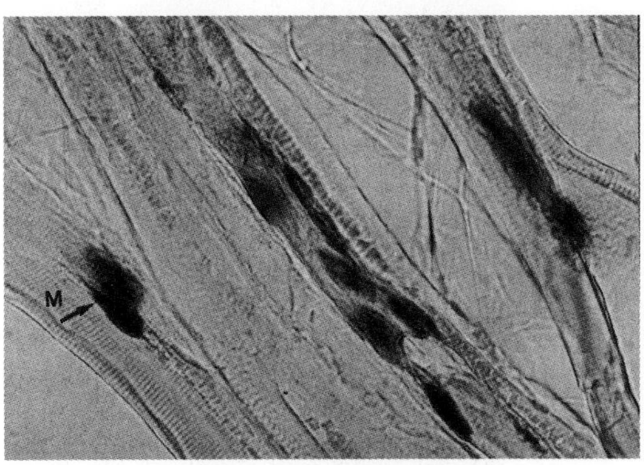

Fig. 3. The thiocholine method staining the thyroarytenoid muscle of the man showing the motor end-plates (M) (400×).

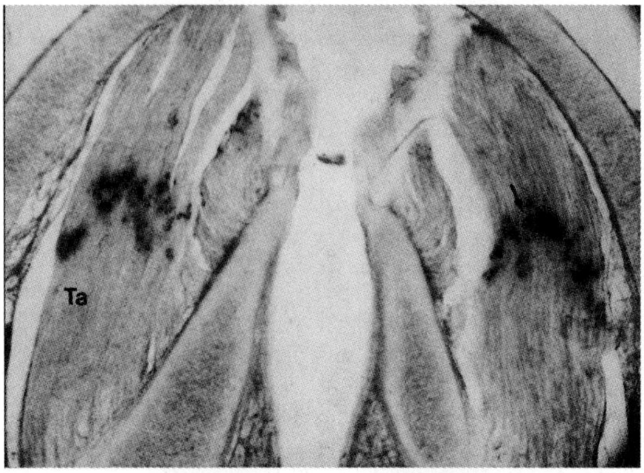

Fig. 4. Motor end-plates of the thyroarytenoid muscle of the rat (Ta) in a transverse middle band (50×).

larynx has potential clinical applications for treatment of neurological disorders at the neuromuscular junction [2].

Rosen et al. [8] have shown that motor end-plates in the human thyroarytenoid muscle have a diffuse distribution with no recognized band or any other cluster arrangement. Rossi et al. [6] found the same diffuse distribution in the human thyroarytenoid muscle, but only in the medial two-thirds of the muscle.

Another study by Guindi et al. [11] revealed no significant differences in the distribution of the motor end-plates, regardless of age or sex.

In contrast with these results, our study shows that in the thyroarytenoid muscle of the rat the motor end-plates are arranged in a transverse middle band, and in human

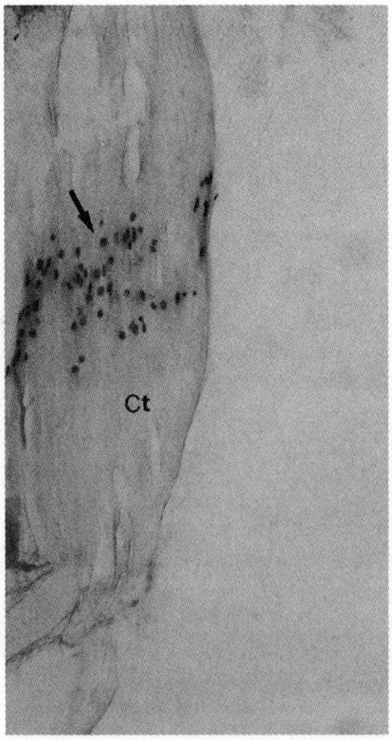

Fig. 5. Motor end-plates of the cricothyroid muscle of the rat (Ct) in a transverse middle band (100×).

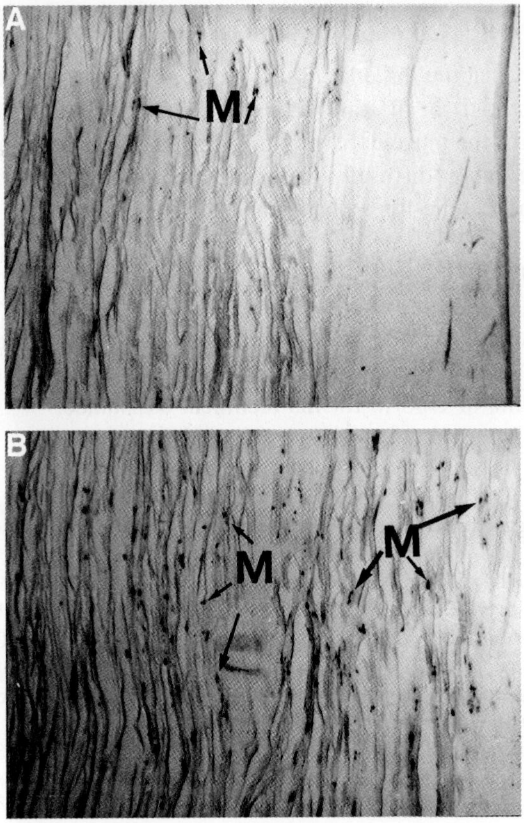

Fig. 6. Motor end-plates (M) distribution of the thyroarytenoid muscle of the man. A: The anterior third zone of the muscle. B: The middle third of the muscle (25×).

thyroarytenoid muscle they have a more diffuse distribution, but clustered in the area corresponding to the transverse middle band of the rat's thyroarytenoid muscle.

The higher concentration of end-plates in the middle-third of the muscle may have clinical significance for intramuscular injection of botulinum toxin, which has been effective in treating certain neurologic disorders, such as spasmodic dysphonia [1]. This voice disorder is thought to be the result of overadduction of the true vocal folds [1,12] and injections of myoneural blocking agents in the middle portion of the thyroarytenoid muscle, where there is an increased concentration of motor end-plates, may have better results with a lower dose of the therapeutic agent.

Hirano and Ohala [13] have described a percutaneous approach to the intrinsic laryngeal muscles using hooked wire electrodes for electromyography. However, it is possible that a modification of this procedure may contribute to the proper injection site in the lateral cricoarytenoid muscle, as well as monitoring its effect on the muscle activity [2].

Conclusion

The motor end-plates at the three laryngeal muscles (thyroarytenoid, cricothyroid and posterior cricoarytenoid) in the rat occurred in a transverse motor region located at the middle portion of the muscle. In human larynx the motor end-plates of thyroarytenoid muscle were more diffusely distributed with a preferential area of higher concentration at the middle-third of the muscle.

Acknowledgements

The authors are grateful to Professor A. Coimbra, Chairman Institute of Histology for his support and scientific advice, and to Professor Pinto da Costa, Director Institute of Forensic Medicine of Oporto for his technical assistance.

References

1. Izdebski K. Symptomatology of adductor spasmodic dysphonia: A physiologic model. J Voice 1992;6:306–319.
2. Freije J, Malmgren LT, Gacek RR. Motor end-plate distribution in the human lateral cricoarytenoid muscle. Arch Otolaryngol Head Neck Surg 1987;113:63–68.
3. Coers C. Contribution à l'etude de la jonction neuromusculaire. II. Topographie zonale de l'innervation motrice terminale dans les muscles striés. Arch Biol (Liege) 1953;65:495–505.
4. Schwarzacher HG. Uber die lange und anordnung der muskelfasern in menschlichen skeletmuskeln. Acta Anat (Basel) 1959;37:217–231.
5. Kupfer C. Motor innervation of extraocular muscle. J Physiol (London) 1960;153:522–526.
6. Rossi G, Cortesina G. Morphological study of the laryngeal muscles in man. Acta Otolaryngol 1965;59:575–592.
7. Kuffler SW, Vaugham Williams EM. Small nerve junctional potentials. The distribution of small motor nerves to frog skeletal muscle, and the membrane characteristics of the fibres they innervate. J Physiol (London) 1953;121:289–317.
8. Rosen M, Malmgren LT, Gacek RR. Three-dimensional computer reconstruction of the distribution of neuromuscular junctions in the thyroarytenoid muscle. Ann Otol Rhinol Laryngol 1983;92:424–429.
9. Sodré-Borges BP. O método de Koelle a pH neutro no estudo da inervação visceral. Folia Anatomica Universitatis Conimbrigensis, vol XL, no. 3, 1970–71.
10. Freije J, Malmgren LT, Gacek RR. Motor end-plate distribution in the human interarytenoid muscle. Arch Otolaryngol Head Neck Surg 1987;113:63–68.
11. Guindi GM, Michaelis L, Bannister R et al. Pathology of the intrinsic muscles of the larynx. Clin Otolaryngl 1981;6:101–109.
12. Aronson AE, DeSanto LW. Adductor spastic dysphonia: One and a half years after recurrent laryngeal nerve resection. Ann Otol Rhinol Laryngol 1981;90:2–6.
13. Hirano M, Ohala J. Use of hooked wire electrodes for electromyography of the intrinsic laryngeal muscles. J Speech Hear Res 1969;12:362–373.

Voice Update.
M. Pais Clemente, editor.

Role of molecular genetics in management of laryngeal cancer (LC) — genetic alterations in LC revealed by FISH analysis: preliminary report

M. Pais Clemente[1], C. Moura[1], M. Ribeiro[1], F. Vales[1], L. Pais Clemente[1], S.R. Wolman[2] and K.J. Flom[2]

[1]*Department of Otorhinolaryngology, Oporto Medical School, Hospital São João, Oporto, Portugal; and* [2]*Oncor®, Inc., Gaithersburg, Maryland, USA*

Abstract. The majority of squamous cell carcinomas are known to have extremely complex chromosomal constitutions, and this probably contributes to the paucity of reports that analyse a large number of tumors. Cytogenetic analysis has identified a great variety of chromosome changes including duplications and deletions, which probably reflect the formation of unregulated oncogenes and tumor suppressor genes. This seems to be an important prognostic factor in the determination of treatment response and survival. The relationship between amplification and deletion of specific regions on a chromosome and numerical aberrations of that chromosome in laryngeal cancer (LC) are often not defined.

We analysed tissues for target sequences using the FISH (fluorescence in situ hybridization) technique on malignant laryngeal tumors and respective lymph node metastases from three patients. The tissues were examined for numerical aberrations involving chromosomes 7, 9, 11, and 21. These data were correlated with the clinical staging, and we verified that the best survival rate case showed the minor aberrant chromosomal alterations.

Key words: FISH analysis, laryngeal cancer.

Introduction

Head and neck squamous cell carcinoma (HNSCC) represents 2–3% of all human malignancies [1], and in Portugal the estimated incidence of laryngeal cancer (LC) in 1990 was 30.3% for males and 5.5% for females [2].

Recent investigations support the concept that laryngeal cancer is a consequence of successive genetic changes, which may include: 1) overproduction of a gene product; 2) production of an abnormal gene product; and 3) loss of a gene product through inactivation by mutation, translocation or deletion of a gene [3].

Abnormal cellular DNA content has been well documented as a hallmark of malignancy in human solid tumors and the great majority of studies showed that aneuploid tumors have a poorer prognosis than diploid ones [3,4].

The extremely complex chromosomal constitutions found on the majority of squamous cell carcinomas (SCC) in conjunction with the technical difficulties

Address for correspondence: M. Pais Clemente MD, PhD, Instituto Português da Voz, Rua Caldas Xavier 38 – 6°E, 4150 Oporto, Portugal.

encountered in cytogenetics, probably contribute to the limitation of our knowledge on karyotype abnormalities and their clinical implications [5–8].

Overall, the chromosome changes observed in solid tumors tend to be losses or gains of chromosomes rather than translocations [8]. In HNSCC, cytogenetic studies have shown structural aberrations involving chromosomal arms 18q, 13p, 10p, 8p, 15p and 22p, and numerical aberrations involving trisomy for chromosome 7 or nullisomy for the 3p and 18q chromosome [3,9–11].

Interphase cytogenetic studies of fixed sections or short-term cultures of malignant laryngeal tissue, are potentially an important means of defining chromosomal gains or losses, and of confirming the previously reported aberrations of chromosomes 3, 4, 7–11, 13–15, 17, 18, 21 and 22 [6,12–15] in laryngeal cancer, which seems to be an important prognostic factor determinant of treatment response and survival.

The genetic alterations that underlie laryngeal tumorigenesis are assumed to comprise gain or loss of specific chromosomal regions, whole chromosome or sequence-specific mutations that probably reflect the formation of unregulated oncogenes and tumor suppressor genes. The relationship between amplification and deletion of specific genetic regions on a chromosome and numerical aberrations of that chromosome in laryngeal cancer and other tumors is often not defined.

This preliminary report describes the analysis of tissues from three patients by using FISH technique (fluorescence in situ hybridization) on malignant laryngeal tumors and respective lymph node metastases. The tissues were examined for numerical aberrations by using five different biotinylated centromere-specific DNA probes to the chromosomes 7, 9, 11, 17 and 21.

Materials and Methods

For purposes of this study, paraffin-embedded tissue sections containing areas of laryngeal carcinoma and respective lymph node metastasis have been selected.

The corresponding paraffin-blocked samples from laryngectomies were serially sectioned into two groups of five micron sections, then applied to silanized slides without coverslips. The slides were allowed to air dry and then baked at 65°C overnight. Every first slide of the group was stained with Hematoxylin/Eosin (H/E) to visualize areas of frank malignancy. These areas were circumscribed with ink and used as templates to examine or excise the same areas from adjacent nonstaining sections. The second section was retained intact and the circumscribed areas were delineated by etching the bottom of the glass slides as mapping for FISH. Storage of the slides for several months had no effect on FISH hybridization.

FISH

The slides were first deparaffined in xylenes with agitation for 10 min followed by two washes in 100% ethanol for 5 min each. The hybridization procedures use a chromosome in situ kit for paraffin-embedded formalin-fixed tissue sections (Oncor®). The biotin-labeled centromeric chromosome probes (Oncor®) used included probes for chromosomes 7, 9, 11 and 17 and a regional probe for chromosome 21 in tissue sections from laryngeal cancer. The hybridization protocol suggested by Oncor® [16] was followed, with a single difference, the hybridization mixture consisted of 2.5–3 μl of the probe and 10 μl of Hybrisol VIII, instead of the 2.0 μl probe volume suggested.

Counterstaining of nuclei was accomplished by incubating slides in 30 μl of propidium iodide/antifade for 5 min. After counterstaining for 3 min in 1X PBD, 30 μl of antifade was added to each slide to prevent fading of fluorescent signal. Analysis was conducted at 10×–100× on a Zeiss epifluorescent microscope fitted with double dichroic mirrors using a FITC filter combination that permits simultaneous blue and green excitation and green and red emission frequencies. Results were recorded using Kodak Ektachrome 400 film.

Initially, 200 nuclei of good technical quality for each probe were scored for the number of positive signals.

A mapping procedure was developed when it became clear that heterogeneity of signal frequency could be found in individual tumors with or without concomitant histologic heterogeneity. By low power (10×) examination of the circled area after exclusion of folded regions, a grid of microscopic coordinates was generated. Areas with sufficient representative malignant epithelium were selected for analysis. Between 15 and 20 coordinates, distributed over the grid encompassing the entire region of interest, were counted as fields at higher power for signals per nucleus.

Results

The tumors were classified according to the WHO classification of upper respiratory tract tumors [17] and were grouped according to the staging of TNM/UICC [18] (Table 1). The correlation with the survival of each patient was performed (Table 1). All of the three tumors were well-differentiated cases and have lymph node metastases, and none of the patients had distant dissemination (M0). The survival varies among 10 months to a T4 tumor and 22 months to a T3 tumor.

The results of FISH analysis for each of the three LC are generically presented in Table 2 and each sample is specifically described in Table 3.

Definition of disomy by FISH

Because direct comparison of normal and tumor cell populations on these sections of laryngeal tumors was not possible, an arbitrarily chosen cut-off of 35% or more has been used to define monosomy in this study, based on previous reports of prostate cancer [19–20]. Considering the generally larger size of squamous tumor cells, this is probably a very conservative estimate.

Frequencies of trisomy or tetrasomy above 10% were defined as true increases in signal.

Discussion

In this preliminary study, we have used the FISH technique to examine biopsy material from three primary LCs and their respective lymph nodes, using five centromeric chromosome-specific DNA probes. The probes chosen for this study are those of chromosomes for which numerical aberrations have been reported in HNSCC [3,9,12]. Case 1 Lt was considered as the control since it contained no identifiable tumor in a lymph node, falling within the expected values for normal tissues, two signals for each probe (except for the heterosomes in the males) representing the paired chromosomes.

The results described in this work provide a detailed view of the numerical chromosomes' alteration occurring in the analyzed samples. We have evaluated the observed chromosomal ploidy patterns in the individual cases (Tables 2 and 3) in the context of the clinical staging of the disease (Table 1).

The findings of FISH analysis suggested that several regions of the genome are preferentially deleted or duplicated. Each tumor showed uniquely different and abnormal patterns of chromosomal losses and gains. To analyze the results, some characteristics of both sample and probe must be considered:

- Slight variations in section thickness may have substantial effects. Major concerns are the average and range of nuclear diameters within each tumor and the extent of heterogeneity within the lesion. The structural characteristics and preservation (fixation) of DNA may vary with cell type.
- The probes are expected to vary in signal size as a function of probe length

Table 1. Patient staging.

Case	Stage	Survival
1	T3 N2 M0	14 months
2	T4 N2 c) M0	10 months
3	T3 N2 b) M0	22 months

Staging according to [18].

Table 2. Genetic alterations: FISH for all specimens.

Specimen	Chromosome				
	7	9	11	17	21
1 CaL	Gain	BL gain	Gain	Loss	Loss
1 Lt	N	N	N	N	N
2 CaL	Gain	Gain	Loss	Gain	Loss
2 Lt	BL gain	Gain	Loss	BL gain	*
3 CaL	Loss	Loss	Loss	Gain	*
3 Lt	Loss	Loss	Loss	Loss	N

Note: N = normal; BL = borderline aberrations; CaL = primary tumor; Lt = lymph node metastasis from primary tumor; * = not analyzed.

(constant for a specific probe) and the number of target repeats (constant for an individual). Similarity of a probe to other genomic sequences can result in cross-hybridization.

– The thinner the tissue section, the smaller the average nuclear fraction available for analysis will be. An average nuclear diameter above 5 μm will usually exceed the thickness of the section. Similarly, as the average nuclear diameter of the tumor cells increases, the average nuclear fraction analyzed will be less, reducing the apparent signal count. Conversely, if the nuclear diameter is small there is a greater likelihood that signals will overlap, also reducing the apparent signal count.

Table 3. Deviation from disomy and monosomy.

Case 1 CaL

	0	1	2	3	4	5	6	Total
Cocktail-7	2	28	84	53	27	5	1	200
Classic-9	14	71	100	12	3	–	–	200
Alfa-11	7	52	107	34	–	–	–	200
Alfa-17	3	103	86	7	1	–	–	200
Cosmid-21	23	84	90	3	–	–	–	200

Note: Sample 1 CaL showed 43% of nuclei with increased signals for the centromeric probe for chromosome 7, a smaller increase for chromosome 11 (17%), and significant losses from chromosome 17 (52%) and 21 (42%).

Case 1 Lt

	0	1	2	3	4	5	6	Total
Cocktail-7	8	41	142	7	2	–	–	200
Classic-9	7	68	122	3	–	–	–	200
Alfa-11	9	47	133	11	–	–	–	200
Alfa-17	3	51	143	1	2	–	–	200
Cosmid-21	8	54	136	1	1	–	–	200

Note: Case 1 Lt contained no identifiable tumor in a lymph node and was considered as the control, falling within the expected values for normal tissues. In normal cells we expected to see two signals for each probe (except for the X and Y in male), representing the paired chromosome.

Case 2 CaL

	0	1	2	3	4	5	6	Total
Cocktail-7	14	52	89	41	4	1	–	201
Classic-9	5	20	64	78	28	–	–	200
Alfa-11	28	78	102	26	3	5	–	237
Alfa-17	11	46	94	42	8	–	–	201
Recount	21	45	106	42	6	–	–	220
Cosmid-21	33	52	88	26	2	–	–	201

Note: Sample 2 CaL showed increased copies of chromosome 7 in 23% of cells and great increases in chromosome 9 (56%), with a loss of signal of chromosomes 11 (50%) and 21.

(*continued*)

Table 3. Continued.

Case 2 Lt

	0	1	2	3	4	5	6	Total
Cocktail-7	—	84	94	21	1	—	—	200
Recount	14	62	97	40	9	—	—	222
Classic-9	2	37	79	60	22	—	—	200
Alfa-11	—	122	72	3	1	—	—	198
Alfa-17	—	103	92	2	3	—	—	200
Recount 1	33	78	83	29	10	—	—	235
Recount 2	25	78	96	23	3	—	—	225
Cosmid-21	—	—	—	—	—	—	—	—

Note: The pattern for sample 2 Lt was very similar to that for 2 CaL with gains of chromosomes 7 (11% – marginal), 9 (41%) and 17 (25%), with loss of 11 (61%). Only one of two readers detected a similar gain of chromosome 17 in 20% of cells in the metastasis.

Case 3 CaL

	0	1	2	3	4	5	6	Total
Cocktail-7	3	155	40	2	—	—	—	200
Classic-9	0	81	113	6	—	—	—	200
Alfa-11	0	45	104	52	—	—	—	201
Recount	21	101	106	1	—	—	—	229
Alfa-17	0	67	103	31	—	—	—	201
Cosmid-21	—	—	—	—	—	—	—	—

Note: Samples 3 CaL and 3 Lt were less abberrant overall than the other tumors. They were similar to one another and showed predominant patterns of chromosome loss involving 7 and 9, with some gain evident only for the chromosome 11 in the primary (3 CaL) lesion. A second reader observed loss for this chromosome in approximately 50% of cells in both lesions. A very small fraction of cells were apparently trisomic for chromosome 17 (12%). Comparisons of data for the cosmid 21 probes were not available for cases 2 and 3 because of insufficient numbers in sections.

Case 3 Lt

	0	1	2	3	4	5	6	Total
Cocktail-7	0	79	104	17	—	—	—	200
Classic-9	0	129	66	5	—	—	—	200
Alfa-11	0	59	129	12	—	—	—	200
Recount	27	109	75	16	—	—	—	200
Alfa-17	0	75	108	17	—	—	—	200
Cosmid-21	0	48	150	2	—	—	—	200

– If the configuration or integrity of tumor DNA differs from that of normal cells, the frequency of cross-hybridization may change. If the degree or tightness of binding to signal is altered, the apparent signal size may also change.
– Larger signal size may result in more overlaps decreasing the apparent counts.

Conversely, smaller but precise signals are easy to read, but if very small, may be so faint that some are not recognized, also decreasing the apparent counting.
- The higher the homology (sequence similarity) between the probe and other sequences, the greater the chances of cross-hybridization, increasing the apparent number of signals. No specific "background" fluorescence can be identified by its appearance over areas other than nuclei.

This is a pilot study and only 200 nuclei per each probe/sample have been counted. When discrepant results were found between tumor and metastatic lesion, a second reader also evaluated the sample. The results are clearly more reliable when a larger number of cells are analysed, by more than one reader per case.

Increases in chromosome 7, noted in cases 1 and 2, have been observed in many other examples of solid epithelial tumors (lung, kidney, bladder) and have been found occasionally in nontumor tissues as well [8,21,22]. On the other hand, the striking increase in chromosome 9 in case 2 was unexpected, as reports of whole chromosome 9 (bladder carcinoma) and focal molecular losses are common [8,22]. This increased DNA content appears to be an indicator of a cell genetic instability, consequence of mitotic abnormalities that may become more prominent as neoplasms develop, and include structural and other numerical abnormalities [23–25]. The previous studies concerning HNSCC showed that ploidy strongly correlated with the prognosis [11,15,26].

Conclusion

Comparing chromosomal analysis of primary tumor and respective lymph node metastases, with the exception of case number 1 Lt with no identifiable tumor, we can conclude that the chromosomal patterns of the metastases were very similar to the primary tumor. This probably indicates that lymph node metastases can act as an individual prognostic factor.

Case 3 had the best survival rate and simultaneously showed the least aberrant chromosomal alterations. These could be remarkable data if confirmed in the sequence of this study.

Survival rates for patients with cancers of the head and neck have not been significantly improving recently [27], and there is a need for new prognostic elements for therapeutic approaches. These can only be developed on the basis of an improved knowledge of the tumor properties and its behavior in vivo and in vitro, and well-characterized cell lines are fundamental for such studies [9]. In this context DNA analysis acquires significant importance in the early diagnosis of laryngeal carcinomas since it allows the clinician to improve the diagnosis of the tumor staging and patient management [28].

References

1. Cann CI, Fried MP, Rothman KJ. Epidemiology of squamous cell cancer of the head and neck. Otolaryngol Clin 1985;18:1–22.
2. Estève J, Kricker A, Ferlay J, Parkin DM. Facts and figures of cancer in the European Community.

International Agency for Research on Cancer, World Health Organization, 1993.
3. Cowan JM. Cytogenetics in head and neck cancer. Otolaryngol Clin North Am 1992;25(5): 1073–1087.
4. Hedley DW, Friedlander ML, Taylor IW. Application of DNA flow cytometry to paraffin-embedded archival material for the study of aneuploidy and its clinical significance. Cytometry 1985;6:327–333.
5. Jin Y, Heim S, Mertens F, Mandahl N, Olegard C, Wennerberg J, Biorklund A, Mitelman F. Chromosome abnormalities in eighty-three head and neck squamous cell carcinomas: influence of culture conditions on karyotyping pattern. Cancer Res 1993;53:2140–2146.
6. Allegra E, Garozzo A, Grillo A, Catalano G. Cytogenetic alterations in laryngeal carcinomas. Arch Otolaryngol Head Neck Surg 1992;118:1320–1322.
7. Van Dyke DL, Worsham MJ, Benninger MS, Krause CJ, Baker SR, Wolf GT, Drumheller T, Tilley BC, Carey TE. Recurrent cytogenetic abnormalities in squamous cell carcinomas of the head and neck regions. Genes Chromosomes Cancer Res 1993;53:2140–2146.
8. Sandberg AA, Turc-Carel C. The cytogenetics of solid tumors. Cancer 1987;59:387–395.
9. Heo DS, Synderman C, Gollin SM et al. Biology, cytogenetics and sensitivity to immunological effector cells of new head and neck squamous cell carcinoma lines. Cancer Res 1989;49:5167.
10. Latif F, Fivash M, Glenn G et al. Chromosome 3p deletions in head and neck carcinomas: Statistical ascertainment of allelic loss. Cancer Res 1992;52:1451.
11. Voravud N, Shin DM, Ro JY, Lee JS, Hong WK, Hittelman WN. Increase polysomies of chromosome 7 and 17 during head and neck multistage tumorigenesis. Cancer Res 1993;53: 2874–2883.
12. Carey TE, Van Dyke DL, Worsham MJ et al. Characterization of human laryngeal primary and metastatic squamous cells lines UM-SCC-17A and UM-SCC-17B. Cancer Res 1989;49:6098.
13. Cowan JM, Becket MA, Ahmed-Swan S et al. Cytogenetic evidence of the multistep origin of head and neck squamous cell carcinoma. J Natl Cancer Inst 1992;84:793.
14. Jin Y, Mandahl N, Heim S et al. Unique karyotypic abnormalities in a squamous cell carcinoma of the larynx. Cancer Genet Cytogenet 1988;30:177.
15. Jin Y, Heim S, Mandhal N, Biorklund A, Wennenberg J, Mitelman F. Multiple clonal chromosomal aberrations in squamous cell carcinomas of the larynx. Cancer Cytogenet 1990;44:209–216.
16. Oncor Chromosome in situ hybridization system. Ed 3.1, June 1994.
17. Shnmugaratnam K. Histological typing of tumors of the upper respiratory tract and ear. World Health Organization. International histological classification of tumors, 2nd edn. Berlin: Springer-Verlag, 1991.
18. TNM Atlas Illustrated Guide to the TNM/pTNM Classification of Malignant Tumours, 2nd rev 3rd edn. New York: Springer-Verlag, 1992.
19. Micale MA, Sanford JS, Powell IJ, Sakr WA, Wolman SR. Defining the extent and nature of cytogenetic events in prostatic adenocarcinoma: paraffin FISH vs. metaphase analysis. Cancer Genet Cytogenet 1993;69(1):7–12.
20. Macoska JA, Micale MA, Sakr WA, Benson PD, Wolman SR. Extensive genetic alterations in prostate cancer revealed by dual PCR and FISH analysis. Genes Chromosomes Cancer 1993;8(2): 88–97.
21. Sandberg AA, Turc-Carel C, Gemmill RM. Chromosomes in solid tumors and beyond. Cancer Res 1988;48:1049–1059.
22. Sandberg AA. Chromosomes changes in bladder cancer: clinical and other correlations. Cancer Genet Cytogenet 1986;19:163–175.
23. Nowell PC. Mechanism of tumor progression. Cancer Res 1986;46:2203–2207.
24. Shackney SE, Smith CA, Miller BW et al. Model for the genetic evolution of human solid tumors. Cancer Res 1989;49:3344–3354.
25. Sobel ME. Metastases suppressor genes. J Natl Cancer Inst 1990;82:267–275.
26. Holm LE. Cellular DNA amounts of squamous cell carcinomas of the head and neck region in relation to prognosis. Laryngoscope 1982;90:1209–1224.
27. Garfinkel L. Cancer statistics. CA, 1987;37:2–19.
28. Ruá S, Comino A, Fruttero A et al. Relationship between histologic features, DNA flow cytometry, and clinical behaviour of squamous cell carcinomas of the larynx. Cancer 1991;67:141–149.

Voice Update.
M. Pais Clemente, editor.

Photodiagnosis of premalignant and malignant laryngeal diseases: A new diagnostic procedure

M. Pais Clemente[1], L. Pais Clemente[1], E. Cardoso[1], R. Pratas[1], K. Svanberg[2], S. Svanberg[2] and I. Wang[2]

[1]*Department of Otorhinolaringology, Oporto Medical School, Hospital S. João, Oporto, Portugal; and* [2]*Lund University Medical Laser Centre, Lund Institute of Technology, Lund, Sweden*

Abstract. The development of fluorescence methods to mark malignant tumors has been closely connected to the application of photodynamic therapy (PDT).

However, recent advances in laser technology gave the possibility to use the same concepts for detection of suspicious lesions of the upper aerodigestive tract and early diagnosis of head and neck tumors.

A fiberoptic fluorosensor was used to record fluorescence spectra of the mucosa during standard fiberscopy examination. The drug fluorescence was induced by the haem precursor ∂-amino levulinic acid (ALA) which was administered orally. When ALA, a nonfluorescing drug, is excessively administered, the regulatory feedback system in the haem cycle is bypassed and an accumulation of Protoporphyrin IX (PpIX) occurs. Due to differences in the content of the enzymes, regulating the ALA transformation, the build-up of Pp IX is enhanced in malignant tumor tissue compared to normal mucosa, and it can be monitored with dual-peaked fluorescence at 635 and 700 nm, using an optical multichannel analyser (OMA System).

This important photobiochemical reaction will facilitate the differential diagnosis of normal vs. pathologic mucosa which needs to be confirmed by biopsy.

Key words: ALA, laser-induced fluorescence (LIF), photodiagnosis, premalignant and malignant laryngeal diseases, protoporphyrin IX, sensitization.

Introduction

Photodynamic therapy (PDT) is an investigational local tumor treatment modality based on the induced activation of various photosensitizing agents which are administered to the body at different time intervals before laser irradiation. The photosensitizing agents exhibit characteristic fluorescence signals and have been used in the development of a new diagnostic procedure for early photodetection or photodiagnosis (PD) of tumors, based on the specific drug-related fluorescence combined with the autofluorescence from tissue chromophores [1–4].

The most commonly used drug is a haematoporphyrin derivative (Photofrin®) which is administered intravenously usually 24–48 h before the procedure. After this time interval the concentration of the drug is higher in the tumor than in normal

Address for correspondence: M. Pais Clemente MD, PhD, Instituto Português da Voz, Rua Caldas Xavier, 38 - 6°E, 4150 Oporto, Portugal.

surrounding tissue, depending upon different factors, such as the molecular properties of the dye and the tumor vascular supply [5].

An unwanted side effect with Photofrin® is the transient skin sensitization, and for this reason it is advisable to keep the patients out of ambient light for a period of about 4 weeks. This adverse reaction has played a major role in the slow clinical acceptance of this agent and its therapeutic application. The skin response is dose dependent and in PD procedures the drug dose can be reduced drastically with the avoidance of the skin sensitization, provided sensitive fluorescence equipment is used [3,4].

Second-generation sensitizers have been developed and some of them have less side effects with much shorter periods of skin sensitization [6]. Recently, a new drug, called ALA (∂-amino levulinic acid), has been introduced for PDT and PD, opening the possibility of topical and oral administration. The local application is of special interest for skin and/or bladder tumors [7–9]. The ALA is a nontoxic white powder, haem precursor, photodynamic, inactive but which enables the synthesis of protoporfirin IX (PpIX), a potent sensitizer with a skin sensitization for several hours.

The ALA is the first step in the haem cycle and is formed in the condensation procedure of coenzyme A and glycine. The formation of ALA in the body as well as the synthesis of haem from PpIX is regulated by feedback systems. When ALA is administered in excess the cell regulation of the ALA formation is disrupted and PpIX is formed during several steps within the cycle [8]. Each step in the haem cycle is regulated by enzymes. Due to differences in the content of these enzymes in normal and malignant tissue some of the steps are facilitated and others slowed down. Thus, the content of the enzymes regulating the first two steps in the cycle is high in malignant tissue, enhancing the formation of tetrapyrole in malignant tumors [10]. On the other hand the content of ferrochelatase is low in malignant tissue and therefore the step from PpIX to haem is slow and an accumulation of PpIX occurs [11].

With lower ALA doses (5–7.5 mg/kg b.w.) the availability of ALA in normal tissue is too low for the enzymatic capability. On the other hand, PpIX can still be synthesized in tumor tissue as the enzymatic pattern is organized to meet the higher metabolic demand from proliferating tissue. Most probably, there is a threshold for the ALA dose which varies from organ to organ for optimal tumor demarcation. The time interval for maximal tumor build-up of PpIX in tumor tissue may also vary with the grade and stage of the tumor as well as with the tumor type. For the evaluation of the optimal time window for diagnosis and treatment, pharmacokinetic studies are important. In vitro fluorescence microscopy investigations have been performed for pharmacokinetics studies of the distribution of PpIX in different tissue types in a few patients [12,13]. The microscopy fluorescence studies revealed a maximum PpIX build-up 4–6 h after the oral administration of ALA.

Laser-induced fluorescence (LIF) is a noninvasive method for real-time in vivo monitoring of the chromophores in the tissues. As the sensitizing agents exhibit specific fluorescence signatures, LIF can be utilized for the drug detection. Although the intensity of the fluorescence signal cannot be directly interpreted in terms of drug concentration, the fluorescence intensity is clearly related to the tissue content. The monitoring of the drug can also be performed by tissue fluorescence microscopy [14] or chemical extraction of the drug content. The disadvantages with these methods, in comparison to LIF, is that they are invasive with tissue destruction and do not provide real-time results. Moreover, during the tissue sensitization for in vitro investigations the photosensitizing agent may be degraded or destroyed.

PpIX fluorescence, as well as background tissue autofluorescence, increase proportionally with the excitation energy. With increased excitation energy the signal-to-noise ratio is improved, but high signal-to-noise ratio does not mean that the tumor demarcation criterion will be improved. Instead, photobleaching of the tissue and photodecomposition of the photosensitizer take place and a photodynamic effect may occur. One way to improve the detection limit is, however, to utilize not only the red porphyrin fluorescence signal but also to take advantage of the information emanating from the blue-green tissue autofluorescence [2]. Forming a ratio between the red fluorescence signal resulting from the PpIX retained in the malignant tissue and the blue-green tissue autofluorescence offers two advantages. First, a dimensionless function is formed, which is insensitive to the excitation and detection efficiency, and secondly, a contrast enhancement is gained due to a decrease in the blue-green tissue autofluorescence parallel with the increase in the PpIX-related fluorescence in the tumor region.

LIF can also be used in the detection of the endogenous sensitization with the transformation of ALA to highly fluorescent substances, which makes it a very useful tool, as it provides prompt in situ results. We have used LIF for real-time in vivo investigations of the PpIX build-up after oral administration of ALA with low doses (5–15 mg/kg b.w.) for the detection of head and neck tumors and other skin malignancies [15,16].

In this study we present some preliminary results obtained with this new diagnostic procedure in patients with premalignant and malignant laryngeal diseases.

Materials and Methods

Patients

For this study seven patients were evaluated (six men, one woman; mean age 50.5 years (range: 27–67 years)) with laryngeal lesions, except one patient with squamous cell carcinoma of the oropharynx. The patients were all investigated on an outpatient basis.

In order to compare the data we have divided the patient population into three groups:

1. Group 1 consisted of two patients with benign laryngeal lesions (hypertrophy of the false fold and laryngeal papillomas).
2. Group 2 presented with premalignant diseases, such as leukoplakia and early stage squamous cell carcinomas (three patients).
3. Group 3 consisted of two patients with malignant tumors (squamous cell

carcinomas), one from the epiglottis and the other from the oropharynx.
All the patients with premalignant and malignant diseases were heavy smokers. Microlaryngoscopy with biopsy was performed in all the patients, except one (hypertrophy of the false fold), to confirm the clinical diagnosis.

Drug

ALA (Porphyrin Products Inc., Logan, Utah, USA) was delivered as a hydrochloric salt dissolved in orange juice. Two different drug doses, 5 and 7.5 mg/kg b.w., were prepared immediately before use and administered orally to the patients. The preparation resulted in a pH below 5 at which level ALA is stable in the solution.

Equipment

A schematic diagram of the optical arrangement required for this study is shown in Fig. 1. As an excitation source a nitrogen (N_2) laser (PRA Model LN 250) or the same N_2 laser pumping a dye laser (Laser Science Model VSL-DCM-3) was used. The lasers emit about 3-ns long pulses at 10 Hz with a wavelength of 337 nm and a pulse energy of 175 μJ for the N_2 laser and any wavelength between 360 and 700 nm at pulse energies up to about 35 μJ for the dye laser. The light energy impinging on the tissue is about 20% of the laser pulse energy, the rest being lost in filters and optics. Bandpass filters are used in front of the lasers to suppress plasma emission lines and broadband dye fluorescence from the N_2 laser and dye laser, respectively [2].

To change the wavelength of the dye laser, the cuvette with the dye solution has to be interchanged with a cuvette containing another solution lasing at a different wavelength and another combination of dichroic mirror and filters may be necessary. Changing the excitation wavelength takes less than 30 s and there is almost full flexibility in the choice of excitation wavelength with this equipment.

The fiber, Fiberguide Inc., Model SFS600N, has a core diameter of 600 μm, a numerical aperture of 0.22, is 3 m long and is made of an almost fluorescence-free quartz. It is protected in a 4-mm diameter plastic tube. A sterilized quartz fiber is connected to the end of the optical fiber carrying the exciting laser light. The fiber is pointed towards the tissue being investigated, the laser light excites the molecules within the sample, and fluorescence will occur. By holding the fiber tip close to the target, the fluorescent light is efficiently collected by the same fiber and guided back to the equipment. A cut-off filter is placed in front of the entrance slit to suppress any stray light from the laser.

Two excitation wavelengths were employed during the investigations: 1) 337 nm, for which a good contrast in the blue-green autofluorescence between the tumor and normal surrounding tissue has been obtained [15,16]; 2) 405 nm, close to the peak of the Soret excitation band for any endogenous porphyrin that might be present in the tissue.

Fluorescence was conducted to the entrance slit of a Jobin Yvon 0.25 m grating

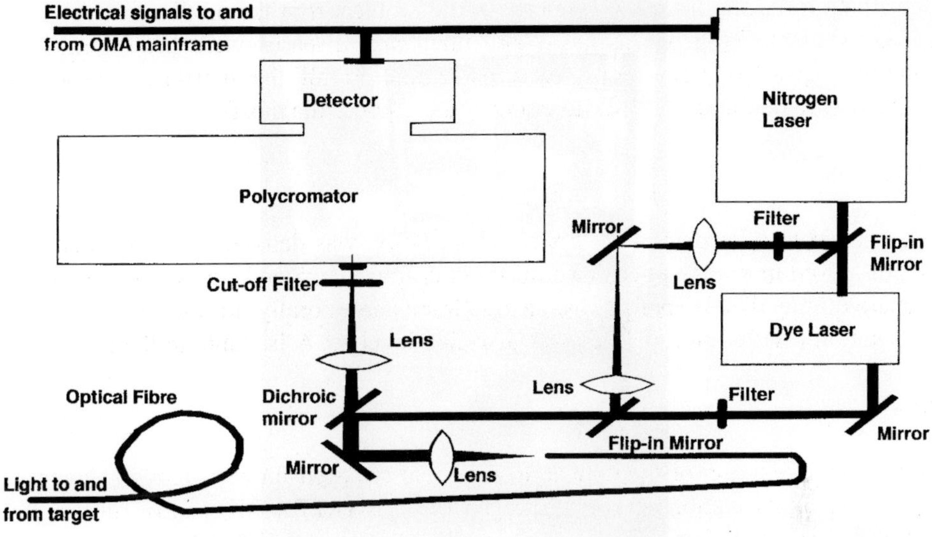

Fig. 1. The optical arrangement for in vivo laser-induced fluorescence recording.

monochromator equipped with an EG & G, Model 1460, gated and intensified linear array detector connected to an EG & G OMA mainframe, where the fluorescent spectrum is displayed in real-time and stored. The signal from 100 laser pulses was averaged during a period of 10 s. The signals were spectrally corrected using a calibrated standard lamp.

The described equipment was assembled on the mobile trolley shown in Fig. 2. The trolley is three-storeyed, one storey for the optical arrangement, another for the OMA mainframe, and the third for cables, dry air supply and storage for optical components and tools. The equipment is enclosed in a plexiglass box for hygienic reasons.

Fluorescence investigations can therefore be conducted with this equipment in ambient room light without any risk of photobleaching of the target tissue due to high excitation energy.

Fluorescence investigations

The fluorescence investigations were performed before and at different time intervals after the ALA administration. The patient sits facing the examiner who is standing. The nasal cavity and laryngopharynx are sprayed with 10% lidocaine (Xylocaine®) spray. The tip of the flexible fiberscope is lightly lubricated and gently inserted into the nose. The flexible laryngoscope is connected to a miniature CCD camera with a C-mount coupler for video recording.

An optical fiber based mobile OMA System was used for tissue fluorescence monitoring. The fiber was placed in the working channel of a flexible laryngoscope

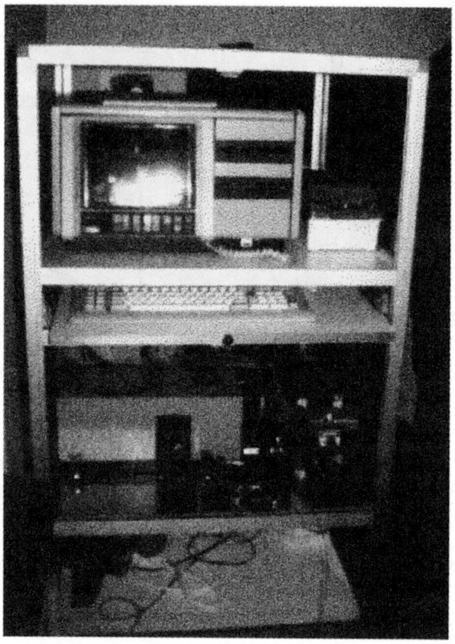

Fig. 2. Equipment arranged on a three-storeyed mobile trolley for laser-induced fluorescence.

for measurement of the tissue fluorescence in the supraglottic and subglottic areas, while the skin of the forearm, the tongue and the mucosa of the oral cavity were used for normal tissue control measurements. All recordings were performed with the fiber tip placed in close contact with the tissues.

Tissue fluorescence investigations were performed in all patients before the ALA intake and every hour until 8 h after ALA administration in skin, tongue, buccal mucosa and, in several cases, nasal mucosa. The fluorescence of the laryngeal lesions of all the patients was monitored during endoscopic procedures, 7—8 h after the ALA administration. In one patient with a malignant tumor (squamous cell carcinoma) of the oropharynx area, the tumor measurements were performed with the same time intervals as for the normal tissue types because of its easy access.

Results

The data from seven patients presented in this study is summarized on Table 1. Two patients (numbers 2 and 4) had benign laryngeal diseases. Premalignant lesions and early malignant tumors were found in three patients (numbers 3, 5 and 7). Two patients (numbers 1 and 6) had advanced squamous cell carcinomas.

The fluorescence intensity at 635 and 490 nm is evaluated and expressed in terms of an internal reference. In all patients a low PpIX-related fluorescence intensity at 635 nm was found in the measurements from normal tissue except in one patient (number 6). In all the patients with premalignant and malignant lesions the

Table 1. Fluorescence data from seven patients with benign, premalignant and malignant laryngeal diseases and carcinoma of the oropharynx.

Patients	Dose ALA	Time post ALA intake	Intensity 635nm	Intensity 490 nm	Intensity ratio 635/490
Patient 1	15 mg	6 h			
Squamous cell carcinoma of the oropharynx			0.62	0.11	5.9
Normal soft palate			0.25	4.95	0.05
Patient 2	5 mg	7 h			
Hypertrophic left false fold			0.69	4.29	0.16
Normal right false fold			0.52	3.02	0.17
Normal bruccal mucosa			0	3.30	0
Patient 3	5 mg	7.5 h			
Dysplasia of the right vocal fold			1.61	0.22	7.3
Carcinoma in situ of the left vocal fold			0.42	1.10	0.38
Normal buccal mucosa			0	3.38	0
Patient 4	5 mg	8 h			
Squamous papillomas of the vocal folds			0	20.80	0
Normal buccal mucosa			0	8.06	0
Patient 5	5 mg	7 h			
Dysplasia of the right vocal fold			0.11	0.13	0.85
Normal epiglottic mucosa			0.19	2.20	0.08
Normal buccal mucosa			0	10.47	0
Patient 6	5 mg	8 h			
Squamous cell carcinoma of the epiglottis			0.15	0.01	15
Normal buccal mucosa			3.74	7.37	0.51
Patient 7	5 mg	8 h			
Dysplasia of the right false fold			0.48	0.73	0.66
Normal buccal mucosa			0	8.53	0

autofluorescence (490 nm) shows lower intensity in diseased tissue as compared to normal tissue. The ratio of the intensity at 635 and 490 nm shows a high value in the advanced tumors. For patient number three with dysplastic tissue a high ratio was also found. The tumor demarcation ratio is high in all patients including the patients with dysplasia. In the patient with benign hypertrophy of the false fold the ratio between the lesion and normal tissue does not show any demarcation.

Figure 3 shows the fluorescence spectra from a patient with dysplasia of the vocal fold and from a normal buccal mucosa recorded at the same time. As seen in the spectrum the dysplastic area of the vocal fold is characterized by a marked fluorescence in the red wavelength region with a dual-peaked light emisson at almost 635 and 710 nm and a very low autofluorescence peaking at 490 nm. On the other hand, the spectrum from the buccal mucosa shows a high autofluorescence intensity and no sign of PpIX.

Also a typical dual-peaked PpIX-related signal and a weak autofluorescence

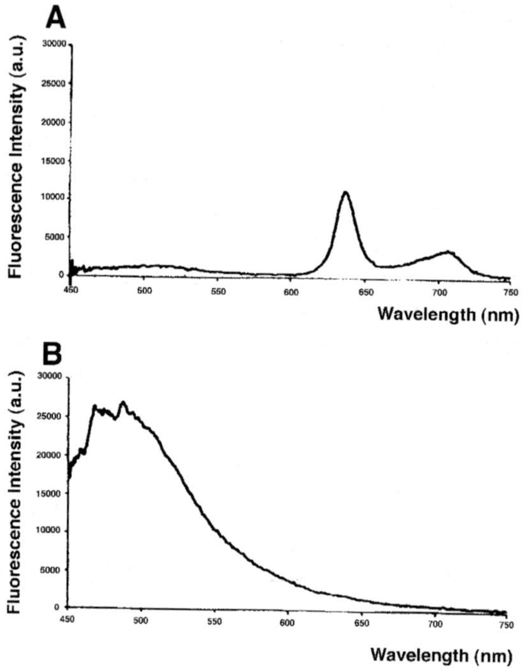

Fig. 3. Fluorescence spectra from a dysplastic area of the vocal fold (A) and the buccal mucosa (B) in a patient sensitized with oral ALA.

intensity is observed in the fluorescence emission from the patient with a carcinoma in one of the vocal folds (Fig. 4). The other normal vocal fold exhibits no sign of

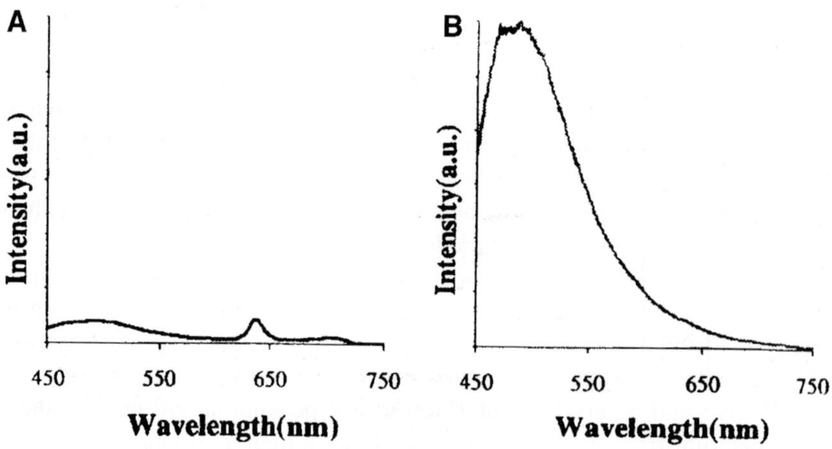

Fig. 4. Fluorescence spectra recorded from the surface of a squamous cell carcinoma of the vocal fold (A) and from the normal vocal fold (B) on the opposite side in a patient sensitized with oral ALA.

PpIX and a very high autofluorescence intensity.

The fluorescence recordings from the patient with a squamous cell carcinoma of the oropharynx during 8 h after the ALA administration are presented in Fig. 5. Spectra are shown from the tumor area with its surrounding mucosa as well as from the nasal mucosa and the tongue. The tumor area was investigated by the fiber tip monitoring the tumor and its border as well as the mucosa tissue 5 and 10 mm outside the tumor borders. All tumor spectra is characterized by a low auto-fluorescence signal and PpIX-related fluorescence is strongest in the tumor center. However, the spectra from the tongue and the nasal mucosa also exhibits PpIX-related signals, although of lower intensity but with a normal autofluorescence. Consequently, the ratio of the intensity at 635 and 490 nm shows any demarcation when compared with the higher ratio observed in the tumor area.

Discussion

Laser-induced fluorescence (LIF) is a technique for real-time, noninvasive tissue characterization. The fluorescence emission from tissue exhibits alterations in the spectral signature very early in the biological process when normal tissue is affected by different kinds of diseases. Besides the utilization of the tissue fluorescence,

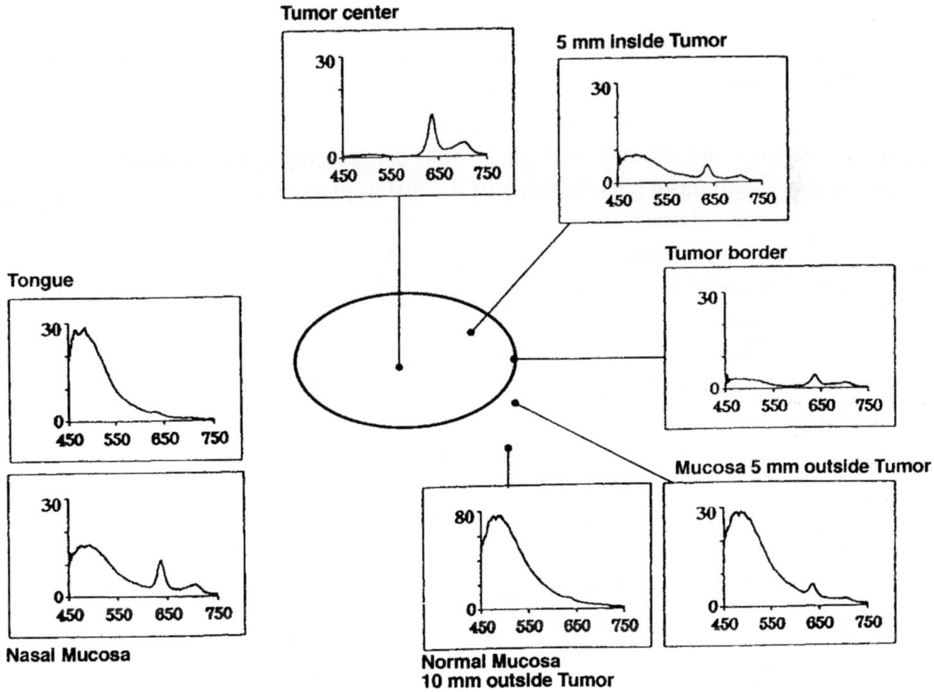

Fig. 5. Fluorescence spectra from a patient with a carcinoma of the oropharynx area sensitized with oral ALA. The tongue and nasal mucosa spectra were used for normal control measurements.

different photosensitizing agents can also be used. Recently, the endogenous sensitization utilizing the haem cycle in the body for the ALA-induced PpIX sensitization was introduced [13–16]. The PpIX build-up is enhanced in tumor tissue as compared to normal nondiseased tissue due to an altered enzyme pattern in malignant tissue. For a maximal tumor demarcation using ALA sensitization the administration dose has to be kept low; otherwise the bioavailability in normal tissue is too high. In this study we have identified an ALA dose of 5–7.5 mg/kg b.w. to be optimal for tumor demarcation.

In tumor diagnosis, early identification of tumor growth is important. As LIF is noninvasive, with the potential of being a technique for the detection of early changes in biological tissue the method is promising. The concept of utilizing spectral tissue identification has been called "optical biopsy". The correlation between the spectral signature and the histopathology is very important for the evaluation of the selectivity and sensitivity of this technique. In this study we found a perfect correlation between the data obtained with the LIF and the histopathology results, which means a great accuracy for this new diagnostic procedure. It is important to develop this method as a guiding tool for the biopsy sampling, which in many clinical conditions is blindly performed. In such cases, early tumor growth might otherwise be overlooked and misdiagnosed. Consequently, the use of LIF in early tumor diagnosis in conjunction with oral administration of ALA might also have a great potential.

Conclusions

1. A new tumor sensitization for photodiagnosis (PD) of premalignant and malignant laryngeal lesions has been studied using ALA, which is a new, nontoxic promising photosensitizer and the only one so far that can be administered orally.
2. The knowledge of laser spectroscopy of the different human tissues, including their autofluorescence characteristics and their spectral properties after being sensitized by different photosensitizers, is very important for this new diagnostic procedure.
3. The tip of a fiberoptic fluorosensor was used to detect the fluorescence spectra from mucosa vs. disease tissues giving results on real-time.
4. These preliminary results suggest that it may be possible to discriminate between premalignant and malignant laryngeal lesions and their surrounding normal mucosa.
5. A clear demarcation between normal tissue and premalignant and malignant tissue areas was obtained, which makes it possible to guide biopsy specimens for early stage malignant tumors and to look for occult tumors.
6. In the future, combining the features of photodiagosis with the advantages of CO_2 laser surgery, it may also be possible to monitor the CO_2 excision of premalignant and malignant laryngeal diseases.

Acknowledgements

This study was supported by a grant from the Portuguese National Council for Smoking Prevention.

References

1. Profio AE, Balchum OJ. Fluorescence diagnosis of cancer. In: Kessel D (ed) Methods In Porphyrin Photosensitization. New York: Plenum Press, 1985;43.
2. Andersson-Engels S, Elner Å, Johansson J, Karlsson SE, Salford LG, Strömblad LG, Svanberg K, Svanberg S. Clinical recording of laser-induced fluorescence spectra for evaluation of tumour demarcation. Feasibility in selected clinical specialities. Lasers Med Sci 1991;6:415–424.
3. Lam S, Palcic B, McLean D, Hung J, Korbelik M, Profio AE. Detection of early lung cancer using low dose photofrin II. Chest 1990;97:333–337.
4. Baert L, Berg B, Van Damme B, D'Hallewin MA, Johansson J, Svanberg K, Svanberg S. Clinical fluorescence diagnosis of human bladder carcinoma following low-dose photofrin injection. Urology 1993;41:322–330.
5. Lin CH. Selective localization of photosensitizers in tumours: a review of the phenomenon and possible mechanisms. In: Kessel D (ed) Photodynamic Therapy of Neoplastic Disease, vol II, Boca Raton: CRC Press, 1990.
6. Andersson-Engels S, Ankerst J, Johansson J, Svanberg K, Svanberg S. Laser-induced fluorescence in malignant and normal tissue of rats injected with benzoporphyrin derivative. Photochem Photobiol 1993;57:978–983.
7. Kennedy JC, Pottier RH. Endogenous protoporphyrin IX, a clinically useful photosensitizer for photodynamic therapy. J Photochem Photobiol 1992;14:275–292.
8. Svanberg K, Andersson T, Killander D, Wang I, Stenram U, Andersson-Engels S, Berg R, Johansson J, Svanberg S. Photodynamic therapy of non-melanoma malignant tumours of the skin using topical δ-amino levulinic acid sensitization and laser irradiation. Br J Dermatol 1994;130:743–751.
9. Stepp H, Baumgartner R, Beyer W, Knuchel R, Rick K, Steinbach P, Stepp HG, Kriegmair M. Bladder tissue diagnosis utilizing protoporphyrin IX fluorescence detection. Proc: Progress in Biomedical Optics. SPIE 1994;2324:20–31.
10. Leibovici L, Schoenfeld NILI, Yehoshua HA, Mamet R, Rakowski R, Schindel A, Atsmon A. Activity of porphobilinogen deaminase in peripheral blood mononuclear cells of patients with metastatic cancer. Cancer 1988;62:2297–2300.
11. Dailey HA, Smith A. Differential interaction of porphyrins used in photoradiation therapy with ferrochelatase. J Biochem 1984;223:441–445.
12. Grant WE, Hopper C, MacRobert AJ, Speight PM, Bown SC. Photodynamic therapy of oral cancer: photosensitization with systemic aminolaevulinic acid. Lancet 1993;342:147–148.
13. Loh CS, MacRobert AJ, Bedwell A, Regula J, Krasner N, Bown SC. Oral versus intravenous administration of δ-aminolaevulinic acid for photodynamic therapy. Br J Cancer 1993;68:41–51.
14. Bedwell J, MacRobert AJ, Phillips D, Brown SG. Fluorescence distribution and photodynamic effect of ALA-induced PpIX in the DMH rat colonlc tumor model. Br J Cancer 1992;65:818–824.
15. Svanberg K, Wang I, Rydell R, Elner Å, Wennerberg J, Pais Clemente L, Cardoso E, Pratas R, Pais Clemente M, Andersson-Engles S, Svanberg S. Fluorescence diagnostics of head and neck cancer utilizing oral administration of δ-amino Levulinic Acid. Proc: 5th International Photodynamic Association Biennal Meeting. Amelia Island, Florida, 1994.
16. Svanberg K, Pais Clemente L, Pais Clemente M, Wang I, Warloe T, Andersson-Engels S, Berg R, Moan A, Peng Q, Svanberg S. Pharmacokinetic studies of δ-amino levulinic acid-induced protoporphyrin IX build-up in some malignant tumours. Proc: Advances in Laser and Light Spectroscopy to Diagnose Cancer and other Diseases II. SPIE 1995;2387:30–42.

Acknowledgements

This First World Voice Congress was made possible by generous support from some governmental and private sponsors whose help is gratefully acknowledged, mainly the following institutions:

Totta & Açores Bank
Luso-American Development Foundation
Gulbenkian Foundation

Index of authors

Keyword index